Psychiatry, Mental Institutions, and the Mad in Apartheid South Africa

African Studies

History, Politics, Economics, and Culture

Molefi Asante, *General Editor*

Kwame Nkrumah's Politico-Cultural Thought and Policies
An African-Centered Paradigm for the Second Phase of the African Revolution
Kwame Botwe-Asamoah

Non-Traditional Occupations, Empowerment and Women
A Case of Togolese Women
Ayélé Léa Adubra

Contending Political Paradigms in Africa
Rationality and the Politics of Democratization in Kenya and Zambia
Shadrack Wanjala Nasong'o

Law, Morality and International Armed Intervention
The United Nations and ECOWAS in Liberia
Mourtada Déme

The Hidden Debate
The Truth Revealed about the Battle over Affirmative Action in South Africa and the United States
Akil Kokayi Khalfani

Britain, Leftist Nationalists and the Transfer of Power in Nigeria, 1945–1965
Hakeem Ibikunle Tijani

Western-Educated Elites in Kenya, 1900–1963
The African American Factor
Jim C. Harper, II

Africa and IMF Conditionality
The Unevenness of Compliance, 1983–2000
Kwame Akonor

African Cultural Values
Igbo Political Leadership in Colonial Nigeria, 1900–1966
Raphael Chijioke Njoku

A Roadmap for Understanding African Politics
Leadership and Political Integration in Nigeria
Victor Oguejiofor Okafor

Doing Justice Without the State
The Afikpo (Ehugbo) Nigeria Model
O. Oko Elechi

Student Power in Africa's Higher Education
A Case of Makerere University
Frederick Kamuhanda Byaruhanga

The NGO Factor in Africa
The Case of Arrested Development in Kenya
Maurice Nyamanga Amutabi

Social Movements and Democracy in Africa
The Impact of Women's Struggle for Equal Rights in Botswana
Agnes Ngoma Leslie

Nefer
The Aesthetic Ideal in Classical Egypt
Willie Cannon-Brown

The Experience of Economic Redistribution
The Growth, Employment and Redistribution Strategy in South Africa
Clarence Tshitereke

The Role of the Press and Communication Technology in Democratization
The Nigerian Story
Aje-Ori Agbese

The Politics of Ethnic Nationalism
Afrikaner Unity, the National Party, and the Radical Right in Stellenbosch, 1934–1948
Joanne L. Duffy

Mobutu's Totalitarian Political System
An Afrocentric Analysis
Peta Ikambana

Indigenous Medicine and Knowledge in African Society
Kwasi Konadu

Africa in the 21st Century
Toward a New Future
Edited by Ama Mazama

Missions, States, and European Expansion in Africa
Edited by Chima J. Korieh and Raphael Chijioke Njoku

The Human Cost of African Migrations
Edited by Toyin Falola and Niyi Afolabi

Trans-Atlantic Migration
The Paradoxes of Exile
Edited by Toyin Falola and Niyi Afolabi

African Minorities in the New World
Edited by Toyin Falola and Niyi Afolabi

The Ancient Egyptian Family
Kinship and Social Structure
Troy D. Allen

The African Origins of Rhetoric
Cecil Blake

Balancing Written History with Oral Tradition
The Legacy of the Songhoy People
Hassimi Oumarou Maïga

African Discourse in Islam, Oral Traditions, and Performance
Abdul-Rasheed Na'Allah

Heroism and the Supernatural in the African Epic
Mariam Konaté Deme

Psychiatry, Mental Institutions, and the Mad in Apartheid South Africa
Tiffany Fawn Jones

Psychiatry, Mental Institutions, and the Mad in Apartheid South Africa

Tiffany Fawn Jones

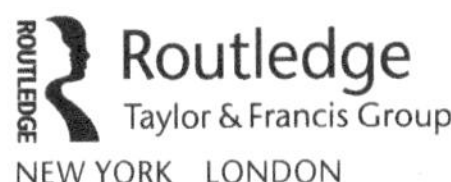

NEW YORK LONDON

First published 2012
by Routledge
711 Third Avenue, New York, NY 10017

Simultaneously published in the UK
by Routledge
2 Park Square, Milton Park, Abingdon, Oxfordshire OX14 4RN

First issued in paperback 2014

Routledge is an imprint of the Taylor and Francis Group, an informa company

Typeset in Sabon by IBT Global.

Library of Congress Cataloging-in-Publication Data

Jones, Tiffany F. (Tiffany Fawn), 1972–
Psychiatry, mental institutions, and the mad in apartheid South Africa / Tiffany Fawn Jones.
p. cm. — (African studies: history, politics, economics, and culture)
Includes bibliographical references and index.
1. Mental health services—South Africa. 2. Mentally ill—Commitment and detention—South Africa. 3. Mentally ill—Abuse of—South Africa. 4. Mental health policy—Social aspects—South Africa. 5. South Africa—Race relations. I. Title. II. Series: African studies (Routledge (Firm))
RA790.7.S66J66 2012
362.2'10968—dc23
2011033434

ISBN13: 978-0-415-88667-3 (hbk)
ISBN13: 978-0-415-75448-4 (pbk)

To all those who were institutionalized and those that were not.

Contents

Figures

Tables

Abbreviations

AIDS	Acquired Immune Deficiency Syndrome
APA	American Psychiatric Association
BAD	Department of Bantu Administration and Development
BOSS	Bureau of State Security
CCHR	Citizens Commission of Human Rights, Church of Scientology
CHP	Centre for Health Policy
DI	Department of the Interior
DOH	Department of Health
DPH	Department of Public Health
ECT	Electro-Convulsive Therapy
EEG	Electroencephalography
GALA	Gay and Lesbian Archives
HIV	Human Immunodeficiency Virus
ICRC	International Committee of the Red Cross
MASA	Medical Association of South Africa
MEDUNSA	Medical University of South Africa
MP	Minister of Parliament
MRC	Medical Research Council
NP	National Party
SADF	South African Defence Force
SAMC	South African Medical Corps
SANA	South African Nursing Association
SANC	South African Nursing Council
SANCMH	South African National Council for Mental Health
SASOP	South African Society of Psychiatrists
SPNSA	Society of Psychiatrists and Neurologists of South Africa
SPSA	Society of Psychiatrists of South Africa
TB	Tuberculosis
WHO	World Health Organization

Timeline of Major Events Pertaining to Mental Health in South Africa, 1916–2002

1916	Mental Disorders Act No. 38
1920	South African National Council of Mental Health established
1939	World War II begins
1944	Mental Disorders Amendment Act incorporates a section on "temporary" patients
	The administration of mental institutions is transferred from the Department of Interior to the Department of Public Health
1945	World War II ends
1946	Tara Hospital opens
1948	The National Party is elected and begins implementing apartheid strategies
1949	South African National Council of Mental Health registrars as a welfare group
1950	Immorality Amendment Act No. 21 prohibits all "immoral" sexual acts, including adultery, between blacks and whites
1951	Separate Representation of Voters Bill places coloureds on a separate voters role than whites
	University of Natal accepts black students into its medical school
	Bantu Authorities Act No. 68 enables the establishment of black homelands with eventual goal of self-government
1953	Tara Hospital initiates the first outpatient program in South Africa
1957	Mental Disorders Amendment Act removes the class of "social defective" and changes the name of the Commissioner for Mental Disorder to Commissioner of Mental Hygiene.
	Immorality Amendment Act No. 23
	Hubbard Association of Scientologists International opens offices in Johannesburg and Durban
1961	South Africa becomes a Republic
	Mental Disorders Amendment Act includes a category for outpatients and extends free treatment to voluntary patients who cannot afford services
	Interdepartmental Committee Report on the construction of mental institutions in homelands

1963 Smith Mitchell opens its first long-term care institution
1966 Society of Psychiatrists and Neurologists of South Africa officially formed
Prime Minister H. F. Verwoerd assassinated
1967 Commission of Inquiry to Inquire into the Responsibility of Mentally Deranged Persons and Related Matters (Rumpff Commission)
Committee of Inquiry into the Care of Mentally Deficient Persons
1968 Immorality Amendment Bill on homosexuality criminalizes all public homosexual activities and bans sexual devices
South Africa leaves the Commonwealth
1969–
1974 Aubrey Levin joins the South African Medical Corps of the SADF and begins "aversion therapy" on homosexuals in the military
1970 Bantu Homelands Citizens Act
1971 Bantu Homelands Constitution Act (National States Constitution Act) No. 21
1972 Commission of Inquiry into the Mental Disorders Act, 1916 (Act No. 38 of 1916, as amended) and Related Matters (Van Wyk Commission)
1973 Mental Health Act No. 18
The American Psychiatric Association removes homosexuality from its *Diagnostic and Statistical Manual of Psychiatric Disorders*
Commission of Enquiry into Scientology
1975 Proclamation on Rehabilitation Institutions in the Bantu Homelands
1976 Government rules that medical schools at universities can no longer admit black students. Sets up the Medical University of South Africa for black students
1976 Mental Health Amendment Act prohibits publication of any photographs, sketches or information pertaining to mental institutions
1977 World Health Organization reports on South African mental institutions
1978 American Psychiatric Association investigates and reports on Smith Mitchell facilities
1981–
1990 Stanley Platman conducts bi-annual reviews of Smith Mitchell facilities
1983 Royal College of Psychiatrists conducts an investigation into Smith Mitchell institutions
1984 Tricameral parliamentary system initiated
1990 Nelson Mandela is released from prison
1994 First democratic elections in South Africa
1997 Truth and Reconciliation Commission, Mental Health Workshop held
2002 Mental Health Care Act No. 17

Preface

When I arrived at the Esda Retirement Home in Springs, Gauteng, in 2002 to interview Dan Sable[1] about his experiences in Sterkfontein Mental Hospital where he spent most of his life, I was struck by the poor conditions in which he lived at the time. At the age of seventy, he had spent many years within mental hospitals in South Africa. He was now housed at the end of his life in yet another state institution with no one other than myself to visit him. He complained about his poor treatment and his lack of freedom within the retirement home. Entrenched with ideas about abuse within mental hospitals, I asked him about his earlier life within Sterkfontein, expecting to hear stories of mistreatment and neglect similar to his present circumstances. He began by telling me about how much he had enjoyed his stay at the mental hospital, his fond memories of the food and how he had earned R150 ($116.17) a month, enough to buy the few things he needed.[2] Although he recognized some problems within the mental institution, he claimed that it was very good for him, and compared with the life he experienced in the retirement home where he currently lived, he found it far more enjoyable. I thought that Sable was an anomaly in the history of apartheid South Africa's mental hospitals, so I continued my interviews and research, setting his story aside. Numerous reports emerged in the 1970s and 1980s that discussed the mistreatment of patients in South Africa's mental hospitals and accused practitioners of being agents of the state. When I began the research for this book, I thought I would find evidence of such terrible human rights abuses in mental hospitals, especially against South Africa's black population. Moreover, my own personal experience as an ex-patriot South African in a psychiatric wing of a Canadian hospital had left a bad taste in my mouth. If I had felt abused within a Canadian hospital, what would a black patient have felt like in a South African hospital during the racial segregationist years of apartheid?

From 1948 when the National Party won its election and began implementing its strict racist policies, segregating people according to their race and ultimately inciting abuses among the majority of its population, the potential certainly existed for psychiatrists to perpetrate human rights abuses. Initially I set out to find evidence of cruelty and mistreatment.

Reading the few patient letters and files I could find, combing through the archives, people's personal collections and various psychiatric writings, I attempted to track down other individuals who had been housed in South African mental institutions—a very difficult task because the stigma of mental illness continues to prevent people from disclosing their histories. I also scanned South African government statistics about patients in mental hospitals. Some of the stories I read about or heard made me weep, but persistently I was struck by the intense focus by practitioners and government officials on white men in institutions. After months of compiling a breakdown of the number of patients in mental hospitals and an analysis of their race, gender, and occupation, I was taken aback to find that from the early twentieth century onwards, per capita, it was poor white men that were housed in mental hospitals in higher numbers than women and those called "non-whites." Could Sable then really be representative of South Africa's mental health system during apartheid? Sable was a fellow psychiatric survivor, who although had worked for the gold mines and the railways, had ended up involuntarily in a mental hospital for most of his adult life, stigmatized with the diagnosis of schizophrenia. He was a white man, and ironically in the context of apartheid South Africa, it was this fact that had most likely resulted in his institutionalization. The majority of South Africa's female and "non-white" populations who had been deemed "mad" rarely saw the inside of a state mental hospital. Most were simply neglected. What this meant, however, was that after 1939 in South Africa, institutions and practitioners focused on the very people that the apartheid government wanted to uplift—poor white men.

Yet, worldwide we see evidence that mental hospitals were places where historically minorities, women, and anyone deemed deviant were housed. Over the past century, accusations of human rights abuse in mental institutions around the world have become more prevalent. Throughout colonial Africa, racism pervaded the practices of practitioners and Africans were often the victims of terrible abuse in mental institutions. In Soviet Russia, psychiatrists were involved in schemes to imprison individuals who expressed opposition to the government in mental institutions. In Nazi Germany, practitioners used mental patients as test subjects in scientific experiments and partook in their execution. In the United States and Canada, high incidences of women and minorities have been, and continue to be, housed in mental institutions. Scholars have also documented the abuse of indigenous peoples in mental hospitals in New Zealand and Australia. Today, cases of psychiatric abuse of minority and female patients continue to emerge.

If South Africa's focus was on treating white men, how do we account for the numerous accusations of human rights abuse against Africans that arose against practitioners during the apartheid years? When interrogating the origins of these allegations, to my surprise, I found that it was not independent international organizations, rogue practitioners, or former patients that had continuously highlighted maltreatment, but the South African division of the Church of Scientology that had played a crucial part in spreading these charges. In the 1960s, Scientology, a zealous anti-psychiatric organization, had become increasingly concerned about what they deemed were human rights abuses in South African mental hospitals and were sending press reports to South African newspapers and around the world, hoping not only to bring attention to what they deemed were human rights abuses, but also to themselves. They were somewhat successful. Reading the published accusations of mistreatment in South Africa advanced by the Church of Scientology in newspapers, organizations such as the World Health Organization, the International Red Cross, the American Psychiatric Association, the Royal College of Psychiatrists, and individuals all conducted studies into conditions in South Africa's mental hospitals for over a decade thereafter. Although these investigations found some evidence of abuse within the institutions, for the most part they found the specific allegations initially raised by the Church of Scientology to be unfounded.[3]

The Church of Scientology's current publications on racism and psychiatry continue to promote their role in uncovering abuses during apartheid South Africa. When they first began publishing their criticisms, Scientologists' accusations against South Africa's psychiatrists and medical practitioners played on the growing anti-apartheid sentiment that existed throughout the world. Whereas psychiatric practitioners were far from ideal global citizens, they were not the literal communist demons, horns and all, as depicted by Scientologists. Certainly, South African mental institutions were spaces where human rights abuse occurred and where the state detained some of its opponents. Indeed, there were instances of these abuses that we should not ignore. Practitioners sometimes contributed to, and at times facilitated, mistreatment. But mental health practitioners as a group did not give blanket support to the racialized ideas of apartheid.

Today South Africa's mental health system is overloaded and understaffed. Makeshift solutions have done little to deal with the overcrowding and overall lack of services in general. It is a convoluted and ineffective system that is desperately in need of an overhaul. Moreover, the inequity of treatment and services along racial, gender, and class lines persists and reports continue to emerge of abuse within the system. Staff shortages, lack of sufficient beds, and limited funding for mental health all have contributed to these human rights violations. But if we do not have a thorough understanding of the origins and historical perceptions that are so ingrained in the system, how do we then know what the solutions are? A more nuanced understanding of South African mental health views and practices in the period leading up to and during the height of apartheid South Africa therefore is desperately needed.

Acknowledgments

The research for this book has not been an easy feat. Sources were scattered in back offices, individual garages, and makeshift archives. Much has been destroyed. Moreover, the writing of this book was often an emotional journey into the lives of those patients who were affected by South Africa's mental health system. Their experiences cannot be possibly appreciated in the confines of these pages, but it is my hope that I have at least captured their context. It is to them that this book is dedicated.

A project such as this could never have been completed without the selfless support of countless of individuals who helped along the way. First and foremost, I owe the utmost gratitude to Alan Jeeves. His thoughtful guidance, patience, and understanding during the research of this project was always much appreciated. Much thanks also to Jane Parpart, Robert Shenton, Alison Goebel, Jacklyn Duffin, Sally Swartz, Villia Jefremovas, Karen Dubinsky, Marc Epprecht, Shula Marks, Glen Elder, and Cherstin Lyon whose suggestions and comments at different stages of research encouraged me to seek beyond the obvious. Their advice was always poignant and helpful. The failures of this book are, however, all my own. Thanks also to the Social Science and Humanities Research Council, Timothy C. S. Franks Travel Award, and Queen's University for funding the original research.

Over the last ten years, this research took me to various places in South Africa and North America where numerous individuals opened their homes, their offices, and their lives to me. Philip Bonner and the University of Witwatersrand History department offered me a most welcome place to hang my proverbial hat during research and I am much obliged. Stanley Platman and his wife, Vera Thomas, in Baltimore gave me access to a plethora of information about Smith Mitchell institutions from their personal archives and offered me numerous cups of tea. Lennart Eriksson opened up part of the archives of Lifecare in Randburg to me and recognized the historical importance of the Platman reports. Melvyn Freeman at the Department of Mental Health made sure that I was able to obtain recent department records not yet housed at the archives. Janis van der Westhuizen, and Eddie and Margie Hattingh opened up their homes to me while researching.

Thanks to all those practitioners and patients who took the time to sit down with me and talk about their experiences. I was always struck by their openness and willingness to discuss difficult issues. Also thanks to the staff at the South African National Archives in Pretoria, the Cape Town, Durban, and Pietermaritzburg archive repositories, the Centre for Health Policy, the South African Historical Archives, and the Gay and Lesbian Archives at the University of Witwatersrand.

Special mention must be made of Mawulom Kuenyehia, Matthew Herrington, Victoria van Eyk, Thomas Hagen and particularly Godfrey (Roy) Dlulane for all their research, interview, translation, indexing and transcription assistance, even when it sometimes became tiresome.

On a personal level, I am extremely grateful and indebted to Gail and the late Brian Heal, who supported me every step of the way and made sure I always had a sanctuary to come home to while researching. Thanks so much to Fred Jones, Dominic Jones, and Samantha Davies, who encouraged me to do what I love. Most importantly, however, I owe an incredible debt to my husband Michael Heal and my two daughters, Devon and Rowan, for giving up their time, supporting me, and essentially living this book along with me. Their smiles, encouragement, and cheers have made the journey all the more enjoyable.

Introduction

In 1975 the Johannesburg *Sunday Times* published a one page opinion article by Fleur de Villiers entitled "Millions Out of Madness." Basing her expose on testimony given by Jan Robbertze, head of Clinical Psychology at the University of Pretoria and Chairman of the South African National Council for Mental Health, she claimed that a private company was making a profit from the mental illness of black individuals and operating "Dickensian workhouses" that were "an uncomfortable reminder of the bad days of Bedlam." De Villiers argued that expenditures on patients were minimal and suggested that the company had a vested interest in keeping patients within these "human warehouses."[1] A few months later, the Church of Scientology's *Peace and Freedom* magazine investigated these allegations further. They claimed that thousands of Africans were forced to work and die in these mental health "labour camps," abuse was rampant, and patient well-being was usurped by economic profit.[2] They then sent press reports to various news outlets in the world. This was merely the beginning of investigations of South African state and private mental hospitals. Throughout the 1970s and 1980s, reports emerged of South African mental institutions housing black political opponents to the government, excessively using electrotherapy, conducting pharmacological experiments on patients, forcing them to work as slave labor, and allowing high rates of sexual abuse by staff against patients.[3] Academics, politicians, journalists, ex-political detainees, international organizations, and religious groups documented human rights abuses by mental health practitioners during apartheid South Africa. The World Health Organization, the American Psychiatric Association, the International Red Cross, individual psychiatrists, patients, and newspapers worldwide all condemned the inhumane treatment of black patients within South Africa's mental hospitals. Their conclusions are somewhat analogous to reports of psychiatric abuse in colonial Africa, Soviet Russia, and Nazi Germany.

In 1997 during South Africa's Truth and Reconciliation Commission, scandals about psychiatric abuse of young, gay white conscripts in the South African Defence Force (SADF) came to the fore. Aubrey Levin, now known as "Dr. Shock," who headed up the SADF's psychiatric wing, administered electroshocks to gay men while showing them nude pictures in order to "cure" them of their homosexuality. In August 2010, these stories were reiterated in newspapers worldwide when Levin, who left South Africa in 1998 to practice psychiatry in Alberta, Canada, was charged with 21 counts of sexual assault against Canadian male patients under his care. At the time of writing this, Crown lawyers estimated the number of Levin's Canadian victims to be even higher. South Africa's psychiatric sector has a long, sordid history of being associated with abuse.[4]

There is credibility to these accusations and certainly there are horrid instances of psychiatric mistreatment that occurred during the racist years of apartheid that are comparable to those in Soviet Russia, Nazi Germany, and other areas of Africa. Some psychiatric practitioners supported the mandate of the racist and heteropatriarchal government and most mental patients, particularly African patients, were treated abysmally. Rudimentary tales of abuse in South Africa's mental hospitals, however, fail to account for the fact that not all South African practitioners partook in abuse and they were not simply oppressors. We need to understand that mental health practitioners' roles were not simply the agents of the racist apartheid government. Their positions were a lot more complex.

Delivery of mental health services in apartheid South Africa was diverse, multi-layered, and often makeshift. South Africa's mental health infrastructure consisted of disconnected components, such as state institutions, prisons, general hospitals, courts, military institutions, semi-private institutions, social welfare offices, and the community. Psychiatrists, general practitioners, superintendents, psychiatric nurses, district surgeons, social workers, and other professionals such as psychologists and indigenous healers treated mental patients on a daily basis. In addition, government officials, magistrates, prison wardens, judges, mental hospital board members, family members, patients, private psychiatrists, and privately owned facilities all had influence in their administration. The mental health sector during apartheid South Africa was not a static and cohesive unit. Individuals' views were often ambiguous, incongruent, and contradictory. Indeed, the disparity among practitioners and the fluidity of practitioners' beliefs, along with the disjointed mental health infrastructure, not only enabled the diffusion of state control, but also permitted practitioners to adopt ideas concurrently that were contradictory to each other—ideas that may have supported and/or challenged apartheid ideologies. This complexity of views was due to the amorphous nature of the psychiatric profession itself and the diversity of the individuals who provided services to patients. Influenced by varying spiritual beliefs, international psychiatric trends, local political events, economic shifts, and advances in pharmacology and neurology, ideas of madness continuously changed. International pressures also played a role in shaping psychiatric practices. Moreover, patients themselves affected the approaches and methods of the country's mental health services. Their important perspectives on the national mental health system during apartheid should be acknowledged.

Certainly South African mental health institutions were spaces where human rights abuse occurred and opponents of the state were detained. Moreover, practitioners often contributed to, and at times facilitated, these abuses. But it is not enough simply to dismiss psychiatrists as a homogenous group of actors explicitly directed by a well-organised and monolithic state. Instead, complex relationships existed between practitioners, patients, and government officials and we should place the meanings of and practices pertaining to madness within their specific historical contexts. South Africa's psychiatric views and mental health policies did not exist in a vacuum. They were highly influenced by local socio-political events and changing international trends. Indeed, South African practitioners and government officials' perspectives of the mad often followed those of their European and North American counterparts, while they also frequently adapted to local pressures. In an examination of the views and practices of practitioners and patients within a changing political structure, one sees the multiplicity of the mental health system, a multiplicity that has often been overshadowed by stories of abuse.

Whereas the reports that emerged of abuses in South Africa's mental health services importantly highlighted the failures of the system, they neglected to recognize its multifarious and contradictory nature. Nor did they appreciate the full historical context or the complex position of those within it. While not contesting the belief that human rights abuses occurred within South Africa's mental hospitals, we need to acknowledge that the South African mental health system during apartheid was far more complicated than what might at first glance appear to be simple cases of patient abuse. Unlike Soviet Russia, the apartheid government never used mental hospitals as its principle means to control its political dissidents.[5] Nor did it use mental hospitals to specifically rid itself of those it deemed racially inferior as in the case of Nazi Germany. Instead, in South Africa, officially sanctioned mental health institutions and services for the black majority were largely lacking. Although this neglect of mental health services during apartheid was in itself a form of abuse, it was also positive in that mental health services were not simply the instruments of the apartheid government. For the most part, practitioners focused on treating white men and hospitals housed more white men per capita than women, Africans, Indians, or coloureds. White men occupied about 20 percent of the beds in the hospitals, while they only made up about 5 percent of the population. Black men and women made up about 80 percent of South Africa's population, but made up only fifty percent of the patients. Black women in particular only made up only 18 percent of the occupants in hospitals.[6] In order to understand why this was the case, we need a more nuanced understanding of the South African mental health system in the period leading up to and during the height of apartheid.

Table 0.1 Number of Beds and Patients in Mental Institutions by Race and Gender, 1935–1970

Type of Patient Resident on 31 Dec	1935		1940		1945		1950	
	Patients	Beds	Patients	Beds	Patients	Beds	Patients	Beds
White	4,153	3,991	4,701	4,495	6,674	6,454	7,056	7,953
Male	2,196	2,119	2,428	2,383	3,354	3,308	3,535	4,142
Female	1,957	1,872	2,273	2,112	3,320	3,146	3,521	3,811
Non-White	5,831	4,928	7,856	5,894	9,117	6,389	10,038	8,189
Male	3,970	3,406	5,226	3,953	6,120	4,464	6,737	5,625
Female	1,861	1,522	2,630	1,941	2,997	1,925	3,301	2,564
Total	9,984	8,919	12,557	10,389	15,791	12,843	17,094	16,142
No. of institutions	9		9		12		13	

Type of Patient Resident on 31 Dec	1955		1960		1965		1970	
	Patients	Beds	Patients	Beds	Patients	Beds	Patients	Beds
White	7,342	7,774	7,651	7,844	8,054	8,762	8,251	8,543
Male	3,734	4,207	3,870	3,818	4,112	4,173	4,259	3,931
Female	3,608	3,567	3,781	4,026	3,942	4,589	3,992	4,612
Non-White	11,577	9,373	12,563	7,305	13,899	8,747	15,598	11,720
Male	7,978	6,665	8,752	5,244	9,647	6,123	9,784	7,249
Female	3,599	2,708	3,811	2,061	4,252	2,624	5,814	4,471
Total	18,919	17,147	20,214	15,149	21,953	17,509	23,849	20,263
No. of institutions	13		13		15		18	

Numbers for 1935 and 1940 are compiled from statistics South Africa and include Voluntary Boarders, but do not include numbers for institutions for feeblemindedness. Numbers from 1945-1970 are from Mental Health Commissioners' annual reports and include institutions for feebleminded and voluntary, observation, temporary and inebriate patients. A few Commissioner's reports had addition errors in them. These have been corrected in the above table.

THE ANOMALY OF APARTHEID MADNESS?

The specific racialized and heteropatriarchal nature of apartheid South Africa does suggest that a power structure existed that would have encouraged a climate of human rights abuses by practitioners and where Africans, particularly African women, were the victims, both physically and mentally, of this oppression. Actions on the part of states to fashion and legitimate particular models of social norms are common. The very process of state formation is intrinsically tied to organizing notions of normality and morality. For example, in their analysis of the rise of the English state between the eleventh and late nineteenth century, Philip Corrigan and Derek Sayer argue that state creation is part of a "cultural revolution" that normalizes specific "forms of social order" so that they become accepted rules.[7] The state adopts a process of what it calls "moral regulation," that is "a project of normalizing, rendering natural, taken for granted, in a word 'obvious', what are in fact ontological and epistemological premises of a particular and historical form of social order." In so doing, the state sanctions some ideas, while "suppressing, marginalizing, eroding, [and] undermining others."[8] Linzi Manicom, through her application of Corrigan and Sayer's arguments to South Africa, shows how the everyday administration of the state, such as the "recording of demographic information, the application of dress codes, the bureaucratic procedures, the regulation of labour, marriage and schooling" all allowed the state to establish political subjectivities and regulate difference.[9] If we extend this argument to include state sanctioned regulations concerning madness, the legitimating of a set of mental health standards, legislation, categorizations, and overall policy in nation states is indeed part of the larger political process of hegemony and subjectification. One could argue further that states are directly concerned with governing the mentality of their populations.

Michel Foucault has written extensively about the influence that the state has historically had on the regulation and order in various social institutions, such as mental institutions, clinics, and prisons. In *Madness and Civilization: A History of Insanity in the Age of Reason*, he examines the confinement of large numbers of poor, mad, and homeless people in Europe in state mental institutions during the mid-seventeenth century. This period of "great confinement," he argues, was due directly to economic and social pressures faced by the state and its need to retain social control. He asserts that a new medical discipline developed that, while couched in terms of scientific humanitarianism, was actually a means by which to enforce existing power structures and to legitimate dominant social positions.[10] This power, which he later calls "disciplinary power," is a tool used to organize and control a population as a means to create productive "docile bodies."[11] Medical professionals therefore "subjectified" patients in the sense that medical and psychiatric discourse imposed certain notions of normality upon them, whereas psychiatrists also objectified patients so that they became "objects of science."[12] In his 1991 essay on government, Foucault also shows how states fashion a patriarchal (and this can be described further as a heteropatriarchal) social structure, similar to that of a father to his family.[13] The state becomes a disciplinarian and regulator of populations, but is not simply concerned with imposing its laws.[14] Simply stated, he argues that in order to fulfill its mandate, a state will often "dispose" or remove those deemed socially deviant, such as those deemed insane or criminals, from society. States can classify and confine patients indefinitely with the semblance of concern about social and individual wellbeing, even if its goal may be to control its labor force, manage the actions of certain of its citizens, or even to simply perpetuate its ideal of a modern, sanitary living space free from vagrants.

Early studies on relationships between colonial states and psychology/psychiatry in Africa tend to emphasize the connection between the state and the mental subjectification of its population. Three key African scholars of the 1950s, Octave Mannoni, Franz Fanon, and Albert Memmi, all have examined the effect of the colonial state on the African mind. They theorized the mental abuses perpetrated by colonialists and practitioners alike in colonial West and North Africa and pointed to the psychopathological nature of colonial control and the negative mental impact of colonialism on all involved. Mannoni, for example, argued that in the African colonial state, two opposing types of psychological complexes existed—the "dependency complex" and the "inferiority complex," the former of which Africans adopted during colonialism as a means to gain "security and protection" from the colonizer.[15] This, he argued, resulted in a reciprocal relationship whereby "the master has a servant, the servant likewise has a master."[16] The colonizer, which included practitioners, in turn, in fulfilling the oppositional role, developed an "inferiority complex." To compensate for their own inferiority, they willingly created dependents.[17] While accepting Mannoni's Hegelian master-slave dichotomy, Fanon, however, challenged Mannoni's contentions of the insecure colonizer and dependent colonized as intrinsic characteristics of each group, and questioned his disregard of the socio-economic affect of colonization on the colonizers. Africans and Europeans did not possess these complexes inherently, he argued, but they were produced by the colonial system.[18] Likewise, Memmi also accepted Mannoni's basic explanation, but challenged Mannoni's failure to account for the economic underpinnings of colonialism.[19] For Memmi, the colonizer lived in a state of "inherent contradiction," which, if left unrecognized, would "disfigure the colonizer." The cure to this "disease" affecting the colonizer is "difficult and painful treatment, extraction and reshaping of present conditions of existence."[20] If this was not done, he argued that the colonized would then force the end of colonialism.[21]

In Fanon's later works, *Wretched of the Earth* and *A Dying Colonialism,* he implicates colonialism as being the "fertile purveyor for the psychiatric hospital." Fanon also argued that colonial psychiatrists were representatives of the state.[22] Fanon himself was a psychiatrist at the Blida-Joinville Hospital in Algeria between 1953 and 1956. He was well situated to present such a criticism. Western medical science in general was, he argued, "part of the oppressive system" and "the doctor always appears as a link in the colonialist network, as a spokesman for the occupying power."[23]

Fanon, however, was concerned with the liberation of the colonized from the constraints of colonial alienation, of which he saw psychiatry as part. He argued that it was necessary for the colonized first to recognize their own subjectivity and become liberated from themselves, be aware of their own difference, and then embrace this difference as a means for emancipation from colonial rule.[24] Lynette Jackson, in her book on the Ingutsheni Mental Hospital in Zimbabwe adopts this aspect of Fanon's argument and applies it to colonial Rhodesia. She contends that the hospital indeed played a disciplinary role in Rhodesian society and became a microcosm for colonial society in general. When Zimbabwe gained its independence, the transformation of the Ingutsheni Mental Hospital became symbolic of removing the very shackles of colonization.[25] What we need to understand though, and what is striking is in Fanon, Memmi, and Mannoni's arguments, is that they recognized that the colonial state fashioned psychological complexes, not only in the colonized, but in the colonizer as well. This may potentially explain why South African mental institutions focused on white men.

These authors focused mainly on the construction of racial difference, but race was not the only factor that influenced colonial policies in Africa. Changing conceptions of class, sex, gender, and sexuality were also central components of colonial segregationist policies. Governments systematically divided their landscapes into hierarchical, racialized, and gendered spaces that set up specific roles for women and men all based on a white heterosexual model. Anyone who moved outside this model was generally marginalized or sanctioned in some way.[26]

Since the late 1960s, feminist scholars all over the world have called attention to and rejected the gendering of psychiatry. They point to how psychiatry is inherently patriarchal and skewed against women, mostly because the main diagnostic characteristics use men as the standard of normalcy, and society expects women to have more passive and less valued roles in society. Any woman who steps outside of her assigned social role can be deemed as mentally disordered. [27] Even the indigenous men in colonial societies played a role in inciting this view of women. Jackson, for example, has shown that in colonial Zimbabwe, any "stray woman" who was no longer being watched by their fathers or husbands was seen to be "pathological."[28] We see this during apartheid South Africa as well, where the apartheid government consigned the position of black women to rural areas through the construction of "homelands" and the implementation of pass laws. When single black women began to move to urban centers, many state officials and some state practitioners declared these women as being the cause of moral decay. As the Minister of Native Affairs, E. G. Jansen, stated, "it is constantly being said that the Natives in the cities deteriorate. The undesirable conditions are largely caused by the presence of women, who in many cases leave their homes contrary to the wishes of their fathers and guardians."[29] Heteropatriarchal conceptualizations dominated South African understandings of normality and mental disorder, with all notions of mental normality based on the white heterosexual male. In turn, blacks, coloureds, Indians, and women were seen as fundamentally disordered. Some feminist scholars have even argued that because psychiatry and society often depict women as irrational beings, women have become the very image of madness.[30]

One can extend these arguments to include conceptions of homosexual men. Worldwide, governments and psychiatric practitioners often deemed gay men who exhibited what they perceived as "abnormal" or "unnatural" sexual behavior as mad. Indeed, it was only in 1973 that the American Psychiatric Association removed homosexuality from its *Diagnostic and Statistical Manual of Psychiatric Disorders* to which practitioners worldwide subscribe.[31] In South Africa, the government classified homosexuality as both a criminal offence and a mental disorder. In the 1960s and 1970s, the apartheid government became increasingly concerned with the "spread" of homosexuality among urban white males, and some military practitioners, such as Levin, even reverted to the use of "aversion therapy" where they administered electric shocks to young conscripts in order to "cure" them of their disordered behavior. They also used hormone therapy and conducted sex change operations.

As the 1950s African writers pointed out about the negative psychological effects of colonialism on the black African mind, feminists and queer theorists have pointed out that the very restrictions placed on women and men to maintain social morality may actually have facilitated concepts of mental disorder. The pressures placed on homosexual men certainly caused them distress. Denise Russell cautiously points out that depression in women is sometimes a reaction to their limited role within society; a sign of the dissatisfaction they feel towards their lives.[32] Julie Parle, in her book on the history of colonial Natal mental health also suggests that the incidences of *indiki* or hysteria were a response by Zulu women to restraints within their own communities.[33] Some scholars, however, have moved even beyond these assertions by actually celebrating those classified as mentally ill. Scholars such as Hélène Cixous and Xavière Gauthier commemorate those women who exhibited hysterical tendencies "as champions of a defiant womanhood, whose opposition, expressed in physical symptoms and coded speech, subverted the linear logic of male science."[34] Forms of mental disorder can be seen as a form of protest against the heteropatriarchal system—a means for individuals to express their frustration—although there may also be some other social factors underlying its cause. Given the stigma attached to mental illness, however, and the sub-standard conditions within mental institutions worldwide, it is unlikely that scores of women and men adopted ideas of mental illness as a form of protest. As Showalter aptly states, ideas of mental disorder as resistance come "dangerously close to romanticizing and endorsing madness as a desirable form of rebellion rather than seeing it as the desperate communication of the powerless."[35]

South Africa shows the difficulty of representing mental diagnoses as either a corrective mechanism or a form of resistance particularly well. As Megan Vaughan points out in her examination of whether Foucauldian accounts of medical "disciplinary power" could be applied in a colonial African context, she argues that the colonial state had no need to create an "Insane Other" in order to detain its opponents. It already had an "Other" in the form of an "African."[36] In other words, Europeans, influenced by ideas of social evolutionism, saw the mad in general as being racially degenerate; that is, madness was already depicted as primordial and racialized. Scientific practitioners represented mad individuals as being "savage," "uncivilized," and having "black" features. Racial degeneration and madness were therefore interconnected. Yet in a world where Europeans saw Africans as inherently inferior and primitive, paradoxical and unstable ideas of madness developed because it was difficult for colonists to seek out, in the words of Anne McClintock, the "mad, the bad and the dangerous, when all were mad, bad or dangerous." So, "if . . . colonised people, especially Africans, were figured as *inherently* bereft of reason, as inherently mentally 'abnormal', how then in the colonies, were 'normal' Africans to be distinguished from the mentally ill?"[37] This is not to argue that psychiatric othering did not occur. Rather, contradictory views could be held simultaneously, so that "anachronistic spaces" remained, that is, spaces where "certain groups and certain spaces within modernity . . . were figured as existing in an earlier, more primitive, prehistoric time." These spaces could survive together with modern ideals, but were somehow separate.[38] To put it in yet another way, layers of "othering" or "madness" could certainly exist within a society at a given time, so that one could be "normal abnormal" and "abnormal abnormal."[39]

Whereas apartheid South Africa was not a true colonial state per se, as Mahmood Mamdani has argued, the National Party's apartheid policies were indicative, if not the epitome, of indirect rule tactics purported by colonialists such as Frederick Lugard in the early twentieth century.[40] Indeed, much of the divide and rule strategies adopted by the National Party built on existing segregationist practices initiated during the years of British colonial rule. One could certainly expect that the actions of practitioners in apartheid South Africa would have echoed those earlier practices in other colonial African countries. Like Vaughan and McClintock point out for colonial Africa, apartheid South Africa had notions of difference that were convoluted and multi-layered, and variations of earlier colonial views of madness endured throughout the apartheid years. Far from being instruments of control for the government or a means of escape for individuals, mental institutions, and those associated with them played a complex role. Contrary to popular opinion, there were only a small proportion of women and Africans who were actually admitted to psychiatric hospitals. Beds for Africans and women, particularly black women, were limited. This is somewhat different from histories related about colonial mental institutions from elsewhere in the continent and indeed the world. Because of the importance of these distinctive gender and racial ratios within South Africa's mental institutions, an explanation for them is overdue.

Why did the racist and fascist South African government not use its institutions as a means of social control as scholars have argued existed elsewhere? And what role then did practitioners and patients actually play during apartheid? Why was apartheid South Africa different from other countries in the world where the most common people institutionalized were women and those with darker skin?

Key to understanding the reasons for apartheid South Africa's difference in comparison to admittance trends in the rest of the world is recognizing the complexity of apartheid itself. As Philip Bonner, Peter Delius, and Deborah Posel have pointed out, apartheid was not a monolithic, well-designed plan.[41] They argue that "the complex patterns of proletarianisation [initiated by apartheid policies] which accompanied . . . processes of migrancy and urbanization, and the intense social dislocation that they entailed, produced distinctive forms of society and struggle which proved far more recalcitrant to state direction and control than much of the earlier scholarship has comprehended." Moreover, the forms of resistance that the government encountered were "far more wide ranging and amorphous" than the larger political movements. Instead, it was the "small-scale acts of non-compliance" that proved more difficult for the government to control and curtail.[42] Within the microcosm of discussions of mental health, we can particularly see the complexity and amorphous nature of apartheid policies and the smaller battles waged, albeit often unsuccessfully, against some of the government's discriminatory practices. Practitioners and patients certainly were not cohesive groups that passively accepted government restrictions.

What we also need to recognize is that apartheid South Africa, while seemingly sharing characteristics of earlier colonial rule elsewhere on the continent, existed in a different historical period where race and gender relations had transformed and international pressures played a larger role on South Africa's domestic policies. Apartheid policies were being devised at a particular moment in history. The National Party implemented its strict racial segregationist practices that divided the population along racial lines and dictated every aspect of South Africans' lives after the Second World War when Adolf Hitler's policies had shown the world the gruesome effects of racism and discrimination. After 1945, although racism continued in new forms, the world no longer blindly accepted overt racialist and social evolutionary thinking as the norm. Moreover, the distinctive nature of the Cold War and the decolonization of most of Africa in the 1950s and 1960s were drawing South Africa further into a world where international pressure played an increasing role in domestic policies. In this political climate, it is not surprising that those that worked for the state had disagreements and policies frequently changed, which in turn resulted in contradictory and inconsistent social practices. We particularly see disagreements among those who worked and were embroiled in the mental health system, many of whom saw themselves as being part of a global community. Internationally psychiatry was becoming more deinstitutionalized, while locally the state had become increasingly militarized. International and domestic pressures were pulling South African practitioners in two competing directions and practitioners shared different ideas about how to deal with those deemed mad. Patients also saw themselves as connected to larger global concerns.

We need to understand how various and changing socio-political forces affected individuals involved in South Africa's mental health system. To date there is no broad historical study of South African mental health that extends throughout the apartheid years.[43] Whereas pre-1948 studies are vital to understanding the development of practices during apartheid, they do not answer the question, what impact did apartheid policies have generally on the treatment of the mad in South Africa and how did the mad react? It is interesting that the mental health history during a period of intense human rights abuses and racism has remained unwritten until now. Perhaps in the past there was an assumption that after the World Wars, psychiatry became a more scientific and politically disaffected field. Because most patient case files were destroyed, perhaps scholars have thought that writing such a history was impossible. Regardless, apartheid South Africa was unique in the sense of the period in which it existed, and although it shared similarities to colonial rule, we can not remove it from its particular historical circumstances. Just as colonialism changed after the Second World War, mental health policies also changed and became increasingly tenuous throughout the apartheid years. Apartheid was a makeshift, complex entity that although it was about segregation, was more concerned about shielding white (Afrikaner) men from foreign (be it local or international) encroachment—we particularly see this when it came to policies regarding madness.

WHAT IS "MENTAL HEALTH" AND "PSYCHIATRY?"

When one begins to write a book about the role that mental institutions and psychiatric practitioners did or did not play in human rights abuses in any part of the world, it is vital to understand what "mental health" and "psychiatry" is. While numerous studies have discussed these issues, to date there is no consensus, probably because psychiatrists themselves cannot agree. Although psychiatry is often classified as a science, what many studies have shown, and I emphasize in this book, is that psychiatry is not simply a science that follows a systematic and ever progressive path, but is instead a fluid construct that is influenced by and influences socio-political events. Moreover, notions of madness are variable and are often based on dominant and imposed notions of social norms. These norms, however, can be negotiated, manipulated, and contested. Thus, the history of madness directly alters with changing social definitions, political intent, and intellectual contexts. By adopting this view, we can see how views of madness in South Africa were historically shaped, but we can also begin to understand the socio-political climate in which they were applied. Thus, we are able to gain a greater understanding of the wider story of apartheid.

Our views today of madness are shaped by the psychiatric discipline. The discipline as we know it, however, is relatively new. The term "psychiatry" has been in use only since the eighteenth century when Johann Reil coined it to describe an emerging popular field of study that dealt with ideas of madness.[44] But from where did this discipline originate? The question of the origins of psychiatry is intrinsically connected to the question of what exactly psychiatry is. If one defines psychiatry as a scientific discipline, then one traces psychiatry's origins to the beginnings of medical science. On the other hand, if one were to expand the definition of psychiatry to include non-systematic ideas of mental and spiritual health, as some scholars have recently begun to do, the definition and origin of psychiatry becomes more complex.[45] Understanding psychiatry and mental health is tied therefore to debates of science, biology, spirituality, and social conditioning.

Earlier histories of psychiatry view it as an evolving science—a science moving on a linear progressive path towards an ultimate goal of understanding the human mind and ridding it of all its defects. Influenced by positivist notions of scientific truth, early psychiatric histories privilege the role of individuals, usually men, who forwarded knowledge of the brain. Erwin Ackerknecht's *Short History of Psychiatry*, for example, reads as a description of those men who progressively advanced the discipline through their theories and experiments. Psychiatry, he argues, is the objective "science of mental diseases."[46] Thus, he rejects any non-systematic forms of psychiatry because he feels that they do not contribute in any way to the practice of the profession.

More recently, scholars have questioned the positivist notions of psychiatry put forward by an earlier generation of historians of science. Beginning in the 1960s, anti-psychiatrists interrogated the validity of scientific psychiatry's basic approach. Arising out of the larger debate concerning the unassailable repute of science, technology, and medicine in particular that arose in the 1960s, the anti-psychiatric movement challenged the scientific validity of psychiatry.[47] Although the anti-psychiatric movement is made up of individuals and groups that have varying arguments and different mandates, it has some shared ideas. Anti-psychiatrists, whose very name suggests their antithetical stance, reject the notion that the discipline is a science that emerged with Western civilization. Instead, they see psychiatry as a modern social construction devised by practitioners in order to support existing power structures and promote their own personal authority. Thus, individuals such as Thomas Szaz and R. D. Laing, many of whom were former disillusioned psychiatrists, reject the notion that mental illness is caused by internal biological forces. They instead argue that it is created by external economic, social, and political conditions. Most of these anti-psychiatric writings are influenced by Foucault's notions that psychiatry is a disciplinary tool of the state. Anti-psychiatrists claim that psychiatric diagnoses are societally driven and question the validity of diagnoses. They argue that diagnoses are merely categorizations used by psychiatrists to perpetuate hegemonic social control.[48] More recently, some scholars have moved beyond simple criticisms of psychiatric control and have begun to point out the role that patients themselves, although often unconsciously, have played in shaping diagnostic categories. Although these arguments underestimate the practitioner's role somewhat in the shaping of patients' identities, they do recognize that diagnoses are not necessarily simply the creations of psychiatrists, as many of their critics would suggest, but are also shaped, albeit often unwittingly, by patients themselves.

Although anti-psychiatrists and those influenced by them have gone far in moving historical studies of psychiatry away fróm ideas of inevitable scientific progress, theories concerning the biological basis of mental illness have continued to be at the forefront of research. Numerous studies on psychopharmacological drugs and neurological surgery are indicative of this trend. Biological explanations are still apparent in some writings of psychiatric history. For example, Edward Shorter's *A History of Psychiatry* (which really should be called *A History of Psychiatry in the Western World*) specifically denounces anti-psychiatric criticism. In response to the anti-psychiatrists' critique of psychiatry, he promotes psychiatric history as an evolution towards more advanced biomedical science, with psychology as simply a temporary diversion from the somatic path.[49] Indeed, his approach is reminiscent of that of Ackerknecht's.

Shorter's attack on the anti-psychiatric movement is not surprising, for it merely reflects the larger struggle between biomedical and psychodynamic or social approaches to mental health that has existed, and continues to exist today. Yet, arguments supporting both scientific psychiatry and its critics have their pitfalls. Scientific psychiatrists fail to recognize that alternative, including indigenous, approaches have for many years coexisted with Western practices, often overlapping, competing, and even working in conjunction with each other. Scientific psychiatry tends to be very Eurocentric and dismissive of anything viewed as "uncivilized" or "primitive." Moreover, it bases its arguments on the idea that mental illness can be explained solely on biomedical factors and rejects the notion that psychiatric disorders also have origins in the social circumstances of the patient.

Likewise, the critics of scientific psychiatry go to extremes but at the opposite end of the spectrum. Their portrayal of psychiatrists as puppets of the state and designers of madness overlooks the disparity in the discipline. In addition, their very conception of mental disorder as a social construct neglects the welfare of the patients.[50] They dismiss the notion of mental illness, and in turn disregard the very real suffering that many patients experience. Moreover, despite their contentions that mental illness is a social construct, anti-psychiatrists have not been able to account for the success of biological treatments that have restored mental stability to many patients. The view of mental illness that privileges its social origins has proven to be a powerful tool of historical analysis. However, its critics have tended wrongly to view the profession as monolithic and all-controlling. This dominance attributed to psychiatry paradoxically ignores opponents within the profession, many of whom assert anti-psychiatric views, but also dismisses the agency of alternative practitioners, such as healers, shamans, and religious guides, as well as the patients themselves.

The embittered struggle outlined here creates the impression that practitioners and scholars fall into two opposing camps. Indeed, the vehemence of the arguments often compels practitioners to adopt a particular perspective. However, the psychiatric profession has itself historically been less definitive than either of these groups has contended. Not only are practitioners a disparate and heterogeneous group, we cannot easily divide their views into these categories. For instance, in practice, most practitioners accept biomedical explanations for mental illness, but they also recognize the effect of social conditions.[51] Thus, it is important that we do not simply reduce their history to the progress of biomedical approaches or to a narrative that privileges social factors involved in conditioning mental disease. The historian must consider both dimensions, recognizing their inter-relationship and integration. A balanced approach is particularly important in a country like South Africa where indigenous practitioners, applying holistic and non-Western approaches, were treating far more patients. As we will see, practitioners trained in Western psychiatric practices grappled with understanding and incorporating these indigenous approaches into their own practice, while also maintaining well-developed biomedical concepts of mental illness.

THE ORGANIZATION OF THE BOOK

Because notions of mental health touch on many aspects of peoples' lives, and because of the convoluted and often multifarious nature in which madness was treated, it is impossible to organize this book in a purely systematic way. I have therefore organized it in two ways: chronologically and by subject. Because trends in psychiatric ideology and practice were not always uniform or limited to one period, some overlap occurs. I begin with a chapter that examines the reasons why in the 1930s and 1940s South African practitioners moved away from simply locking up patients and began to focus instead on releasing them into the community. It looks at the adoption of new, potentially progressive views by practitioners at the end of the World Wars. While practices for most of the early twentieth century had been custodial, the onset of the First and Second World Wars meant that new attention was being paid to white men seen to be suffering from adverse effects of the war. Practitioners applied hereditarianist, psychoanalytical and behaviorist policies, as well as experimented with new radical therapies, in an attempt to discard custodial practices and effectively treat their patients. Racial segregationist policies, however, contradicted the emerging ideals of humane treatment and those working within state institutions, constrained by government policies, tended to ignore black patients and focus on their more treatable white patients.

In order to better understand the apartheid government's views, and how practitioners and patients fit within the system, the second chapter examines the apartheid government's early policies towards the administration of those deemed mentally disordered between 1948 and 1966. Such a discussion reveals the racialized and gendered nature of mental health policy, but more importantly, it shows how, in practice, it was contradictory, inefficient, and ad hoc in nature.

Understanding ideas of mental health in South Africa cannot be complete without examining the views of the very people they affected. The third chapter therefore describes the views of those involuntary institutionalized patients and their confrontations with staff and government officials from 1939 to 1961. Based on the few remaining patients' letters and interviews that describe their experiences, it provides a very important forum for patients' voices during this period. It depicts the alienating nature of the system, while also highlights patients' ability, albeit limited, to contest their positions. Whereas patients suffered in the oppressive mental health structure, they were not ignorant of the world around them and did not simply accept their imposed alienation.

To see the complex position of psychiatric practitioners and the various challenges they encountered in the context of apartheid policies, the fourth chapter looks at the case of Demetrio Tsafendas who assassinated Prime Minister H. F. Verwoerd in 1966. The assassination resulted in a public debate about mental health practices. The chapter considers the attempts by practitioners to advocate for better services, incorporate notions of deinstutionalization and cross-cultural psychiatry that were becoming increasingly popular, and ultimately challenge government policies on mental health in the wake of Verwoerd's death. What we see, however, is practitioners' continued focus on white men and the government's skewing of popular psychiatric views as a means to promote a two-tiered mental health system—one that offered modern services to whites, and another that suggested that blacks, coloureds, and Indians could be treated in the community by "traditional" means. This supported the government's segregationist strategies. Thus, practitioners, some inadvertently, facilitated an even larger divide in the application of services for blacks, whites, coloureds, and Indians.

The idea of practitioners as advocates and the very heteropatriarchal views of apartheid are examined further in the fifth chapter, which discusses the debates from the late 1960s to the 1980s about homosexuality and mental health. Contextualizing these debates within international struggles for sexual freedom, this chapter examines how practitioners played a vital, and not always supporting, role in how the state approached the treatment of homosexuals. The Society of Psychiatrists and Neurologists of South Africa and individual practitioners directly opposed stricter criminal penalties for homosexuals. In the 1970s, however, a few practitioners in the South African military took it upon themselves to conduct experiments on young homosexual white men and human rights abuses did occur. However, even within the South African Defence Force, disagreement existed about the treatment of those deemed mad. Patients also usurped state power in various ways.

The sixth chapter discusses how in the 1960s through to the 1980s, the government, realizing that its policy of repatriating mentally ill blacks was not working, contracted their care to a private company, Smith, Mitchell & Co. These mainly custodial institutions offered little form of therapy. The chapter examines the contradictory role that these institutions and those that worked in them played within the country. Practitioners and staff were often dissatisfied with the atrocious conditions within the institutions, and when scandals of abuse in these institutions erupted in the 1970s, many were able to challenge the system somewhat through international investigators.

The seventh and final chapter of this book examines the origins of the Church of Scientology's attacks in the 1970s on Smith Mitchell institutions and state practitioners, which resulted in an international backlash against South African practitioners. Placed within the context of the Cold War and debates about communism and resistance, the chapter problematizes the affect of various international players on mental health policy in South Africa. While showing how practitioners were ostracized by the international community in the 1980s, it also recognizes the overt attempts by some practitioners to challenge apartheid policies and the emergence of a new awareness among practitioners of their political roles.

A NOTE ABOUT TERMINOLOGY

When discussing how people are depicted, there is a danger of reifying the subjects about which one writes; that is, in writing about perceptions, one creates a system of statements—an object that objectifies the subject. Through the writing about psychiatric discourse and practice, for instance, I may simply be reinforcing existing ideas of difference. Historical analysis, however, is not objective and inevitably reflects the views of the researcher. I do think that it is necessary not to treat perspectives as reality or absolute. As seen throughout this book, theoretical factors such as class, race, gender, normalcy, identity, and power are not fixed, and we should therefore study them within their historical context without set pre-conceived boundaries.[52]

This leads me to a brief explanation about the terminology I use in this book. Race is a flexible, historically conditioned construct. Up until the 1920s, race in South Africa was not always necessarily associated with color, but also depicted tensions between the two main white language groups, English and Afrikaans. In the mid-1920s, race became more strongly related to skin color and this became more established in the decades following.[53] The terms "white," "black," "coloured," and "Indian" or "Asian" are therefore problematic because their meaning throughout the colonial and apartheid process was irregular and ever changing. The government consistently changed its racial categorization scheme so that, for example, "black" sometimes meant "Africans," while at other times it included those later classified as "coloured" and "Indian." Moreover, during the latter part of apartheid, politically conscious "blacks," "coloureds," and "Indians" favored the term "black" to represent their political unity against oppression. I have used the terms "black" (sometimes interchangeably with "African"), "white," "coloured," and "Indian/Asian," all of which were ascribed by the colonial government and used by government officials, practitioners, and patients themselves. This is not because I subscribe to this racialized terminology, but because the terms themselves show the racialized realities of the period. Because of the racialist nature of South African society, it has been necessary to use these terms extensively throughout the book. Thus, I have opted to forgo quotations on these terms. Sometimes I use the collective term "non-white"—also a racialized construct—to include black, coloured, and Indian. "Non-white" was commonly used throughout much of the twentieth century, but is problematic in the sense that it defines individuals by what they are not and suggests that "white" is the norm. I have used this term sparingly only to show the context in which it was used.

Terminology about the mind is also extremely subjective and historically conditioned. Before World War I, words such as "lunatic," "imbecile," "insane," "idiot," "mad," "defective," and "feebleminded" were readily used. By the mid-twentieth century, these words persisted, yet the official records reflected less harsh descriptions of the mental patient. Individuals were now "retarded," "neurotic," "disordered," "unhygienic," and "unstable." With the introduction of psychopharmacological drugs in the 1950s and 1960s, terms became more specialized so that one was "schizophrenic," "depressed," "psychotic," and more recently, mentally "ill." This movement away from somewhat obscure and ill-defined psychiatric terms such as "lunatic," "feebleminded," and "mad" towards specific designations such as "schizophrenic," "depressive," "psychotic," and mentally "ill" is reflective of psychiatry's move towards a more specialized and biologically based viewpoint. However, none of the previous terms disappeared and many were used concurrently. Throughout the book I use the terms of the particular period in order to give the reader a better understanding of the views of the period. Terms were applied depending on the race of the person. Diagnoses and general terms often fell along racial lines. Moreover, it is necessary to note that practitioners often did not make a distinction between those seen to be born with a serious mental "defect" and those with less serious "illnesses." Thus, this book is about all types of individuals who ended up in homes for the mentally disordered and the feebleminded.

For the purposes of this book, a "patient" is anyone who had been at one point under the supervision or treatment of a practitioner. However, even the term "patient" itself is problematic as it infers passivity and brings with it ascribed power dynamics between patient and practitioner. Indeed, as many scholars have pointed out, the very notion of "doctor" and "patient" reflects an imbalanced relationship between a "healthy" practitioner and the "unhealthy" patient. As there is a lack of appropriate alternative, I have chosen to retain the term "patient," recognizing that it has limitations.

Because of the social conditioned nature of terms, translating the various documents is difficult and in turn may reflect the translator's understanding or biases. In most places, I have attempted to retain the integrity of the original text by using the terms of the appropriate period in which they were written. I have also included the original in the notes. I have, for the most part, allowed the words of patients, practitioners, government officials, and family members to speak for themselves. Although I have offered my own interpretation and translation of their writings, my reading is in no way meant to supersede their voices.

1 Prospects of a Progressive Mental Health System in South Africa Before Apartheid

Tara Hospital and Psychobiology, c1939–1948

In 1946, a modern, innovative neuropsychiatric hospital opened on the outskirts of Johannesburg. Tara Hospital, renamed Tara, the H. Moross Centre in 1969, was the first of its kind in South Africa. It was an open, therapeutic hospital that combined new notions of psychoanalytical, behaviorist, hereditarianist, and somatic approaches in the treatment of its patients. For the first time, a mental hospital in South Africa claimed to offer promises of cures for previously neglected mental patients within a relatively hospitable environment.

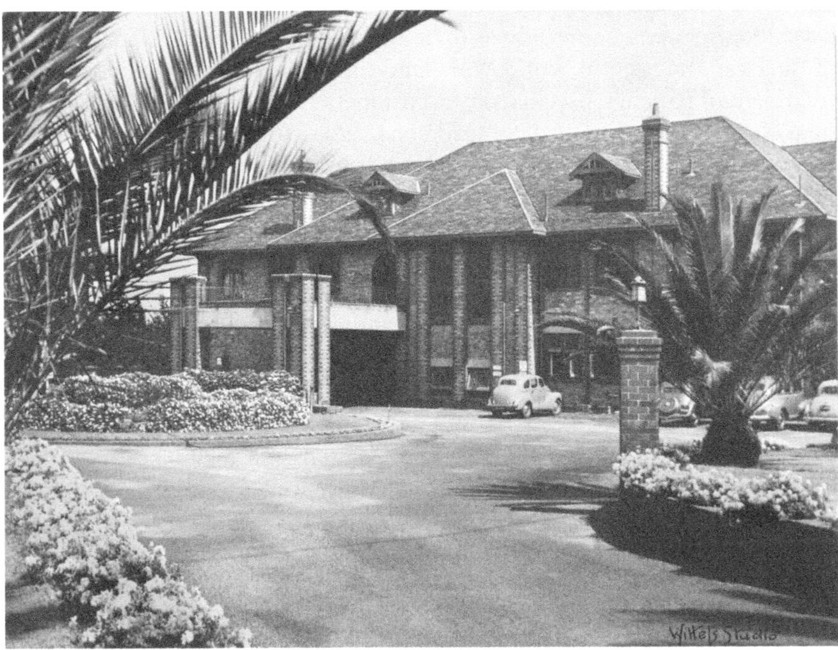

Figure 1.1 Main building of Tara Hospital, c1960s. Photo © Adler Museum of Medicine, Faculty of Health Sciences, University of Witwatersrand, Johannesburg.

Tara was the embodiment of innovative international approaches towards mental health care that challenged a previous custodial system. Before the First World War, like in most of the rest of the world, South African psychiatric practitioners had simply detained mental patients. Yet by the 1940s, new ideas about the treatment of mental patients that were emerging in Europe and North America were changing the way South African practitioners approached mental health care. Psychiatrists began to suggest that patients could actually be cured. This revolution in approach towards mental health care in South Africa was precipitated by new views of psychiatry and the First and Second World Wars, which produced large amounts of soldiers said to be affected by psychoneurosis. International ideas on psychoanalysis and behaviorism, coupled with existing hereditarianist ideas and new radical therapies, for the first time offered hope of restoration to patients and their families.

Conceptualizations of progress are relative, however, and although practitioners in the early twentieth century believed that South African psychiatry was progressing into a therapeutic field where they could actually treat patients, how one measures such progress is subjective. In the eighteenth century, psychiatry emerged as a separate field within the medical sciences, but few viewed it as equal to biological medicine. Even when numbers of patients increased throughout the nineteenth and early twentieth centuries, and more institutions opened, the government rarely saw psychiatrists and psychologists in the same light as their medical counterparts. With the onset of the First and Second World Wars, and the emergence of new ideas about treatment of patients, psychiatric practitioners felt the need to advance their own status within the medical field. Their goal seemed in line with South African government officials, who wanted to regulate the behavior of the public and maintain a semblance of social control. What becomes apparent through an analysis of this period, however, is that psychiatrists neither were simple lackeys of the state nor were they a homogeneous group. South African psychiatrists held disparate views about the cause and treatment of mental disorder. Not all of these views supported those of the state. Indeed, in the 1930s and 1940s genuine attempts at reform originated from within the mental health profession, even if these endeavors mainly targeted white patients. Although their efforts for change often resulted in unanticipated consequences and psychiatric practice in the 1940s ended up perpetuating racial and gender inequality in South Africa, we also need to acknowledge that most state-sanctioned psychiatrists genuinely wanted to reform a previous dismal mental health system.

Because many of the practices set up during and immediately after the First and Second World Wars formed the foundation for future mental health policies, understanding practitioners' perceptions of treatment of mental illness during this period is important. New views towards patients informed later practices. Although apartheid, implemented in 1948, changed mental health services somewhat, the foundation had been laid for future inequities. The opening of Tara Hospital reflected the complexity of these new psychiatric views. It promoted an emerging therapeutic psychobiological ideal among practitioners, but also reflected the very gendered and racialized structure of South African society and psychiatry in general.

THE TREATMENT OF MADNESS BEFORE THE FIRST WORLD WAR

To fully comprehend the complex role of the South African psychiatric profession and their actions after the First World War, we need to understand the state of mental health services in the years leading up to the twentieth century. Tracing the origins of apartheid South Africa's mental health policy is somewhat problematic because of the diverse and ambiguous nature of mental science both as a profession and as a medical specialty. The inception of the actual discipline in South Africa is difficult to determine.[1] Most historians begin their history of South African psychiatry with the establishment of the Cape of Good Hope settlement in 1652.[2] They usually discuss the movement from makeshift beds for lunatics during early colonialism to the establishment of permanent institutions for the mentally disordered in the late nineteenth century. However, the question of the origins of psychiatry is intrinsically connected to the question of what exactly psychiatry is. If one defines psychiatry as a scientific discipline, then one traces psychiatry's origins to the beginnings of medical science, and in South Africa's case, the beginning of colonial occupation.[3] On the other hand, if one were to extend the definition of psychiatry to include unconventional ideas of mental and spiritual health, as some scholars recently have begun to do, the definition and origin of psychiatry becomes more complex.[4]

Conceptualisations of mental health and mental disorders may have existed in South Africa before the advent of colonialism. The lack of pre-colonial written sources renders this history mostly inaccessible. Some scholars have suggested looking at African views of mentality during colonialism as indicative of pre-colonial views. Indigenous healers' understanding and treatment of mental disorders certainly have their roots in pre-colonial times. Anthropologists have suggested that Africans had terms to describe and distinguish between mental complaints.[5] However, one must recognise that notions of mentality among African groups are not universal, static and separate from that of the body.

Whether madness is a universal phenomenon irrespective of culture remains under debate.[6] Understandings of deviancy and madness should however be seen in relation to their socio-political context. In the early years of Dutch and British rule in South Africa, institutions for the mad were non-existent and they were left to the devices of their families or arbitrarily placed in wings of hospitals, prisons or on the convict station of Robben Island.[7] The first institution solely designated for the detention of the mad opened in Grahamstown in the Eastern Cape in 1876. Later known as Fort England Hospital, Grahamstown Lunatic Asylum materialized out of the abandoned structures of a British military post. Four years later, Town Hill Mental Hospital in Natal, then known as Pietermaritzburg Lunatic Asylum, was built. A few years after, Bloemfontein or Oranje Hospital in the Orange Free State and Valkenberg in the Cape opened its doors. The first institution to open in the Transvaal was Pretoria Asylum (now known as Weskoppies), which in 1892 was specifically built for the purpose of housing mental patients.

Much debate exists about why institutions and psychiatrists became the means to care for the insane at this particular juncture in history. South Africa was highly influenced by trends in the western world. The nineteenth century in Europe and in the United States, as Andrew Scull points out, was a period of dramatic change. Perceptions of the mad transformed from the idea that they were simply part of the larger group of social miscreants, towards a more defined view in which they were seen to have a specific condition that could only be determined by experts. It was a period in which larger amounts of individuals were restrained within isolated institutions and where the psychiatric profession arose as the legitimate and legal manager of the insane. Force, abuse, and suffering were commonplace within the institutions and explicitly accepted.[8]

There are many reasons for this increased institutionalization. Scull argues that exiling the mad to institutions in western countries was connected to the rise of the industrial economy.[9] Indeed, the nineteenth century was a period when increased industrialisation was causing a breakdown between rural and urban areas and previous practices of dealing with the insane were no longer viable. At the same time, there was also an increased concern with humanism that was propounded by a desire for modernity and scientific rationalism. Within this institutional structure, however, contradictions existed between the ideas of humanism and authoritarianism.[10] Institutions were therefore in paradoxical positions—on the one hand signifying the increased concern with protecting and treating the insane, while on the other regulating and disciplining patients.

Johann Louw and Sally Swartz have demonstrated how trends within Europe influenced South African perceptions of the insane. They show how there was a strong desire to replicate British institutions. The rise of humanism in Britain certainly played a part in the colonial office's decision to build Valkenberg Mental Hospital in the late nineteenth century. They point to how staff within the institutions were placed in a contradictory position, wherein they had to "tread a fine line between freedom and confinement, domesticity and institutionalism, recreation and labor, and treatment and simple incarceration."[11] British influence inevitably penetrated the practices of practitioners, as most of those working within the institutions were either British or trained in England. Before 1922, South Africa did not have its own medical or psychiatric training programme, and many of those practitioners interested in medicine and psychiatry took courses, albeit rudimentary courses, on psychoses in Europe. Up until 1932, mental nurses also had to take the Royal Medico-Psychological Association of Great Britain and Ireland test, which was administered in South Africa and graded in Great Britain.[12]

In South Africa, however, the choice to open mental institutions at this particular juncture can not only be ascribed to international trends in humanism. South Africa was experiencing its own era of industrialisation. At the end of the nineteenth century, when gold and diamonds were discovered in the interior and South Africa experienced rapid industrialization and urbanization, family relationships changed. It became increasingly difficult and more of a nuisance to take care of a deviant family member. The previously "eccentric" aunt or the "wandering" sibling became more noticeable and inconvenient.[13] In the growing urban areas, the control over and the safety of such individuals was also less assured. Moreover, the large exodus of single black men to work on the gold mines and the lack of family members to care for them in the vicinity meant that more beds, even if just used temporarily before repatriation, were needed to control those exhibiting abnormal behavior.

In 1910, South Africa unionized. The various republics and colonies came under the unitary rule of an Afrikaans and English-speaking coalition government that continued to enforce segregationist practices against Africans. Whereas racial exclusion of black Africans from the vote was not initially legislated, the socio-economic restrictions meant that the majority of the black population had no franchise. The Union government established a Ministry of Native Affairs and passed a series of legislative acts that enshrined segregationist practices.[14] Mental institutions were microcosms of the state reflecting its desire to enforce a universal social norm, while simultaneously promoting exclusion and differentiation, particularly along the lines of race and gender. In the late nineteenth and early twentieth century, psychiatry reinforced segregationist structures by perpetuating its racist and gendered rhetoric. Practitioners depicted Africans as more childish and less susceptible to treatment than Europeans. They also classified individuals and used differential diagnoses to maintain and rationalize the inequalities of the facilities.[15] Indeed, white men obtained significantly superior accommodation than black men and women, although treatment for all patients was limited.

In 1910, South Africa had eight mental institutions roughly fashioned along their European counterparts that accommodated approximately 1,692 European and 1,932 non-European patients.[16] Pre-union legislation regarding the insane differed provincially, with each province or colony having its own, albeit similar, Act governing mental services.[17] In 1914, the Union government passed the Lunacy and Leprosy Laws Amendment Act to ensure that certifications of mental patients were recognized cross-provincially. Shortly thereafter, it implemented the Mental Disorders Act of 1916 to further unify mental health services of the country.[18] Under the

1916 Act, the administration of psychiatric patients, practitioners, and mental hospitals now fell under the jurisdiction of the Commissioner for Mental Hygiene in the Department of the Interior (DI), a department also responsible for overseeing prisons in the country. After 1919, the DI also accommodated the Department of Public Health, which was in charge of a few public hospitals that mainly handled infectious diseases.

The connection between prisons, infectious disease, and mental institutions had always been close. Jail cells had always housed those deemed mad. Even when permanent mental institutions had been erected, they were quickly filled, and prisons continued to serve as temporary holding areas for the mentally disordered. The DI also housed tuberculosis (TB) and leprosy patients in wings in mental hospitals, or sanatoriums next door. Moreover, mental hospitals and TB sanatoria were very like prisons. They were closed detention centers that mostly housed the underprivileged, disorderly, and miscreant.[19]

Poor treatment within the institutions was exacerbated by the lack of available nursing staff. Mental nursing was extremely demanding and there was always a high staff turnover rate. For most of the early years of the asylums, white English-speaking male nurses, many of whom were discharged soldiers, were the main custodians of patients. Institutional work involved physical constraint and was generally considered unsuitable for women, yet some widows served as supervisors of a few coloured female attendants, and black male attendants were later hired to attend to the few institutionalized black female patients.[20] With the onset of the World Wars, the shortage of practitioners and nurses would become more critical as white men were called to partake in the war and the numbers of traumatized patients increased.

M. Minde, a psychiatrist interested in the history of psychiatry in South Africa, fittingly calls the period from the nineteenth century up to the 1930s as the "custodial period," when practitioners simply housed patients in institutions and had few alternatives for the treatment of their patients.[21] Indeed, few therapeutic options were available to practitioners who acted mainly as wardens, and patients were left to spend the rest of their days within the bleak walls of the institutions. South Africa had insufficient trained psychiatrists. Medical practitioners with an interest in mental disorders mainly oversaw the care of the mentally insane. In 1922, physician superintendents at Valkenberg Mental Hospital began training students. Two years later, the University of Witwatersrand began offering a course on psychiatry led by the Commissioner for Mental Hygiene, J. T. Dunston. Both of these courses were poorly attended.[22] Interest in psychiatry was limited and the discipline was imprecise and subjective. Practitioners rarely understood the distinction between certain diagnoses and psychiatric diagnoses were constantly confused and changing.[23] Psychiatry as a discipline in general in the late nineteenth and early twentieth century was not highly regarded. Psychiatrists lagged behind their medical counterparts in innovations and they had made little progress in the treatment of the insane.[24]

As some scholars have pointed out, a few practitioners at times used psychiatry as a means to control threatening African responses to the colonial government's racist policies.[25] Robert Edgar and Hilary Sapire write about the life of Nontetha Nkwenkwe, a female prophet in the 1920s, who preached the unity of all Africans, encouraged the boycott of white churches, and gained a large following. White authorities were concerned that her actions would result in a repeat of the 1921 Bulhoek massacre of African Israelites, where police and defense force officers had killed 183 and injured 100 African Israelites. The Bulhoek incident had caused heightened paranoia and suspicion among the white community about black independent religious movements and they were afraid that Nontetha was a political radical. In an attempt to undermine her authority and avoid making her a luminary among her followers, the government ended up housing her in Fort Beaufort Mental Hospital and later Weskoppies Asylum, where she remained for the rest of her life. Nontetha's institutionalization, which corresponded with the emergence of psychiatry as a new medical discipline, shows that although psychiatry was couched in terms of scientific humanitarianism, it at times enforced colonial hegemony.[26] But Nontetha's story was an anomaly and after the World Wars, for the most part, practitioners' positions became increasingly multifaceted. They were particularly concerned with treating former soldiers, most of whom were white men.[27] When South Africa joined the war efforts on the side of the Allies, Africans supported the government's controversial decision, but they were not allowed to hold combat roles. Thus, they were neither seen as the main victims of post-war trauma nor the focus of practitioners. For the most part, concern about Africans after the war was limited and practitioners concentrated on treating white men rather than constraining the "African mind."

COMING OUT OF THE SHADOWS: NEW POST-WAR EXPLANATIONS AND THERAPIES FOR MENTAL DISORDERS

The onset of the World Wars, in conjunction with growing eugenic fears about the rise of white poverty during the Great Depression, gave South African psychiatrists the impetus to move out of the shadows of detention into the forefront of medical science. With large numbers of white male soldiers experiencing mental trauma and high numbers of whites living in poverty-stricken multiracial slums, concerns about racial degeneration became more prominent. Seemingly normal white individuals, most of whom were men who had never previously shown any indications of mental disorder, suddenly were affected by psychoneurosis. The recognition that anyone could be affected by a mental disorder given adverse circumstances brought attention to the field as a whole. Officials and practitioners were reminded that environmental stress played a vital part in the mental health of individuals and the government was being pressed by family members and practitioners to effectively deal with former soldiers experiencing trauma. At the same time, however, the twentieth century worldwide saw a return to biological explanations for mental disorders. Influenced by these trends, for most South African practitioners, difference in genetic traits was a key reason why some soldiers experienced mental trauma while others did not. Recognition of recessive genes made some practitioners believe that environmental conditions could invoke mental problems that normally lay dormant, such as those showing up in soldiers. For psychiatrists and officials who had been wanting change within the mental hospital, the period of war offered them a valiant excuse to promote the mental welfare of their patients. There was, as Andreas Sagner points out, "a genuine reform-will within parts of the state administration. Officials who had tried hard to improve social and health services for a long time, finally gained a hearing within their departments."[28] War images of the struggle for liberty were transferred to discussions of mental treatment. As many of those needing treatment were former soldiers, government officials invoked the image of soldiers and freedom in debates about the need for further mental hospitals and changes in treatment. "We are face to face with the treatment of large numbers of our soldiers who have suffered during the war and have become temporarily mentally disordered," MP for Pinetown, M. Marwick argued, "I consider that our duty is not lightly to allow the liberty of these men to be treated as if it were not of first class importance to everyone of us."[29]

Even though war veterans were predominantly from the poor Afrikaans-speaking working class, veterans held some power within the community. After the war, ex-servicemen, many of whom had previously been unemployed, had high expectations for employment and "the act of volunteering and wearing a uniform created a special, albeit precarious, relationship of obligation and entitlement between soldiers and the state."[30] However, increased industrialization after the war led women, blacks, Indians, and coloureds to take over previously white male dominated jobs. Former soldiers and their families became incensed with the government's failure to provide for them. Pressures placed on the United Party by veteran advocacy organizations such as the Springbok Legion did at least make some members of the government acknowledge the problems that veterans faced.[31] Moreover, the promotions of practitioners, many of whom had worked as medical doctors and psychiatrists in the war, to provide for former veterans meant that the government began to investigate the possibility of opening up more beds in mental institutions. Mental hospitals offered the government a means by which to dispose of those men who could potentially arise against it. The threat of insurgency among ex-servicemen was not so far-fetched. Just over twenty years earlier in 1924, Jan Smuts, leader of the South African Party before he became Prime Minister and leader of the United Party, had been driven out of office by incensed Afrikaner nationalists and the white poor. At the same time, the government came up with the Soldier's Charter in 1944 that acknowledged the state's responsibility towards providing adequate social services for former soldiers so that they could reintegrate back into society.[32]

Practitioners sought new ways to deal with patients who had previously been abandoned within the confines of the institution. New psychotherapeutic approaches to nervous disorders made popular by Freudian notions of the unconscious, and concepts of behaviorism that promoted the idea that if one changed one's environment one could be conditioned as one practitioner put it to be "a genius or an idiot," were spreading rapidly throughout Europe and America.[33] Influenced by these trends, some South African practitioners readily debated the application of psychoanalysis and behaviorist theory to their patients. Probably one of the most staunch, and most controversial, advocates of a form, albeit a somewhat obscure religious form, of behaviorism was J. J. de Villiers, a psychiatrist who had been admitted as a patient in a mental institution himself. De Villiers had been a psychiatrist during the war in Egypt from 1941. In 1943, the South African Defence Force (SADF) sent him to North Africa for service. However, in 1944, he was detained in a mental hospital first in Geniefa, Egypt, and then transferred to the Union's No. 134 Military Hospital in Potchefstroom, South Africa, where he stayed on and off for approximately two and a half years. After release, he continued to practice without a valid medical certificate, which led to his arrest in 1947 and his admission to Weskoppies hospital as a governor general decision patient, that is, an involuntary patient, until 1949. He thereafter obtained conditional discharge, was placed under the care of a cousin, and lived off his meager military pension.[34] With his psychiatric license revoked, de Villiers struggled to clear his name for most of the decade, to no avail, but he continued to promote his theories, some of which the *Edinburgh Medical Journal* and the *South African Medical Journal* eventually published. De Villiers argued that psychiatrists had no understanding of the etiology of mental disorder, and it was for this reason that errors in diagnoses would be made and its incidence would continue to rise. Taking on the Afrikaans word for mental disorder, *sielkunde* or *sielsiekte*, which he translated as "knowledge of the soul" and "derangement of the soul," he argued that mental illness was caused by a "sickness of the soul—and not primarily with a sickness of the brain."[35] A "sick soul" he argued could have been caused by being sinned against, or by actually sinning:

> the sick soul, torn between the socially-sound advice of its conscience on the one hand, and the asocial, amoral, unethical urgings of the "Id" on the other, is liable to lose his or her clear understanding of right and wrong and to commit crimes like theft, or murder, or sex-crime, under the impression that by such means the mental conflict will be resolved, and that, in his or her case, such behaviour would be right.[36]

Although he adopted psychoanalytic terminology, de Villiers opposed Freudian methodology, arguing that Freud advocated for a sinful world "where 'the social order no longer forbids the seduction of young girls', and where girls and women willingly seek to be seduced."[37] Rather, the etiology of "a sane person," he argued, was "a healthy-minded, clean-thinking, honourably-living, truth-speaking human being, who believes in Jesus Christ and practices His teaching."[38] Anyone not living up to these standards was thus mentally disordered.[39]

De Villiers is an extreme example of the adaptation of behavioral and psychoanalytical theories that went on among practitioners in South Africa. But other practitioners promoted forms of behaviorism and psychoanalysis to treat patients, although often with a heteropatriarchal and racialized tinge. The underlying ideas of psychoanalysis and behaviorism seemed to support the government's racial and gendered segregationist ideals. As feminist scholars have shown, Freud founded his ideas on a male prototype. Freud had specific notions of women that R. E. Facher has shown were not always consistent and often were contradictory.[40] Thus, they are difficult to summarize. Simply stated though, he based his ideas on the notion that women were biologically inferior to men. For example, one of his arguments was that women were merely "castrated" males, suffering through many obstacles in their sexual development, so much so, that they were unable to have any energy for anything intellectual. This view, as feminists have pointed out, entrenches gender stereotypes and suggests that a woman is "less moral, has little sense of justice, is submissive, emotional and makes no cultural contributions."[41] Additionally, Freud's arguments pertaining to what he called "savages" suggested that Europeans were inherently superior. His *Totem and Taboo* suggested that "primitives" in Africa, Asia, and Melanesia were indicative of the pre-history of the European world. They simply had a less-developed superego that failed to restrict their sexual practices. It was therefore necessary for Europeans to restrict their sexual activities in order to stop them from damaging themselves.[42] Freud's writings are, as Jock McCulloch points out, "rich and complex" and "it would be wrong to reduce Freud's argument to a handful of quotations emphasizing the ethnocentrism [and patriarchalism] he inherited from thinkers such as Comté, Darwin and Frazer."[43] A few practitioners interested in psychoanalysis and the mental processes of the African, however, espoused the ethnocentric views implicit in his theories. Indeed, psychoanalysis in South Africa tended to promote a white masculine ideal.

Wulf Sachs's *Black Hamlet*, for example, a particularly popular book published in 1937 and then again in 1947, was an example of the ethnocentrism of psychoanalysis in South Africa.[44] Sachs, who worked as a practitioner at the Pretoria Mental Hospital in the late 1920s, wrote the book in an attempt to determine whether psychoanalysis could be applied to African cultures. Psychoanalyzing a "normal" Manyika indigenous healer identified as "John Chavafambira" for a period of two and a half years, Sachs claimed to enter the life of an African and gain a clear understanding of the "African mind." Sachs's conclusion was that Freudian analysis could be applied to Africans and that Africans' mental constitution was equal to that of whites.

Sachs's views were similar to those forwarded by B. J. F. Laubscher, a state psychiatrist with an interest in psychoanalysis, who published *Sex, Custom and Psychopathology* also in 1937. Examining the psychopathology of the Tembu and Fingo of the Eastern Cape, Laubscher argued that although Africans experienced the same mental disorders as Europeans, they may have expressed or explained them differently. Whereas Africans saw their mental disorder as stemming from "spiritual" sources, Europeans were more "rational" in their explanations of mental illness.[45]

Laubscher's views were more overtly racist than Sachs's, for he specifically argued that Africans were inherently inferior to whites. Sachs's arguments, as Saul Dubow points out, were "conceived in a far more sophisticated fashion because . . . [he] was innovative in attempting—albeit by his own admission not always successfully—to accept John as a fellow human being and as an individual, rather than the exemplification [*sic*] a collective type."[46] Nevertheless, both Laubscher and Sachs were universalists in the sense that they believed that mental disorder, even if represented differently, was a universal phenomenon that existed in all societies regardless of cultural distinctions.[47] Universalist arguments, however, fail to recognize that their own cultural environment skews their views. Moreover, they tend to suggest that their notions of Western analysis are the standard, and in turn, perpetuate racial stereotypes.

Psychiatric behaviorist approaches were also based on these universalist notions and promoted the view that white male behavior was the norm. In turn, they reinforced rigid and stereotypical racial and sex roles in which individuals were expected to act, promoting the notion that if Africans changed the way they acted, and adopted specific behavior, they would be able to alleviate their disorders. Behaviorists often used these views to suggest that those Africans who moved to urban centers and encountered urban stressors could alleviate their distress by relocating back to rural areas, an idea that the government used to justify segregationism.

Those South African practitioners actually applying psychoanalysis and behaviorist techniques in their treatments, however, were somewhat of a rarity.[48] Both were time-consuming, subjective treatments that many practitioners felt had little empirical foundation. As Lewis Hurst put it: "In South Africa, unlike in America, we have preserved our intellectual integrity against the shallow environmentalism of the psychoanalysts and behaviourists."[49] Indeed, in the late 1920s, P. J. G. de Vos pointed out that many felt that psychoanalysis had been "over-sold, and that more materialistic treatment would be popular."[50] Mental institutions were terribly overcrowded and practitioners had limited time to spend with each patient, never mind dedicating extensive amounts of time delving into the childhood, dreams, behavior, and sexuality of a patient. In 1940, there were no more than fifty medical practitioners working in mental hospitals in South Africa, only twenty-six of whom were registered psychiatrists.[51] These numbers declined during World War II, when many practitioners enlisted in the South African Medical Corps (SAMC). Moreover, language and culture barriers seriously impeded psychoanalysis and behaviorism's effectiveness in black patients, and their usefulness was usually limited to the neuroses, which were seen as border-line cases that did not require long-term care.

Other theories such as hereditarianism were a little more popular. The fact that the majority of those housed in institutions were poor and white supplemented racial degeneration fears. Influenced by early twentieth century hereditarianist ideas, many South African practitioners equated madness with an inherited defect and confounded fears of societal degeneration. Although seemingly at odds with psychotherapy and behaviorism, hereditarianism was often adopted in conjunction with these views as a means to deal with patients. Unlike psychoanalysis and behaviorism that was not widely accepted or respected by practitioners, hereditarianism enabled practitioners to promote their field as a "science" and depict themselves as doctors, rather than caretakers.

One of the key proponents for hereditarian views was L. A. Hurst, the Medical Officer at Pretoria Mental Hospital who would become Chair of Psychiatry at the University of the Witwatersrand and Chief Psychiatrist at Tara Hospital from 1959 to 1975. Because of the "unscientific" nature of psychoanalysis and behaviorism, he staunchly rejected them both. Neither "Psychoanalysts nor Behaviourists," he argued, "accepted the recent genetic findings" and their views were "artificially bolstered up by two scientifically untenable tendencies;" (i) "the general human tendency to rebel against the idea of determinism in human behaviour" and (ii) "the tendency of the physician to stress the manipulable aspect of disease." Instead, he argued that all mental disorders were biologically determined and thus "scientific genetics" was of more "practical significance to psychiatrists and general practitioners" than behaviorism or psychotherapy.[52] Hurst was strongly influenced by a German eugenicist, Franz J. Kallmann, whose studies of schizophrenia in twins made him one of the leading psychiatric geneticists in the world.[53] Kallmann argued that the etiology of mental disorders could be traced to a single recessive gene and constitutional, not environmental factors, contributed to its materialization. Solutions therefore should be biological in nature. Hurst indeed focused on empirical solutions and strongly eschewed psychoanalytical theories. He was one of the first in South Africa to begin using the electroencephalography (EEG) that measured the rate, shape and amplitude of brain waves in order to determine biological explanations for mental disorder and assess certain drugs' effect on a patient. For Hurst, the significance of these tests was to prove the underlying organic causes of mental disorder and negate any psychoanalytical or behaviorist interpretations.[54]

During much of the twentieth century, hereditarianist theory was influenced by social evolutionists and eugenic thought. Saul Dubow has done extensive work on the role that hereditarianist scientists, specifically eugenicists, had on racial segregation in South Africa in the late nineteenth and early twentieth century, particularly in the 1920s and 1930s. After dramatic industrialization in South Africa at the end of the nineteenth century and into the early twentieth century, a few medical professionals adopted eugenic views as a means to deal with some of society's disorders such as crime, poverty, and disease. Concerned with the prevalence of mental disorder among "poor whites," particularly poor Afrikaans whites, coupled with fears of mental and intellectual degeneration of the white race, eugenicists began promoting compulsory segregation and/or sterilization of the mental defective.

Central to the promotion of eugenics were ideas of gender roles and the control over procreation. Susanne Klausen, like Dubow, has effectively shown how English-speaking eugenicists in early twentieth-century South Africa linked their fears of racial degeneration among rising numbers of "poor whites," particularly poor Afrikaans whites, during World War I to ideas of "feeblemindedness," a vague term used to describe an individual who was, according to the 1916 Mental Disorders Act, "incapable of competing on equal terms with his normal fellows or of managing himself and his affairs."[55] She shows that eugenicists tied their theories about mental degeneracy to ideas about motherhood, placing importance on the procreative role of women as a means to ensure the future of the white race.[56] Eugenicists relied on controlling the sexual activities of women and detaining those deemed genetically weak, thereby reinforcing the patriarchal role of practitioners. However, like psychoanalysts and behaviorists, eugenicists were a small group who had limited influence in South Africa. They became increasingly unpopular as their ideas contradicted with ideas of white domination, especially their views of the "poor whites" as being inherently inferior and genetically weak. Moreover, the Holocaust revealed the potentiality of their beliefs and they were not too popular with politicians who were very concerned with disassociating themselves from any suggestion of "racial cleansing" and needing assurance of white (Afrikaans) superiority.[57] Nevertheless, their idea of the "mad African" as being genetically inferior did resonate within the field of psychiatry and would continue to do so, as we will see, for decades after.

Although the theories of psychoanalysis, behaviorism, and hereditarianism were rarely popular in their pure forms in South Africa, they undoubtedly pervaded many practitioners' thoughts, particularly as psychiatry was such an undefined and experimental discipline. In their quest to rationalize their scientific positioning, practitioners would apply prospective treatments to their patients, often at the same time, regardless of whether they contradicted each other or not. Hereditarian notions were often fused with behaviorist ideas, so that while hereditarianists urged for staunch restrictions on the procreation of the mad, they also stressed the important duty that individuals, particularly white women, had towards creating a nurturing and healthy environment for their children. Thus, combined notions of hereditarianism, psychoanalysis, and behaviorism became the means to deal with mental disorder. If mental deficiency was passed on through genes, they were supplemented by environmental factors. In turn, the environment could affect biological functions and inner mental processes. Indeed, the late 1940s saw a rise in the number of medical practitioners who began to discuss the affect of the mind on the body, and argued that that environmental stress and emotions could affect bodily responses and create psychosomatic disorders. Even de Villiers, who had promoted his unique form of religious behaviorism admitted that the sick mind might manifest itself biologically.[58]

New international radical treatments also offered an alternative to the vast hereditarianist, psychoanalytical, and behaviorist approaches and allowed psychiatry to gain more credence among the medical community. Championed as "miracles of the century," these new treatments had the potential to cure a patient relatively quickly, even if they were usually ad hoc experiments that frequently had disastrous effects.[59] The rise of microbiology brought about the awareness of bacterial infections and their effect on the brain. Practitioners worldwide began experimenting with contagions and fever-inducing agents on their patients. They used malarial parasites to treat "general paralysis of the insane" brought about by syphilis. They induced African relapsing fever and administered typhoid vaccines, metallic anti-luetic treatment, tryparasmide, and radiotherm as a means to produce fever in patients. Practitioners also experimented with arsenic and bismuth medication, despite the fact that doctors recognized arsenic as a poison that could actually cause depression.[60] They utilized hydrotherapy, placing patients in cold-water baths or running cold water over the wrists and ankles in attempts to reduce a patient's metabolic rate and in turn create change in their mental state. They also employed sleep-therapies, mainly by administering high levels of insulin twenty to fifty times to produce comas. Results of sleep-therapy were anything but peaceful, with patients experiencing confusion, muscular twitching, and in some cases, seizures. Practitioners considered seizures progressive in that they were believed to interject mental disturbances. Cardiazol, otherwise known as phrenazol, was given to produce violent epileptic fits that practitioners believed produced improvements in schizophrenics. They also introduced electro-convulsive therapy (ECT), initially without any anesthesia, which remained extremely popular for many decades thereafter.[61]

Many of these therapies left broken bones, dislocations, and deaths behind in their wake, but they did seem to work more quickly and better than anything else previously tried. South African practitioners often administered these treatments in conjunction with existing behaviorist or psychoanalytical approaches, but no longer did they have to rely solely on these techniques, or even wait a few generations through limitations on reproduction to alleviate mental illness. Morris J. Cohen, for example, advocated for the use of these new biological therapies, but also argued for the use of psychotherapeutic techniques in addressing psychoneurosis.[62] J. S. du T. De Wet, a major in the SAMC, also argued for a combined approach of convulsive therapy and psychotherapy for the treatment of military officers experiencing neurosis.[63] G. F. Langschmidt maintained that mental health should recognize the psychological effects of the war, while also treating a mental illness as a biological entity.[64] Doctors and psychiatrists began pressing for a "psychobiological" approach to medicine that recognized the interrelation between the mind and body.[65]

These views and treatments challenged the notion that a mental disorder was a permanent failing and offered hope for the future, not only for veterans, but for the psychiatric discipline as well. Psychiatry now promoted itself as a therapeutic medical occupation and not a sub-section of the prison system; no longer were psychiatrists merely keepers of the insane but they saw themselves as medical practitioners able to remedy patients. As the Minister of Health stated, "the introduction of these new methods have served to bring the mental hospitals nearer to the general hospital services, which produce treatment and cure for the physically ill."[66]

In 1944, the government transferred the administration of mental hospitals from the DI to the Department of Public Health (DPH), a sub-department of the DI until 1946. This, according to the Minister of Health, signaled a change in the government's viewpoint towards the mentally ill from one of "compulsory detention" to treatment.[67] That same year, Parliament amended the 1916 Mental Disorders Act to reflect what the President of the Medical Council and Member of Parliament, D. Bremer, called "an advance in our conception in this country of mental disorder." Amendments showed, he argued, that "mental defects are capable of treatment scientifically, that they are not what the ordinary layman's conception of them is, namely something really incurable."[68] The 1944 Amendment did indeed reflect the move away from notions of permanency in mental disorder towards one that recognized the possibility of short-term patients. A new section encompassing temporary patients was introduced that allowed individuals to voluntarily take advantage of the services offered by the mental hospitals without being certified by a magistrate—an option that also moved the burden of temporary patients away from medical practitioners in general hospitals to psychiatrists in mental institutions and private practice. Mental hospitals, government officials argued, should no longer be places of detention.

Yet long-term involuntary patients still made up the majority of the patients in mental institutions. Mental hospitals were overcrowded. Continued urbanization brought substantial numbers of Africans to the urban areas and demands for more mental health beds from officials were increasing. In 1944, black, coloured, and Indian wings were overcrowded by approximately

2,574 patients, while white sections only had an overabundance of about 176 patients.[69] Yet, the government's interests were on supplying beds for white men and beds for Africans remained a lesser priority. The Mental Health Commissioner, William Russell, admitted to the dire need for further accommodation. He suggested that two mental hospitals be built in the Cape—one that would offer 1,500 beds for whites and another housing 1,500 coloured patients. He also called for the completion of the Krugersdorp Mental Hospital for 800 white and 800 non-whites, and wanted two new mental hospitals that would provide 3,000 beds for Africans, one in the Transvaal and another in Natal. In addition, he suggested the replacement of condemned buildings at existing mental hospitals. These suggestions revealed what he saw as the "desperate situation" in psychiatric care.[70]

Yet government funding was poor both during and after the war. Financial support of mental hospitals never became a main priority of the government. Nevertheless, the desire to promote psychiatry as a therapeutic discipline and to support white male soldiers returning from the war led practitioners to make a distinction between those with impermanent mental illnesses who could quickly be cured and those with long-term disorders. Mental deficiency, psychoses, and schizophrenia, or dementia praecox as it was formerly known, were considered long-term illnesses, especially if not identified in the earlier stages. Depression, mania, and neuroses were seen as curable and thus temporary.

The differentiation between these lesser and more chronic illnesses manifested itself along racial lines. Practitioners often diagnosed white patients with less chronic illnesses and black patients with more long-term diagnoses. David Perk, a Medical Corps officer, for example, argued that "the more highly developed and integrated racial types, break down into a psychoneurosis more often than a psychosis and, conversely, the less advanced racial types tend to break down into a psychosis"—psychosis being a more serious mental illness.[71] When examining the annual breakdowns of diagnoses reported by state practitioners to the Commissioner of Mental Hygiene, we see that they diagnosed whites predominantly with manic-depressive psychoses, neurosis and defective mental development, and blacks, coloureds, and Indians with schizophrenia, paranoia, and/or epileptic psychoses. The predominance of whites diagnosed with defective mental development was mainly due to the fact that no separate wards or institutions for black mental defectives existed, and only a few were housed in state hospitals. For the most part, however, whites were diagnosed with the less-critical diagnoses, while blacks were accorded the more permanent disorders, a differentiation that most certainly reflected the racial bias among both services and practitioners. Many psychiatrists working within state-run institutions argued that Africans and coloureds were not able to experience depression at all. Because they saw depression as inextricably linked to guilt, and argued that Africans and coloureds experienced considerably less guilt—particularly sexual and criminal guilt—than Whites, the rate of suicide and depressive

Table 1.1 Main Diagnoses of Patients by Race, 1939–1950

	1939	1940	1944	1945	1950
Manic-depressive psychoses and involutional melancholia*					
Whites	488	469	454	477	455
Africans	362	399	348	399	350
Coloureds	123	123	123	130	102
Asiatics	18	30	17	18	20
TOTAL	991	1,021	942	1,024	927
Defective Mental Development					
Whites	2,267	2,270	2,394	2,428	2,710
Africans	614	588	671	640	691
Coloureds	334	345	371	387	394
Asiatics	20	14	24	30	45
TOTAL	3,235	3,217	3,460	3,485	3,840
Dementia Praecox/Schizophrenia and paranoid conditions and paranoia**					
Whites	2,189	2,262	2,390	2,410	2,509
Africans	3,733	3,857	4,439	4,570	5,255
Coloureds	784	778	939	948	1,027
Asiatics	110	112	121	128	144
TOTAL	6,816	7,009	7,889	8,056	8,935
Epileptic psychoses					
Whites	446	460	411		
Africans	642	655	765		
Coloureds	126	128	122		
Asiatics	9	9	15		
TOTAL	1,223	1,252	1,313		

*Involutional melancholia was not a classification until 1953 when it was added to the category
**Dementia Praecox changed to Schizophrenia in 1953

psychoses applied was considerably less than that for whites. Schizophrenia, a more severe and ambiguous illness than depression, became the most prominent diagnosis for black patients. This trend, as we will see, would continue into and throughout the apartheid years.

The reason given by practitioners for this racial difference in diagnoses was that while behavior and environment played a role in the manifestation of mental disorder in blacks, heredity was a more dominant factor for them than for whites. Perk claimed that "constitutional and environmental factors played complementary roles in producing both neurotic [mainly white] and psychotic [mainly black] breakdowns; [with] the constitutional factor playing the predominant role in the latter and the environmental in the former."[72] Where environmental or behaviorist factors played a part in Africans, it was in influencing hereditarian dynamics. Michael Gelfand argued that cultural factors explained why there was a lower number of Africans presenting themselves with disorders seen to be predominantly caused by recessive genes, such as neurosis:

> It is not easy to know how great a part heredity plays in mental disorders of the African. Obviously it is important, but as a greater degree of exogamy is practiced amongst them than amongst the European, traits which depend on expression of rare recessive genes and likely to appear with parental consanguinity tend to be uncommon in the African.[73]

Similarly Hyman Moross, the superintendent at Tara Hospital, contended that beliefs such as "fears of supernatural forces" that could say "interfere with dietic habits and the satisfactory nutrition of a tribe" could essentially lead to a change in tribal hereditary constitution.[74] Most practitioners however spent very little time with black, coloured, and Indian patients and it was only those who seriously disrupted the social norm who were placed in institutions. The less-disruptive individuals rarely made it into the system. Whether it was simply racial bias on the part of the practitioners, or the inadequacy of the official system to diagnose non-white patients with less critical mental disorders, or both, the recognition of temporary disorders in non-whites never manifested. For the most part, practitioners continued to focus on curable white patients.

TARA HOSPITAL: THE EMBODIMENT OF WHITE THERAPY

In 1946, Tara Hospital opened its doors. Because of the emphasis placed on treating former soldiers with psychoneurosis and the racialization of mental diagnoses, it is not surprising that Tara Hospital in Johannesburg initially catered to white, mainly male patients. According to the Annual Report of the Johannesburg Hospital, Tara only admitted patients if they were not "likely to be a disturbing influence to the community" and if they were not "uncooperative in regard to treatment or unwilling to undergo the treatment."[75] However, because practitioners were less likely to diagnose blacks with neurosis and more likely saw them as "disturbing influences to the community," the likelihood that they would diagnose non-whites with neuropsychoses was very low. Thus, the need for black beds within Tara or a separate neuropsychiatric hospital for blacks was never seen. The government expected Johannesburg General, Baragwanath, and Coronation Non-European Hospital to offer basic psychiatric and neurological coverage for them. Custodial state institutions were to continue to house those more acute black patients. In 1949, a year after the apartheid government came into power, Moross estimated that the Johannesburg General Hospital saw 1,372 new white neurosis cases and had about 8,500 previously diagnosed patients. In its non-European section, these numbers were only at 162 new cases with 170 former cases.[76]

Tara's origins lay in the Union Defence Force's No. 134 Military Hospital in Potchefstroom.[77] In 1944, Moross was commander of the hospital, and in 1943, Alice Cox joined him as chief psychiatrist. They both were formidable proponents for the establishment of a medical facility that would integrate new psychological, behavioral, and biological medical treatments to cater to non-certifiable, that is, temporary patients. After the closure of No. 134 Military Hospital at the end of the war in 1945, the government transferred staff and about a third of the patients to the new Tara Hospital, which initially was under the authority of the Red Cross but would later be taken over by the Transvaal Provincial Authorities.[78] In a joint meeting of Union, provincial, and Johannesburg Hospital officials, the decision to appoint the provincial authorities, not the Union government, to take over the administration of Tara was made so that the centre could avoid the stigma of a mental hospital. Moreover, the Minister of Health, Henry Gluckman, argued that psychoneurotic cases, which were not certifiable in the same sense as other mental illnesses, could not be accommodated at general hospitals partly because of "lack of accommodation and partly because of close propinquity with other 'general' cases tend[ed] to militate against rapid recovery."[79] With this guise, Tara could also address public concerns about the erection of a mental hospital in a more urban setting by assuring the population that admissions would be less-dangerous neuropsychiatric patients, and not general psychiatric patients as would have been the central government's obligation.[80] Tara was therefore associated with the Johannesburg General Hospital, which had both administrative and financial responsibility for the hospital and its staff.

Moross was Tara's first Medical Superintendent and he, along with Cox, began initiating a new psychobiological approach in the centre.[81] According to Moross, neurosis was caused by both physical and "circumstantial factors," and was essentially a problem with adaptation. Heredity, family, social, and racial factors all played a role in the onset of neurosis.[82] Similarly, Cox argued that both underlying biochemical and psychological factors contributed to the onset of more serious mental illnesses and it was the (in)ability of one to adapt that explained why some were affected and others not.[83] Thus, it was important to enable patients to learn how to adapt and to repair the disturbed social and biological functions in an appropriate environment such as the following:

> In the static and confidential atmosphere of the consulting room it is not possible to see the patient in the social situations, which a group environment makes possible. Such an environment should permit observation of spontaneous behaviour, thus providing a background for living diagnosis and prognosis. Furthermore, the difficulties of manipulating circumstances in the home and occupational environment of the individual are temporarily avoided if the patient is placed in a flexible controlled experimental environment, where the organization is fluid and adaptable and which can be modified to meet the needs of any particular patient or generation of patients.[84]

Tara was heralded as such a place. It was indeed very different from other mental institutions in the Union. It was located on 30 acres of land, had recreational facilities such as tennis courts, a swimming pool and a soccer field, and offered physical training, relaxation therapies, arts and crafts, and occupational therapy along with the latest in convulsive and biomedical treatments. Tara was meant to be the ideal combined therapeutic and medical hospital for temporary patients. A closely allied diagnostic and therapeutic team consisting of social workers, psychotherapists, psychiatrists, occupational therapists, recreational therapists, career counselors, physiotherapists, and dieticians was set up to treat patients. It was a place where practitioners allowed patients to roam around the premises and socialize with other patients. They encouraged families to visit patients with flexible visiting hours. Patients were also gradually released for weekends in order to ease them back into the community. The objective of Tara was to rehabilitate patients so that they could return to their daily life. Rehabilitation meant more than mental and physical rehabilitation, but also placing individuals in better jobs. In a 1949 report to the Provincial Secretary of Health, the Medical Superintendent argued that the cause for many of their patients distress was "occupational maladjustment." Therefore, aptitude tests were to be administered and patients would be offered job placement assistance.[85] The occupational therapy department consisted of three workshops, one crafts area, leather and weaving, carpentry, a library and gardening section, five instructors, three occupational therapists and one senior therapist.[86]

The hospital also conducted outpatient clinics where nurses visited patients in their homes. At first, these were mainly diagnostic clinics where patients were ultimately referred to a psychiatrist or other practitioner, but as the service continued, it offered follow up psychotherapy. Since its inception, the hospital maintained a therapeutic social club where former patients could receive support after release and in 1953, the hospital also opened up a day patient service where patients could receive treatment during the day and return to their homes at night.[87]

The number of staff far outweighed those available at state mental hospitals. In 1951, Tara had eighteen medical staff which included neuropsychiatrists, registrars and a medical superintendent, fifty-two nursing staff, one part-time psychologist, one part-time social worker, five occupational therapists, four arts and craft instructors, three physical educational specialists, two psychotherapists, and a number of clerical workers.[88] This meant that the staff patient ratio was exceptionally high. The hospital accommodated approximately 152 patients in eight wards, two of which were for women. As the war years subsided and more women were admitted, female patients continuously complained about not having enough bathroom and toilet facilities. For the most part, however, white men remained the majority of patients.[89] Tara had been a training hospital since its inception and because of its holistic approach, it offered a unique atmosphere where medical personnel including psychiatrists, psychologists, psychiatric nurses, occupational therapists, physiotherapists, and social workers could all train. The South African Medical and Dental Association did not initially recognize clinical psychologists, but in the early 1950s Moross suggested to the President of the South

African Psychological Association that Tara be used as a training hospital for the profession. In 1958, four unpaid clinical psychological internships were granted to students holding the minimum of an honours degree in psychology.[90] In 1956, a full-time chair of psychological medicine was created and the position was officially affiliated with the University of Witwatersrand and the Johannesburg Hospital.[91] Tara was held up as the ideal mental hospital, and there were many discussions about similar hospitals to be established in other provinces. Because of budget cuts and the national government's continued control over mental health, they never came to fruition.

CONCLUSION

Tara embodied the concept of the transitory nature of mental illness and offered therapeutic options to custodial certification, an option that would later transform into notions of deinstitutionalization and community psychiatry, which we will examine in later chapters.[92] However, it also denoted a multi-tiered mental health system that ultimately perpetuated the racial and gendered divide of services. Therapeutic applications were limited mainly to white men. Even after concepts of community psychiatry, where patients were meant to be treated in the community, and the development of psychotropic drugs became prominent in the 1950s, proponents buttressed apartheid ideologies by suggesting that Africans should return to their "traditional" way of life and be taken care of by their own communities. Women, they argued, should be cared for by their families. Thus, for the most part, custodial practices merely continued, now with an increased racial and gendered bias. South African practices were constrained by political, racial, and gendered differentiation. In attempts to address the lack of mental health services and to continue to promote their discipline as therapeutic, practitioners created a multi-tiered mental health system determined by biological difference; one for temporary patients, made up mostly of white males, and another for long-term patients, the majority of whom were black or coloured. This racially divided diagnostic practice meant that ideas of racial difference pervaded treatment, and new therapies were limited to whites. We have to be careful not to simply describe the treatments white men obtained as progressive. Those who received the latest treatments did not always improve and in some cases, actually died. Therapies were applied to the elderly, weak, and unhealthy with very little consideration of physical contraindications. Nevertheless, while practitioners treated their short-term white male patients with new therapies, they neglected their long-term patients, particularly long-term black patients. South African psychiatry therefore became simultaneously therapeutic and custodial. Mental health hospitals such as Tara during the 1940s reflected the contradictory nature of a multiple-tiered system, a system that, as we will see, would only be further reinforced during the apartheid years.

2 The "Disordered" State

Government Policies and Institutions for the Administration of the Mad During Apartheid, 1948–1973

Between late May and early June 1948, just days after the National Party won the general election, Johannesburg police officers arrested six black men for strange behavior. The police called in a district surgeon, that is, a state employed doctor, to examine them. He deemed them mentally disordered and transferred them to the Newlands Police Station, which frequently housed black mentally disordered individuals. As they had no registered relatives in Johannesburg, a magistrate ordered their continued detention, pending admission to a mental hospital. No beds for black men were available in any mental institution in South Africa, so they remained in police custody for the statutory maximum of twenty-one days. On the evening of July 9th, they were due to be released unless the commanding officer at Newlands could make alternative arrangements. That afternoon, he telephoned a field officer in charge of repatriation at the Native Commissioner's court to inform him that the men did not have the necessary passes and therefore could not be released. He wanted to know his options. The Additional Native Commissioner instructed one of the messengers of the court to bring the men to the pass office and lock them up for the night in the large wire and metal shed outside in the yard that was commonly used for temporary accommodation for those awaiting repatriation. It was bitterly cold that winter evening, and the shed, with its broken windows and wire door, offered little protection. Two of the men apparently became extremely agitated and demanded to be released. Their appeals were ignored. At around 11 p.m., one of the clerks at the court reported hearing an "alarming" noise that sounded like "the beating about of an instrument the sound of which could be attributed to noise caused by beating an empty tin."[1] Knowing that night duty guards were responsible for looking after the mental patients, he did not bother to check on the noise. The next morning, one man lay bruised and dead. Another died in a non-European hospital in Fordsburg while awaiting transfer.

At first, the investigating detectives and the district surgeon thought that the men had died from hypothermia. Yet they soon realized that the two men had been beaten and strangled to death. The remaining four, who had no signs of injuries, were returned to the Newlands Police Station cells. A month and a half later, one man from the case, who was deaf and mute, once again found himself waiting repatriation in the shelter outside of the pass office while officers unsuccessfully attempted to obtain information about his origins.

The case might have remained unknown except for the fact that it hit the English-language newspapers the next day. The *Star* and *Rand Daily Mail* highlighted the neglect of the men by the Native Commissioner's office and criticized its treatment of the patients.[2] The Native Commissioner for Johannesburg, K. D. Morgan, denied his department's responsibility for the deaths. He blamed the inappropriateness of the accommodation on the premises of the pass offices and the general lack of beds in mental hospitals. While there does exist the possibility of a police cover up, or the anger of one of the individuals in the cage resulted in a deadly fight with his fellow inmates, the record unfortunately remains silent as to who exactly assaulted these men.[3]

This situation was not unique. In a response to an inquiry into the matter, Morgan wrote that "the case is typical of the many that have to be dealt with, almost daily, by this office, and is the second that has come before me today."[4] The situation, and the many like it, were indicative of the arbitrary and brutal nature of South Africa's mental health process. Due to a lack of accommodation, indifferent officials often made impromptu, ad hoc decisions. Arrangements were intrinsically linked to the legal system that failed to offer black individuals any protection at all. In turn, it effected frustrated and often outraged actions by those in its grasp as a means of protest, protest for which they or others paid with their lives.

When the Herenigde Nasionale Party (NP), under the leadership of D. F. Malan, came into power in May 1948, they did so under the mandate of a makeshift policy of apartheid. Unclear as to exactly how to go about implementing the "separate but equal" strategy, the government passed laws that prohibited mixed marriages, reserved jobs for whites, and classified its population into various population groups based on skin color. The apartheid state, however, was a complex, contradictory structure that was beset with stressors caused by "the co-existence of a racially exclusive social and political order with an economic system based on the incorporation of expanding numbers of black workers."[5] Because the government relied on millions of black migrants in order to uphold and expand its industrial economy while simultaneously planning for total racial segregation, it consistently had to deal with irresolvable tensions and contradictions. Indeed, the large numbers of blacks in urban centers placed tremendous strain on the mental health system that for most of the nineteenth and early twentieth century had focused mainly on whites. Yet, with its apartheid strategy, the government was unwilling to invest in treatment or beds for black patients in existing mental institutions because its policy was to send them to the reserves, areas later known as bantustans or homelands. Mental health practitioners, constricted by these policies, tended to continue their focus on beds for white male patients for most of the 1950s and 1960s, while the crisis of overcrowding and neglect among black patients compounded.

The Nationalist government was Janus-faced when it came to the administration of those deemed mad. On the one hand, the pressures placed on the state to effectively deal with the disordered after the First and Second World War had subsided as memories of the war receded. Moreover, practitioners and government officials saw a direct connection between poor whiteism and mental deficiency, that is, they often saw poor whites as feebleminded. As the government began to address the poor white problem, the urgency placed on mental health also abated. Yet, social miscreants remained a disturbing element to the state, and it seemed that the number of individuals exhibiting disordered tendencies was rising as industrialization and urbanization increased. White disordered individuals still needed to be treated and rehabilitated, while those black individuals perceived to be dangerous also had to be dealt with.

With its objective of total social control, the apartheid state saw the mentally disturbed as a dangerous element of instability. The Department of Health's (DOH) strategy to deal with the disordered was institutionalization, which was an immediate and convenient approach. Yet this policy in itself was paradoxical. Mental hospitals not only were meant to provide a means to isolate social miscreants, they were also to be rehabilitative so that individuals, especially white patients, could become productive contributors to the apartheid project. Most institutions were located in remote rural areas, partly due to the objections of the public who found it disturbing to have deranged individuals in their immediate vicinity. But isolation made rehabilitation for patients more difficult. The rural locations also made it increasingly difficult for the government to oversee practices within them.[6] In turn, beds were constantly filled and an accommodation crisis developed that prevented government policies to be effectively implemented. Moreover, despite the apartheid government's aim to detain its black patients and rehabilitate its white patients, its failure to invest in the system meant that it was unable to do either effectively.

THE INSTITUTIONS

In 1948, there were twelve institutions in South Africa with only 13,558 beds, of which 6,680 were for whites.[7] In total, South Africa's mental institutions housed 16,676 patients, over 3,100 more patients than beds; 2,818 of these patients were designated non-white. Overcrowding was particularly severe for blacks.[8] Most of the buildings in which practitioners housed patients dated back to the nineteenth and early twentieth century and were former military buildings. Witrand Institution in Potchefstroom, for example, was originally a nineteenth century British army cantonment. Tower Hospital in Fort Beaufort in the Cape had been an army frontier

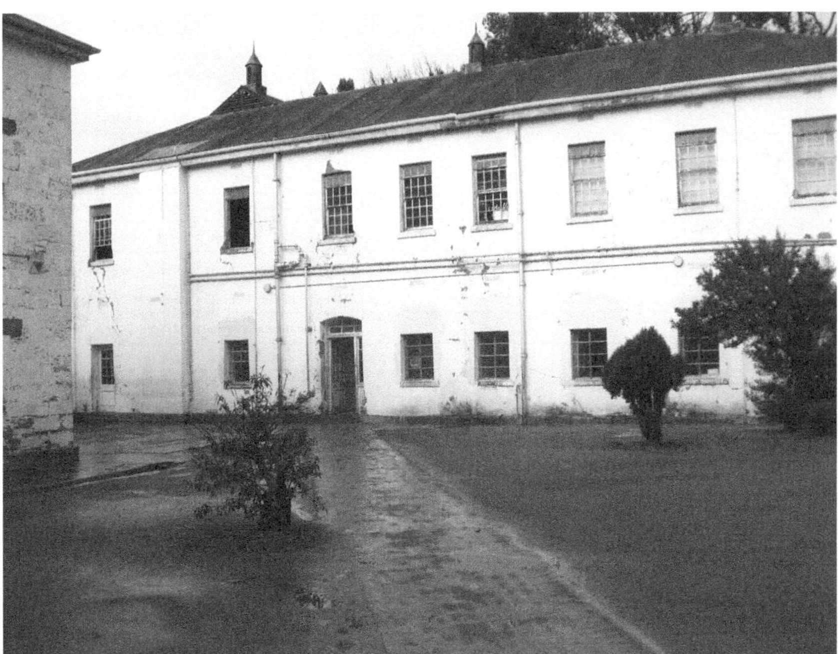

Figure 2.1 Remains of the female infirmary of Old Tower Hospital, Fort Beaufort, 2004 (now a school). Photo by author.

post that was taken over and made into a mental hospital in the 1890s. Fort Napier hospital had transformed from a military fort to a concentration camp during World War I and then became a mental hospital in 1928.[9] With the exception of the newer hospitals such as Tara, Sterkfontein, and Stikland, which had opened in the late 1930s and 1940s, the government had upgraded few of the institutions and most of them remained little more than dilapidated prisons.

In 1958, the Member of Parliament for Durban-Central, A. Radford, after a visit to Fort Napier Hospital in Pietermaritzburg, implored the Department of Public Works to undertake badly needed repairs. He described what he saw: " . . . it is in great danger of falling down. Parts of it are propped up by gumpoles, not just a little support here and there, not just 18-foot and 16-foot poles here and there, but 20 feet to 25 feet long stuck at an angle to stop it from blowing over."[10] The Department of Public Works did little to make the institutions livable. Nine years later, the Commissioner for Mental Health, Alistair Lamont, found conditions just as bad: "the picture is one of grossly overcrowded wards, shabby internally and externally, some in an advanced state of dilapidation and all inappropriately planned for their purpose. Steps taken over the years to meet demands for accommodation have created a sorry state of affairs."[11] Effective treatment was

Table 2.1 Year Opened, Building Date and Type of State-Run Institutions by Province, c1967

Name c1967	*Year Opened*	Buildings Erected	Type of Patient
CAPE			
Fort England, Grahamstown, (Previously known as Grahamstown)	1876	Military post erected in 1816	Whites, male coloured, Asian and Black
Valkenberg, Observatory	1884	Built as a mental hospital 1884	White and coloureds
Port Alfred, Port Alfred (Previously known as Kowie)	1889	Convict station erected in 1869	Black males and females
Tower Hospital, Fort Beaufort (Previously known as Fort Beaufort)	1894	Originally a frontier post	Black males and females
Alexandra, Maitland	1921	Originally a military hospital	Long-term Whites
Komani, Queenstown (Previously known as Queenstown)	1922	Built as a mental hospital	All races
Westlake, Westlake	1962	Originally a military cantonenment.	Coloured Mental Defectives
Stikland, Bellville	c1938	Built in WWII	White and coloureds
NATAL			
Town Hill, Pietermaritzburg (Previously known as Pietermaritzburg)	1880	Built as a Mental Hospital 1880	All races
Fort Napier, Pietermaritzburg	1927	Military fort erected in 1845. Concentration camp in WWI.	All races
Napier Ward, (Part of King George V Hospital), Durban	–		Indians and a few white patients
Umgeni Waterfall Institution, Howick	c1948	Originally founded as a convalescent camp for soldiers in World War II.	White males and females and Black males
ORANGE FREE STATE			
Bloemfontein (later changed to Oranje), Bloemfontein	c1883	Originally built as a military stronghold in 1848	White and Black
TRANSVAAL			
Weskoppies, Pretoria (Previously known as Pretoria)	1891	Built as a mental hospital	White and black
Witrand, Potchefstroom	1923	Originally built as British Army cantonment in the 19th Century	Long-term Whites
Sterkfontein, Krugersdorp (Previously known as Krugersdorp)	c1938	Built as a mental hospital	White and Black
HOMELAND			
Bophelong Homeland Hospital, Boputhutswana	c1966		Black
Madadeni, Kwa-Zulu	c1967		Black

impossible in the circumstances and patients were consigned to makeshift wards fashioned out of storage rooms, staff rooms, cleaning rooms, dining rooms, and enclosed verandas. Rundown, condemned buildings continued in use until they literally fell down, as occurred in more than one hospital.

E. Northover, the Assistant Chief Architect of the Department of Public Works, in his report on Fort England Hospital in Grahamstown, described the use and adding on of verandas as "a local craze" that rendered the "rooms behind almost inhabitable" due to the lack of effective planning and blocking out of sunlight.[12] Mental hospitals already had small windows and poor lighting, and improvised porches left wards dark and ventilation inadequate. Northover deemed most of South Africa's mental hospital buildings and their makeshift add-ons as uninhabitable.

In the early apartheid years, Lamont had requested funds for the rebuilding, maintenance, and restructuring of mental hospitals. The Department of Public Works, which had limited funds allocated to it, however, was reluctant to spend large amounts of money on rebuilding mental hospitals, especially as many of the institutions were in white areas and housed non-white patients. It was cheaper and more convenient simply to deport black patients to the reserves. Thus, for the most part, practitioners had to make do with limited beds in broken down, unsanitary buildings and improvised wards.

In an interview with me, Jan H. Robbertze, a state psychiatrist practicing since the early 1960s and sharp critic of poor conditions in mental institutions, explained that conditions for all patients were deplorable: "You can't say that they discriminated more against whites than against blacks. There were no services at all. They were housed in unbelievably bad conditions."[13] Whereas Robbertze's comments say much about the overall poor facilities, his claim that conditions were as bad for whites as for blacks is not entirely accurate. George Hart, a psychiatrist working in South Africa also since the 1960s, had a different opinion. When visiting Sterkfontein hospital, he was shocked by what he saw:

> I had just been around the wards and I was appalled that the condition that these people, blacks, I have to draw the distinction because they were separated and the black accommodation was appalling. In fact, I'm sure I still have letters in my possession where I wrote saying that I believed that patients were dying because of hypothermia . . . First of all, the windows, many of the windows were non-existent, in other words, there were holes in, if you want to call them a window, holes in the walls. So you can see our temperatures go quite low, so that there was first of all this problem of cold air coming in at will through these holes and there was no heating. So the temperatures in those wards must have fallen to very low degrees. The bathing arrangements were terrible, just like how you might do with cattle, going through a dip, that sort of arrangement. Really, it was quite appalling.[14]

When I asked if the conditions were better for whites he stated, "Yes, the conditions for whites were better. You know mental hospitals are never very decent places, you can go look at them in America, they are not the greatest places, but the wards for white patients were considerably better. The numbers of people were less in many of the wards."[15]

Although there was pressure to move black patients to the bantustans so that practitioners could attend to white patients, many of the buildings in which African patients stayed were in such bad shape that they were deemed unlivable for white patients. Northover, in his report on Komani Hospital in Queenstown, for example, had telling comments about the difference in facilities between white and black patients: "The disappearance of the non-White patients from the site in the future," he argued, "will leave vacant four large ward blocks for which one can see no use. They are totally unfit for White patient occupation; demolition is the solution."[16] In another report on Kowie Hospital in Port Alfred, which was purely for non-white patients, he stated that the dormitories in which patients lived were "almost ideal for their purpose," but then went on to state that the buildings were "not suitable for White patient occupation."[17] In 1958, Radford described the conditions for blacks by intentionally using the words of a report done twenty-two years earlier to show the lack of improvement in the institutions:

> In the case of non-Europeans the position in some of the dormitories is really appalling. Patients are sleeping in absolute contact with one another, not only shoulder to shoulder but feet to shoulder, when patients are placed both transversely and longitudinally in the same dormitory. They really make a solid layer of humanity, so that there is scarcely room to put a foot between sleeping patients.[18]

In 1961, the Department of Public Works established an interdepartmental committee to investigate the issues surrounding the formation of construction of institutions for black mental patients in the bantustans. Headed by J. H. van der Walt, the Secretary for the Department of Public Works, the committee echoed the difference in treatment according to race as expressed by Radford. Based on the idea that the removal of black patients from existing institutions would free up beds for white patients, the committee set out to choose possible locations and strategies for blacks-only institutions. The plans, which were partially, but never fully implemented, continued to support discriminatory practices against black patients and showed the

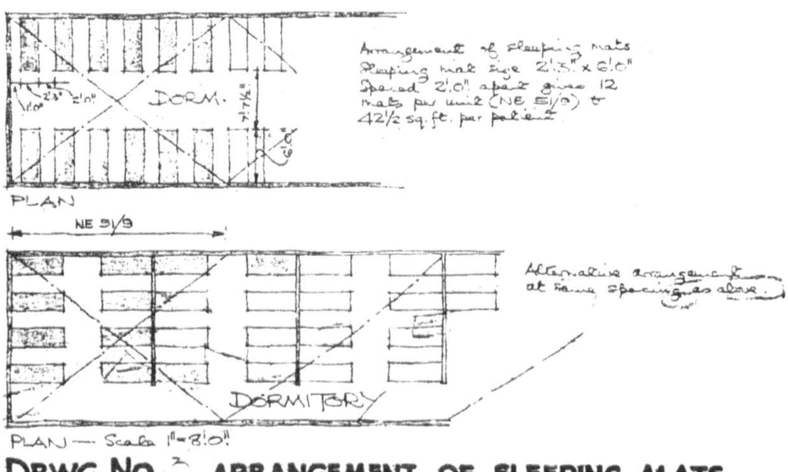

Figure 2.2 Different suggested arrangements of sleeping mats in prospective mental hospitals for black patients in bantustans.[19]

government's intention to spend as little money as possible. For instance, the Department of Public Works designed wards to hold far more patients than in white hospitals; they did not provide patients with beds but gave them mats on which to sleep, and they expected patients to grow much of their own food. Figure 2.2 shows the committee's ideal number of patients that could fit in the designed wards, with little concern over patient privacy or comfort.

In line with apartheid ideology, the committee recommended construction of hospitals for each of the main ethnic groups in the bantustans. In the late 1950s and the 1960s, Prime Minister H. F. Verwoerd's policy of divide and rule through apartheid structures extended even to mental hospitals.[20] The proposal was expensive though. The National Building Research Institute estimated that to build three new hospitals, each of which housed 1,450 black patients, in the bantustans would cost approximately R301,708 ($216,143) each. Whereas the cost per institution was significantly less than what the government spent fifteen years earlier at Tara Hospital for fewer white patients (SA£174,000), it was more than the annual budget of R216,000 allocated to the Department of Mental Health to renovate existing institutions.[21] Nevertheless, if implemented, it was a one-time cost that could have saved the government money in the long run.[22]

Because the Cape had significantly more mental hospitals to provide for the Xhosa population, the government chose to open two new homeland institutions, first in Boputhutswana in circa 1966 and then in KwaZulu in circa 1967. Combined, these institutions had accommodation for 2,708 black patients. The number of new beds was, however, only a small percentage of the total needed and overcrowding simply continued. Because of the shortage of accommodation, practitioners often ignored the policy of ethnic segregation and simply admitted patients to any institution that had space. Moreover, as seen with the case with which I started this chapter, as overcrowding and dilapidation of facilities were chronic, policies outlined in the Mental Disorders Act were difficult to sustain. Patients detained by the police rarely were admitted directly to hospitals, but instead were placed in police cells where they waited for a bed to open up.

According to the Mental Disorders Act, a mental patient could only stay within a police cell for a maximum of 21 days. Thereafter they had to be either transferred to a mental institution or released. For the most part, individuals remained in police cells for the maximum time allowed. Since 1944 in Johannesburg, for example, the Newlands Police Station was used for the detention of mental patients. In 1947, the station noted 411 mental patients, most of whom were black, in the station's cells awaiting transfer to a mental institution or trial.[23] In 1948, the Newlands police cells accommodated about nine or ten mental cases per week. By 1957, there were approximately 460 certified non-white and six white insane housed in police cells, which were themselves overcrowded. Numbers in police cells increased dramatically during the period of resistance crackdown in the

1960s, so much so that by 1965, police stations detained 241 white and 4,398 non-white patients.[24]

MENTAL HEALTH POLICIES

Throughout the apartheid years, the administration of most state psychiatric institutions remained centrally administered through the national government's DOH. Only Tara Hospital in the Transvaal fell under provincial jurisdiction.[25] After 1944, when the management of mental health services shifted to the Department of Public Health (later changed to DOH) from a separate division of the Department of the Interior, mental health policy remained essentially unchanged until 1973, with the exception of two minor legislative amendments.[26] One of them in 1957 transferred responsibility for costs of care for migrant non-South Africans to their home country and changed the name of the Commissioner for Mental Disorder to the Commissioner for Mental Hygiene.[27] Another amendment in 1961 recognized the category of outpatient and extended free treatment to voluntary patients who could not afford to pay for services.[28]

Procedures for the management of the mentally ill remained as set out in the amended Mental Disorders Act of 1916. Figure 2.3 shows the various individuals and departments that dealt with mental patients. The different

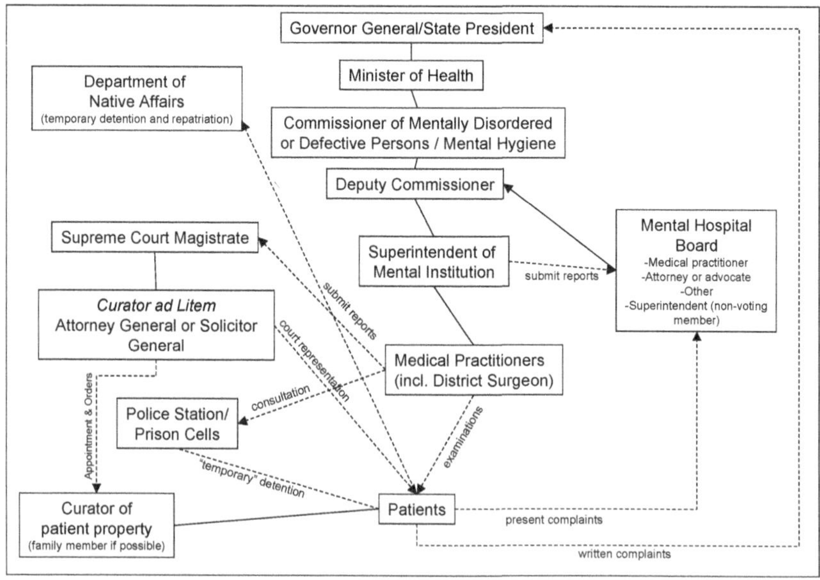

Figure 2.3 Patient and institutional administration, according to the Mental Disorders Amendment Act, 1944.[29]

stages of admission, detention, and release of a patient was a complex and often confusing process, particularly as the resources necessary to effectively implement the policy were limited.

Patients ended up in mental institutions either through voluntary or involuntary admission. Family members, acquaintances, or police officers, who had the authority to pick up any person they thought was mentally disordered, admitted the majority of involuntary patients through an application to a local magistrate. A medical certificate testifying to the mental condition of the individual had to accompany all applications.[30] The magistrate was then, if possible, to consult with one or two additional medical practitioners, one of whom could be a district surgeon, and in turn make a decision as to whether the individual was to be admitted.[31] As medical practitioners were not always readily available, especially in the rural areas, an individual could be institutionalized on the say-so of the original applicant and a single medical practitioner. In the first instance, magistrates could commit individuals for six weeks. Once they were admitted and examined, those whose illness was confirmed came back to the magistrates who had the discretion to order indefinite detention, subject to periodic review, annually for the first three years and every five years thereafter. Patients institutionalized by this means were deemed "general patients" or "ordinary patients" and made up the majority.

Individuals could also be institutionalized through a direct application to a superintendent of a mental institution who would then forward the request to the magistrate within ten days. This was meant specifically for emergencies, where individuals deemed violent or a danger to themselves (usually showing suicidal tendencies) could be hurriedly placed within the confines of an institution. These patients were called "urgent cases."[32]

It is unclear how many involuntary admissions were the result of interventions, respectively, of family members, acquaintances, or police. Surviving applications in the archives, however, are predominantly signed by an acquaintance, employer, police, or court officer. As the definition of mental disorder was vague, one could simply be institutionalized if they were seen to be a public nuisance or an encumbrance to their employers in some way. Even those few applications signed by family members are not always clear as to whether the admission was initiated by them or a police officer. For example, in 1950, Matthew Matabane had been picked up by the local Richmond police near Pietermaritzburg. It is unclear whether his wife requested that the police arrest him, or they did so without her knowledge. The record does show that following his arrest the local magistrate asked his wife to complete a reception order stating that Matabane was "violent and quarrelsome," and "when not tied up" attempted to assault her. After an examination by the district surgeon, the only practitioner available in the area, the Magistrate then confirmed the reception order, consigning Matabane to the Fort Napier Mental Hospital indefinitely.[33]

Table 2.2 Number of Certified General or Ordinary Patients in State Institutions, 1948–1970

Type / Number of Patients on Dec 31st	1948	1950	1952	1954	1956	1958	1960	1962	1964	1966	1968	1970
Certified Ordinary Patients												
Whites	7,404	7,458	7,646	7,881	8,003	8,099	8,455	8,440	8,531	8,801	9,103	9,300
Male	3,739	3,760	3,839	3,996	4,052	4,068	4,245	4,305	4,369	4,516	4,697	4,805
Female	3,665	3,698	3,807	3,885	3,951	4,031	4,210	4,135	4,162	4,285	4,406	4,495
Blacks	7,680	8,008	8,639	9,179	9,511	9,963	10,520	10,935	10,042	10,817	10,676	13,623
Male	5,246	5,528	5,964	6,367	6,677	7,073	7,515	7,747	7,283	7,742	6,850	8,346
Female	2,434	2,480	2,675	2,812	2,834	2,890	3,005	3,188	2,759	3,075	3,826	5,277
Coloureds	2,046	2,096	2,083	2,136	2,259	2,311	2,523	2,738	2,789	3,111	3,093	3,200
Male	1,211	1,247	1,254	1,307	1,404	1,473	1,599	1,769	1,806	1,973	2,001	1,988
Female	835	849	829	829	855	838	924	969	983	1,138	1,092	1,212
Asiatics	253	264	267	259	270	304	346	370	250	245	365	441
Male	167	173	173	164	173	197	227	245	116	144	181	258
Female	86	91	94	95	97	107	119	125	134	101	184	183
TOTAL	**17,383**	**17,826**	**18,635**	**19,455**	**20,043**	**20,677**	**21,844**	**22,483**	**21,612**	**22,974**	**23,237**	**26,564**

Matabane had no criminal charges laid against him but was simply admitted to a mental hospital. For those individuals whom the police arrested and charged with crimes, admission procedures were very similar but were solely at the discretion of the courts and required no family concurrence. At any time during a trial, an attorney general or judge had the authority to call in a medical practitioner or district surgeon to examine the individual's mental state. Once the practitioner made a finding, the individual was either bound over for trial or consigned to a mental institution on a Governor-General's warrant. After South Africa became a republic in 1961 and the position of Governor-General was abolished, the State President signed the warrant. If the practitioner was in doubt concerning the mental state of the prisoner, he or she could be sent to an institution for observation. For instance, in 1959, Brian Musame was arrested and charged with murder. Before he pleaded, his lawyer asked that Musame be removed for medical observation under section 28 of the Mental Disorders Act. Believing his client to have syphilis that caused brain damage, the defense lawyer argued that he was unfit to stand trial. After intensive testimony from practitioners about the possible effects of syphilis and extensive cross-examination of Musame, the magistrate sent him to Fort Napier Hospital for observation. Two months later, a Governor-General warrant provided for his indefinite detention.[34] Whereas his fate is unknown, given the serious charges against him and the fact that he was black, he either was repatriated to a homeland facility or remained in the Fort Napier Hospital for the rest of his life.

After conviction and incarceration, police could transfer prisoners suspected of mental illness to mental hospitals on Governor-General, or after 1961, State President's warrants following examination by two practitioners. The time spent in a mental institution usually counted toward completion of their sentences. Whereas general or ordinary patients could be released from institutions under the authority of the superintendent or hospital board, the release of patients held under warrant of the Governor General required the approval of the Commissioner for Mental Hygiene's office or the Governor General's office depending on the severity of any criminal charges pending or confirmed against them. Patients held under a Governor General's warrant were called "Governor General" or "State President" decision patients.[35]

Whereas the majority of the inmates in mental institutions were involuntary patients, a small number voluntarily admitted themselves. These patients signed forms that hospitals sent to the Minister of Health who authorized their temporary admission. Whereas some of these patients may not have understood the full consequences of their actions, voluntary admission was certainly evidence that they felt unable to cope with life in society.

For the first year of their stay, voluntary patients were known as "temporary patients." They could be discharged upon their own request, unless the superintendent and medical practitioner applied for them to become an involuntary patient. Hospitals could also accept "inebriate" patients with drug or alcohol problems as temporary patients, provided that they signed themselves in for a minimum period of six months. If they left the institution before the end of their treatment, police were allowed to arrest them. After a year, if a temporary patient still chose to remain within the institution, and the medical practitioner had not deemed them an involuntary patient, they became classified as a regular "voluntary patient."[36] The lack of effective treatment, however, especially in the early years of apartheid, meant that hospitals released few temporary patients. Later as the more beds became available when ideas of deinstitutionalization took hold and the state began contracting out beds to private institutions, practitioners began classifying an increasing number of patients as "temporary."[37]

South Africa's Mental Health Act set up a hospital board, similar to a parole board in the prison system, to oversee the discharge of patients. The board was generally made up of a mental health practitioner, an advocate, and one other member, along with the superintendent of the institution, who was simply there as an advisor and not a voting member. Patients only came before hospital boards every few months. The board was meant to act as an independent body standing between the patient and practitioner and the Commissioner, or Deputy Commissioner, for Mental Hygiene. General patients could submit their cases to the board and upon its recommendation secure discharge. The board also made recommendations to the Governor General or State President's office about those patients held under warrants.

Practitioners were to assign patients to one of six classes; (i) a mentally disordered individual; (ii) a mentally infirm individual, (iii) an idiot, (iv) an imbecile, (v) a feebleminded person, and (vi) an epileptic. In 1957, an Amendment to the Act removed a seventh class of a "socially defective" individual, otherwise known as a psychopath or sociopath. The change meant that hospitals moved patients so classified to prisons. Definitions in the remaining six classes were, as the terms themselves suggest, vague, ambiguous, and very much at the discretion of practitioners. The definition of a mentally "disordered" person, for example, managed to be both circular and subject to the opinion of the practitioner making the classification: "a person who, owing to some form of mental disorder, is incapable of managing himself or his affairs." Similarly, a feebleminded individual was, "a person in whose case exists from birth or from an early age mental defectiveness not amounting to mental imbecility [a class which included criminal propensities] so that he is incapable of competing on equal terms with his fellows or of managing himself and his affairs with ordinary prudence."[38]

What constituted "managing" and "ordinary" was astonishingly broad. Illiterate individuals and the physically disabled could fall into these categories. Whereas practitioners rarely used these classes in their own diagnoses, they were meant to be a means by which the government determined to which institution an individual would be sent. The mentally disordered (later known as the mentally ill), the mentally infirm, and some epileptic patients were generally sent to general mental hospitals, while those deemed feebleminded, idiots, or imbeciles (later called mental defectives), were supposed to be sent to institutions specifically set up for them. Yet in this case, the distinction was meaningless for black, coloured, or Indian patients because there were no feebleminded facilities for them. Moreover, the distinction between feebleminded and mentally disordered was never entirely clear and definitions of mental disability, physical disability and mental illness were also confused. Those who could not be taken care of by other government services often found themselves in hospitals for the feebleminded or mental institutions.

GENDER, CLASS, AND RACE IN THE APPLICATION OF MENTAL HEALTH POLICIES

The framers of the Mental Disorders Act intended to introduce a very systematic approach to the administration of mental patients. However, the act also entrenched class, gender, and racial distinctions in the treatment of patients. It is not clear as to whether government regulations created these distinctions or simply reflected those already existing in psychiatric practice, for as we have seen, gender, race, and class played an integral role in the determinations of diagnosis and treatment of patients. Most likely, procedures set out in the Act were both a reflection of existing practices in the mental health system and a product of the biases and prejudices of those who wrote the legislation.

Most institutionalized patients, whether white or black, were from the lower echelons of society. The inmates of mental institutions came disproportionately from the ranks of the unemployed and the poorly paid, and the state, and many of those implementing the policies made a direct connection between economic productivity and the determination of madness. In 1943, for example, one practitioner described the reason for one patient's admission to the Pretoria Mental Hospital as follows: "He has flitted from job to job and says there is no necessity for him to work as long as he can live with his mother."[39] Whereas this particular patient was white, it was precisely those whites from the lower economic stratum of society that were institutionalized. Between 1949 and 1961, most white patients housed in institutions had been unemployed or working in low-waged jobs. The majority of black patients institutionalized were also unemployed. The number of institutionalized mine workers, farm laborers, and commercial workers, most of whom were black, remained low, however, mainly because these individuals were required to return to work or were repatriated to the rural areas. Proportionate to population ratios, black men had significantly less access to beds in institutions. In 1956, for example, the rate of admissions among white men was at eighty-four out of every 100,000, while the rate for black men was much lower at thirty-six out of every 100,000. The admission rate for white women even exceeded that of black men by being approximately sixty-two, whereas the rate for black women was significantly lower at just fourteen out of every 100,000.[40] Whereas the apartheid state made grudging provision for black men needed to serve the urban-industrial economy, it sent the unemployed and those deemed socially deviant, or mentally and physically incapacitated back to the reserves. A smaller number of those viewed as seriously dangerous or threatening were consigned to prisons or mental hospitals.

The legal system of the time depicted women as legal minors, subject to the control of their husbands, fathers, and other male family members. Reflecting this bias, the very language used in the Act was gendered. Those deemed mentally disordered were always men. A mentally disordered person was someone not able to take care of "himself" or "his" affairs.[41] When women were mentioned, they were only referenced in terms of protecting or controlling their sexuality. Any woman who was deemed mentally disordered and "in receipt of relief or assistance from public or charitable funds at the time of giving birth to an illegitimate child or when pregnant of such child" could be institutionalized.[42] Thus having a child out of wedlock was sufficient grounds for practitioners, social workers, and government officers to request their admission to a mental hospital.

Underlying such provisions were remnant eugenic notions that aimed to control the population on the basis of class and gender. Eugenic views never took hold in South Africa as strongly as they did in Europe and North America, but still influenced perceptions of social responsibility. The idea that a woman, particularly a poor woman, could not effectively control her own reproductive activities according to the social standards of the period meant that the government claimed the right to step in and obtain control through institutionalization. Historians of madness elsewhere have documented the connection between class, sexuality, and the institutionalization of women. Yannick Ripa and Elaine Showalter, for example, have shown how single, poor women in nineteenth-century England and France, many with illegitimate children, were more likely to be committed to institutions.[43] Similarly, Phyllis Chesler points out that in the United States of America, husbands, fathers, and male family members feared those women who stepped out of their expected social role, sexually or otherwise, and often "punished" them by placing them in "patriarchal mental asylums."[44] Women were meant to be, to use H. Roberts' words, the "patient patients," and were expected to simply fulfill their roles uncomplainingly.[45]

Once women were institutionalized, the Act continued to restrict their sexual activity in the guise of protecting them. For example, it specifically restricted any male employee to be alone with a female patient, except in emergency cases. If a non-white male nurse was needed, a white male or female nurse had to be present at all times. This meant that white male nurses could be alone with urgency cases. Institutions had to report any male employee working long-term with female patients to the Commissioner for Mental Hygiene.[46] Anyone having sexual relations with an institutionalized female patient, regardless of her consent, could be convicted of a criminal offence.

Whereas these stipulations were in place to protect disordered women from unwanted approaches of male attendants, they also seemed to be representative of early twentieth century paranoia as expressed in hysteria around the "black peril," that is, the fear that black men would rape or sexually abuse seemingly innocent white women. Early twentieth century fears about "black peril" in the wake of the First World War were as much about men feeling emasculated and feeling threatened by a rising-tide of female assertions of public and sexual power than about the threat of black men. In order to maintain white male superiority, it was essential to promote notions of pure white women. As Timothy Keegan points out:

> Defilement of white women threatened the purity of the race. It was unthinkable that respectable women could ever consent to black men being familiar with them. It was essential to the white self-image that black men be seen as bestial villains, and respectable white women as innocent victims.[47]

Indeed, the idea that black male nurses had to be supervised by a white nurse when caring for female patients, most of whom were white (there were practically no beds for black women), reflects the fears of government officials about the overly sexed black man that would take advantage of innocent white women.

Whereas some African women encountered the mental health system before the imposition of pass laws in the late 1950s, the incidences of them doing so thereafter declined. After influx control measures restricted black women from entering urban areas, the government even eliminated a few hundred beds for them in mental institutions. Under apartheid, the objective was to keep black women in the rural areas where they could continue to support, what Glen Elder calls the "procreative economy of apartheid," that is, the way in which the apartheid government expected men and women to fulfill certain roles based on their sex and race.[48] Black women were mostly designated as "mother-rural labourer-black women" whereas black men were "father-miner-black man." Anyone, including the mentally "disturbed," who stepped outside of this role could be sent to the rural reserves where they were expected to be watched over by their community.[49] However, as the apartheid government never recognized the demands placed on women within the bantustans and their need to supplement their income by working in urban areas, black women continued to thwart the apartheid government's procreational economic model and moved, although often temporarily, into urban spaces.

If black women were "mother-rural labourers," then white women were in turn designated as "mother-wife-urban" and white men were "father-husband-provider-urban." Any one failing to support this model could be institutionalized. While there has been limited research into the sexual and socio-political activities of poor white women in the early years of apartheid, as we will see in the chapter to follow, some poor white women did step outside their expected role and were institutionalized. In addition, men who failed to fit the masculine model, such as homosexual men, were deemed disordered. For the most part, black women, however, remained out of the grasp of the medical practitioners.

The apartheid government's failure to invest in the existing mental health structure meant that resources throughout the 1950s and 1960s remained insufficient. Because treatment was minimal, most inmates remained hospitalized for long periods, which meant a chronic shortage of space for new patients. There were never enough beds within the institutions; thus, makeshift solutions were often haphazardly fashioned on a case-by-case basis, depending on the resources available to those who had custody of the patients. Budgetary and other deficiencies worked both for and against apartheid ideology. Resources were sufficient to support treatment of whites, particularly white men, even if not very well, while marginalizing blacks even further from services. The lack of available space in mental institutions meant that black mental patients were often housed in jails, at pass offices, empty buildings, and even outside garages while they awaited beds or repatriation. Sometimes they were left to roam the streets.

CONCLUSION

Although over 4,700 additional beds were made available between 1948 and 1966, most of the increase did not represent new space but resulted from improvised arrangements and makeshift changes to existing structures. The number of beds available fluctuated constantly as wards and buildings were closed for repairs and then reopened. In 1962, because of the closure of grossly inadequate buildings and facilities, the number of beds available actually declined, while the number of patients housed increased. In order to curtail the intense overcrowding, the government came up with a plan to begin "temporarily" contracting out the care of mainly long-term black patients to a private firm, Smith Mitchell and Company (see Chapter 6). Whereas this decision did free up beds, overcrowding persisted within the state system with no letup in the demand for additional beds. In this situation, genuine efforts at rehabilitation became impossible and few patients received worthwhile treatment. Burdened by inadequate funding, overcrowding, and deficient structures, officials struggled to implement policies that were ad hoc and often contradictory. The system left police officers, magistrates, and native commissioners to cope as best they could with those black mental patients for whom there were no beds. The ineffectiveness of the mental health system became a political issue in 1960 when

David Pratt, a "mentally deranged" white farmer made an attempt to assassinate then Prime Minister H. F. Verwoerd. Verwoerd survived that attack but not a second one when former mental patient Demetrio Tsafendas, who somehow secured employment as a parliamentary messenger, stabbed him to death on the floor of the House of Assembly. As examined in Chapter 4, at that point, the state set out to revise its mental health policy.

However, for most of the early apartheid years, the apartheid state's approach to policy had inherent flaws, contradictions, and shortcomings. Inadequate resources placed considerable stress not only on those not able to make it into the institutions, but also on those admitted. Moreover, staff within psychiatric institutions became frustrated and dissatisfied by an increasingly contradictory system that prevented them from treating patients effectively. On occasion, some of them went so far as to challenge official policy. Patients and their families, as we will see in the next chapter, also protested against a system that was negligent, inefficient and left them isolated and untreated.

3 Patient Accounts

Life in State Institutions and Challenging Exile, 1939–1961

> My Deares [*sic*] Darling Father
> Just these few lines to let you know that I am still keeping well only hoping to hear the same from you by return of post. Dear dad I must thank you for your most kind and welcome letter which I recived [*sic*] last week, Dear dad I am very glad to hear that you are coming to see me this month I am looking forward to see you dear dad I must let you know that I feel very unhappy here I realy [*sic*] cant [*sic*] stand this life any longer . . . now dear dad how is my dear old mother getting on please give her my very best love and tell her that I am longing to hear from her I just wish mother could come with you to see me as it is 8 years since I last saw her . . . darling father you want me to tell you every thing in my letter well my darling I cant [*sic*] as our letters get red [*sic*] here but when you come to see me then I will be able to tell you every thing.[1]

This letter written by Anne Waterson, a young white women housed in a mental institution in the 1940s, draws our attention to the impact of being designated as mentally disordered in South Africa. One is immediately struck by her depth of alienation, longing, and feelings of persecution. Waterson's letter is merely one of many that show these thoughts of isolation. Poor conditions, separation from family, and constricted life within institutions meant that for most patients, the feeling of alienation loomed. Life within South African mental institutions, like in the rest of the world during this period, was a lonely and difficult experience. Relegated to the outskirts of society, the institutionalized patient was both metaphorically and physically exiled. State institutions were on the outskirts of society, away from urban centers. This institutional barrier between the sane and the mad meant that patients were consigned to new marginal spaces where their rights and entitlements were extremely limited.

The experiences of patients detained within institutions reveals the very imposing, yet ineffectual nature of psychiatric practices under apartheid. The history of how notions of madness were negotiated and politically shaped cannot be fully comprehended without their perspective. In South Africa, most patient-centered histories have been biographical, which values the individual. To date no collective history of South African patients' views has been written.[2] It is indeed a challenge when attempting to write a collective history from the perspective of the mad. There was not one universal type of mad person or type of madness, but many types and concepts of insanity. Moreover, the ideas and behavior of the mad transformed according to changing situations and relationships. In this chapter, I focus only on those that made it into the institution and were under the care at one time or another of a practitioner. This is in no way meant to suggest that the perceptions and histories of patients were homogeneous, static, or restricted to a specific time and place. Views of patients differed depending on the institution in which they were housed, the length of their stay, their reasons for being there, whether they were mandated to be there or not, their race, their social standing, their gender, their sexuality, their age, their physical health, their diagnoses, and their individual experiences. Within any given time and place, mental patients were affected by changes in society and at the same time were affecting society themselves. Patients' experiences also changed as South Africa's mental health care system transformed. Thus, although I attempt to relay experiences in a succinct and organized manner, I in no way suggest that views of patients or practitioners fell easily into groups and did not change regularly.

My attempt to uncover patients' voices in the history of South Africa's psychiatric practice is challenged, however, by the lack of available sources. Patients' voices are significantly absent from most of the reports about South Africa's mental institutions. The dearth of recorded patients' voices in government and institutional sources reveals the lack of agency placed on patients' views—their voices neither valued nor respected in any way. The powerful stigma associated with mental illness discourages patients from telling their stories. The notion of patients' privacy, while a very valid and necessary practice, tends to perpetuate this stigma by reinforcing the idea that patients have something to hide. The South African government and mental hospitals began after 1961 destroying patient files and letters and few remain. Even before 1961, few records were kept. Because of these limitations, patient voices cannot be exhaustive and I can merely offer a rudimentary study of patients' views.

Despite the difficulty in interpretation of patients' testimony and the gaping silences in the records, it is still possible to gain insight, albeit incomplete, into the lives and views of patients and their relationship with state officials, institutional staff, and society in general during the early years of apartheid. Apart from direct testimony of the afflicted, a few reports sketchily reveal the daily lives of patients. More importantly, however, some patients spoke up, wrote letters, and revealed their perspectives in court proceedings and letters. In order to launch a complaint, a patient could address the board of the hospital and/or write a letter to the Governor General, or later to the State President, if they were held on a Governor General or State President's warrant. The former process was not easy, especially as the superintendent of the institution often sat on its board as an advisor. Although the Mental Disorders Act stipulated that all patients' letters addressed to the Governor General be sent to his (they were all men) office, as Anne Waterson pointed out in her letter, these could be opened by mental hospital staff before mailing. Thus, patients may have restrained their views accordingly. Despite the requirement to do so, hospital staff may not have forwarded all of the letters, particularly those that they considered incriminating.

The state in which the letters of patients remain in the archives is analogous to patients' circumstances. The letters are housed in files under the designation of "mental patient," disengaged from any other data concerning their lives. Other than a few sentences written by the superintendent about the diagnoses of the patients, little background information is offered and the letters are without context. There are few words about patients' social positions, their families, the reasons for institutionalization, their circumstances within the institution, or their fate, unless a patient or their family communicates this information themselves. The estranged, disassociated nature of these letters is akin to the larger process of patient alienation and dehumanization. The lack of information concerning the circumstances of patients and the preoccupation with diagnoses is reflective of the systematic and detached nature of the mental health system that simply objectified patients.

The limited information recorded in these files about patients' lives has meant that my discussion of patient views may at times seem rudimentary and disjointed. Dictated by the deficient nature of the sources themselves, this is unavoidable. Nevertheless, these letters cannot be ignored. Their very existence is indicative of the fact that patients attempted to break out of their isolation and connect to the larger political process.

WRITING PATIENT HISTORIES

Before embarking on a detailed analysis of patient accounts, we need to contextualize them within the broader treatment of patient histories in general, particularly as South African patients were rarely given credence. Experiences and representations of the mad within the written histories of mental health in general have traditionally been eclipsed by discussions about institutional histories and views of practitioners. For the most part, the mad are simply seen as objects upon which practitioners can practice. Overshadowed by the idea that insane individuals have limited consciousness of their surroundings and events shaping their world, histories of madness have often marginalized, ignored, or simply dismissed their views. This may be a consequence of the pervasive view that the state and practitioners hold a systematic dominance and understanding over the minds and bodies of their subjects—a view that is often forwarded by scientific psychiatric histories. The expansion of biological explanations for the etiology of mental illness, the introduction of psychotropic drugs, and the continued specialization of mental diagnoses have reified this view. Indeed, the very practice of compartmentalizing and diagnosing a patient so pertinent to biological interpretations of mental illness denotes a specific behavior and invokes preconceived ideas about their capability, or lack thereof. In turn, the individual voices of the mad are seriously impeded by the terms and language that subjectify them.

The terms used to describe those that deviate from the norm are problematic, not only because they are loaded with preconceptions, but they also usually change depending on the situation. Moreover, the characterization of an individual as mad can differ depending on who is asserting it. The designation of madness is certified by a practitioner, whether or not the person sees themselves as mad, but can every now and then be asserted by individuals themselves.

Similar arguments have been forwarded by historians discussing the changing expressions of cultural, ethnic, racial, and sexual identity within an historical context. Academics have shown that ideas of identity are often fluid and historical constructs that can be, as Saul Dubow puts it, used by individuals to both "name" others and also "claimed" by individuals to identify themselves. When "naming" occurs, it is often done "by one relatively powerful group as a means of defining other less powerful communities," such as in the case of a practitioner diagnosing a patient. "Claiming," on the other hand, is a means by which an individual or group "acquires content and meaning through a process of conscious assertion and imagining," such as when an individual asserts the mad identity for themselves.[3] In a few cases, individuals can *claim* to be insane as a means to escape difficult conditions or to avoid imposed responsibility. Through an examination of South African literary works on madness, Deborah Fontenot argues that the expression of "other worlds beyond known consciousness" is a "metaphorical excuse whereby the harassed citizen finds sanctuary" in an increasingly hostile world.[4] Similarly, Diana Gittins argues that the institution in some circumstances can become a sanctuary for women wanting to escape social expectations.[5] Although not a greatly beneficial endeavor, getting oneself deemed mentally ill could allow one the means by which to remove oneself from an unwanted situation and enable one to express oneself freely through the guise of madness. Most scholars agree that, whether *named* or *claimed*, all forms of identity are social or political constructions that may be invoked or determined at any time or place.[6] Likewise, the claiming or naming of one's status as mad may change depending on political or social motivations and circumstance.

This is not to suggest, however, that madness is always a social construct—biomedical factors certainly play a part, at least for some, in its etiology. Nor is it to suggest that many actively seek to be institutionalized or designated as mad. Indeed quite the opposite is true, for the majority of those institutionalized were involuntarily done so. Moreover, society often ostracized those deemed insane and conditions in mental institutions were atrocious. It is unlikely that many intentionally chose to be institutionalized. Yet there were those few who did voluntarily choose to be admitted. This chapter does not focus on these voluntary patients, but it recognizes the notion that some patients can have some, albeit limited, influence over their positions.

The ambiguous nature of the status of the mad and their history obviously raises questions as to how one goes about presenting such a history. By omission, many scholars have suggested that the indistinctness of the notion of madness and the very unreliable nature of their testimony itself is an impediment to the accuracy and reality of the historical account. Yet all historical sources present their own difficulties when dealing with questions of what is accurate and legitimate. Indeed, as Luise White has pointed out, those voices that have not been given official sanction in historical analysis can in fact offer new perspectives to our understanding of the past:

> What historians might call fantastic can be part of a real and concrete situation. What historians omit in order to make a past "useful" might be what was thought by the actors to be important at the time. An African history that reports local idioms, local rumours, local representations and local misrepresentations reinserts that history into the community that produced it.[7]

Thus, the testimony of the mad and the inclusion of their representations, no matter how difficult, opens up a new perspective of South Africa's mental health approach and the history of patients both within and outside of the institution gains credence. Indeed, a history that includes the views of patients can reveal a lot more about a mental health system and the world in general than one that discounts them.

Recent historians of mental health have been more conscious of including the views and experiences of the insane, and more histories from patients' perspectives have begun to be written, specifically by academics writing psychiatric histories of western countries.[8] These more patient-centered approaches have brought their perspectives and experiences further to the forefront.[9] In South Africa, while most patients were extremely isolated, some played an important role in the transformation of their own treatment and on regulations concerning mental health in general. As we will see, patients attempted to work within and outside the system as a means to challenge and thwart their marginalized position within society.

IN EXILE

Relegated to the outskirts of society, the institutionalized patient was both metaphorically and physically exiled from family and society. During the apartheid decades, the state sometimes disposed of its political opponents, and even occasionally deviant members of the ruling group, in this way. Whereas many political dissidents and those deemed criminally insane were consigned to prisons, and later in the case of the political opposition, driven into exile, those designated as the sick and mentally disordered were exiled to various state institutions and "repatriated" away from urban centers. This institutional barrier between the sane and the mad meant that patients were consigned to new marginal spaces, be it the institution or bantustan, where their rights and entitlements were extremely limited.

Whereas a few patients may have voluntarily admitted themselves to institutions, the majority of patients institutionalized were involuntary. Patients were rarely consulted about their committal, and afterwards seldom included in discussions about their treatment. As patients had no rights (indeed the Mental Disorders Act made no mention of these at all), patients had limited capacity to challenge their situations. As was seen in the last chapter, the process of admission was extremely complex and confusing, especially for patients who did not understand the procedures, were not present at proceedings, or given the opportunity to articulate their own concerns. Most black patients and those caught up in the system of criminal justice frequently had to deal with numerous individuals from different departments, all of whom had little time for them. When patients were present in court, many complained that their voices were obscured or silenced. Carl Van Derkamp for example, a former doctor who was shortly after admission declared to be sane, stated that the magistrate at his hearing for committal had denied him a voice. He pointed out that the magistrate continuously silenced and interrupted him. The magistrate's interventions to stop him from speaking did not appear in the court transcript, creating the appearance that he had not tried to defend himself:

> How could such omissions possibly be perpetrated without prior instructions to the Clerk of Courts; or like a good factotum of the Crown he knew on what side his bread was buttered, however with the people's money. As it is, there is no Court-record to show that the Magistrate's repeated gags of irrelevance and citation threats were true and just . . . nothing to prove that the total absence of defences was my fault and not due to the Magistrate's false interventions. Could such corrupt omissions possibly favour me or the irregularity and illegality of the Court with what it dare not put on record as worse than to make me look absent.[10]

Van Derkamp understood that the court had in effect removed him from the proceedings entirely. He expressed the very real powerlessness that many patients experienced at the hands of the indifferent and arbitrary legal system that incarcerated them. For the most part, those deemed mentally disordered never had the chance to even speak at their own hearings. Their institutionalization was in the hands of doctors and district surgeons' testimony, some of whom had spent very little time with patients.

Patients' feelings of alienation were, of course, amplified once they were admitted to an institution. The reason for their admission was rarely made clear to them and many found themselves institutionalized for extended periods without ever understanding why. Adam Klomp, a German man from South West Africa housed in a South African mental hospital after the war, wrote of the vagueness and lack of consistency in the explanations he was given as to why he ended up in a mental hospital in the first place, and why he could not be released:

> I arrived on the evening of the 7th June, 1944, and the next day I was submitted through [*sic*] a physical examination by Dr. du Plessis, who was at the time the surgeon here. Dr. Crossweight, the Superintendent, who was also here at the time, questioned me on my psychical condition, the nature of the symptoms of my illness, the period of my stay as well as on the causes for the stay at the Bloemfontein clinic. Both gentlemen were officially transferred elsewhere shortly afterwards and could not concern themselves with me any longer.
>
> Meanwhile I have been confined here against my will for over three years. On several occasions I entreated Dr. Delabad, who is working here now, to discharge me and send me home, but I always received an indefinite answer without any further examination. Eighteen times did I address myself to the Hospital Board, which sits here once or twice a month, with the request that I may be discharged and sent home to my dwelling-place and my family, but they also gave me an indefinite answer every time and my efforts bore me no fruit.[11]

The record is silent about the reasons for Klomp's institutionalization, although he does mention a court case and magistrate's decision to institutionalize him after being placed briefly under observation at the Bloemfontein Mental Hospital. As no doctor's report accompanied his letter, the doctors' views remain unknown. As practitioners spent little time with each patient and, as in Klomp's case, rarely re-examined patients after their initial admission, it is unlikely that doctors recognized changes within a patient. Nor was it expected that they take the time to explain to patients their status. Hospital boards, which relied on practitioners' reports, were in turn unlikely to release a patient, especially one detained by a Governor General's warrant, without a practitioner's endorsement. Patients like Klomp could remain within the confines of the institutions for many years.

For most patients, the reason for their exile often eluded them. "I am mentally sound,"[12] wrote one patient. "On no occasion have I been in any way mentally-disordered, mentally-infirm, or socially-defective, despite any psychiatric reports to that effect that have been submitted," wrote another.[13] These words are echoed throughout most patients' and family members' letters who consistently disputed their institutionalization. The arbitrary nature of the system, however, meant that a practitioner could consign potentially sane individuals to the status of involuntary patient with little explanation or evidence other than an initial consultation. It is likely that many patients were institutionalized or remained hospitalized unnecessarily.

Not all patients, however, were unsure about the rationale for their admission. Some patients suggested that they were victims of political persecution. Peter Porter, for example, an inmate of the Pietermaritzburg Mental Hospital who was admitted in 1928, believed that Minister Tielman Roos, the Transvaal Afrikaner Nationalist leader and member of the Hertzog government, had used his influence in getting him admitted because "he heard that he was forming a political party called the Sons and Daughters of South Africa," most likely a party that would support the British empire. Eight years after his institutionalization, Porter wrote:

> I may mention that I am even now undergoing persecution at the hands of Government officials and again appeal to Your Excellency personally for protection. Form [*sic*] what has recently transpired in connection with the police briberies surely the state ministers should realise that similar deplorable attitude and acts can also be done by high officials in other departments. Thanking Your Excellency for your sympathetic consideration of my earnest appeal for justice as the life that I have been subjugated to has become almost unbearable.[14]

In the same way, Marie Short believed it was her husband's political involvement in the *Ossewabrandwag*, a fascist paramilitary group founded in 1939 that opposed the war and asserted Afrikaans values against English influences in government and society, that made practitioners institutionalize him. Writing to the Governor General, she states:

> As you know, he wishes to come back to me, here where I am at home today with his parents. His wish is to get good work and that the two of us may again live happily ever after. He had always taken the wrong path in secret and I did not know. Later, I found everything out and was disappointed that he belonged to the Ossewabrandwag. I am not used to this because I was born and will die for the English. So my husband had worried and my own parents now promise hand and mouth to also be on our side. Will you be so good as to release him so that he is out in October, because as you most certainly have already heard, in which circumstances I am in and I will gladly have him here with me. I promise you that I will look after him, that he will never again take the wrong path and that if he did again, that you can hold him there forever.[15]

Whereas political motives could have played a part in the institutionalization of patients, it is unlikely that the government institutionalized many of its political opponents, particularly as it had means other than psychiatric practitioners with which to control its dissident population. As we saw in the last chapter, accommodation in mental institutions was sorely lacking. Nevertheless, the perception that patients were institutionalized for their political ideas was fostered by the arbitrary nature of the mental health system and the lack of accountability that characterized it. One was judged to be disordered and then removed from society, much like a political prisoner or criminal. It was easy for many patients to feel unjustly persecuted and to accuse officials of manufacturing their charges, or working in cohort with each other to ensure that they remained institutionalized. Ardee Das, for example, a former indentured worker from India, was sentenced in 1919 to six years imprisonment for falsity, a crime that included anything from forging documents to bribery. Four years later, however, just before he was to be released on good behavior, the prison guards requested that a practitioner examine him for mental disorder. He was shortly thereafter transferred to Town Hill Hospital where he remained for the rest of his life. It is unknown if Das was presenting any signs of strange behavior, or whether the guards were trying to ensure his continued detention, perhaps as a means to cover up their own insidious behavior. Das certainly felt it was the latter. Writing from the Town Hill Hospital, he described his experience in a letter to the Governor General:

> I have been in the above institution for the last thirty (30) years, which is absolutely boring. Moreover I am quite old at 66 years. Health poor. Conduct and behaviour—excellent. I have known Dr. Chan for the last 30 yrs. My enemies must have befriended him. I am positive the Dr. must have been bribed by the jail convict Lord . . . I told the Dr. the subordinates [in jail] may use spears to stab me. Then they sent me into the mental hospital after discharge from general law. I was found not to be insane nor guilty. Gaol lord instructed mental authorities to finish me good and solid. I was kept under constant vigilance day and night. Dr. Chan now says I did not complete my sentence after the board of the mental hospital, I have to see heaven. Lies become truth here, vice versa. God is the Supreme being and I swear I will not lie. I plead once more I am not mad. Mr. Jarvis had done me harm by giving electric treatment to my nerves which has wounded me. Their idea was to effect my entrails in the body more than once the Dr and others promised me free.[16]

Das's correspondence does indicate some irrationality, although this may simply be reflective of his lack of facility with English. He was likely diagnosed with dementia praecox (later known as schizophrenia), a diagnosis that as we have seen, was commonly applied to those deemed non-white. Treatment for dementia praecox often entailed the use of electro-convulsive therapy (ECT).[17] Nevertheless, his argument about the cohort between police and mental health officials is compelling, especially as Das was not alone in his persecutory views. Vern Bort also expressed similar feelings of persecution. According to a medical report, he stated that "he had been driven off his head by worry and police persecution" and believed that "the police are all against him, and despite assurances, he thinks we [staff in the mental institution] are in league with the police."[18]

Whereas doctors usually explained away these feelings of persecution as mere paranoia and evidence of patients' illness, these views could equally be evidence of the harsh treatment to which patients were subjected by unsympathetic staff. Relationships with staff were not always hostile, and staff views of patients crossed a wide spectrum. However, even with the fact that patients knew staff read their letters, many of them contained allegations of their corrupt and abusive behavior. While it is difficult to know how much abuse actually took place within the institutions and how many of the accusations of patients are valid, the fact that patients and family members consistently wrote about poor treatment and abuse suggests that mistreatment was widespread. Janet De Porteius, for example, described the handling of her daughter in Witrand Institution:

> . . . and the [*sic*] make the child sick up there that we can't get her, and the more she stay there she be sicker and sicker. She will be beter of [*sic*] here than there, if she is by me, in a months time she will be better and full of health. They treat her like a dog, they treat her very badly and they are very cruel to her.[19]

Having spent some time in the Witrand Institution herself as an inmate, De Porteius certainly had first-hand experience of the abusive treatment by staff and her concerns were echoed in other patients' letters. Kobes Wilhelm Tobias, a patient at Valkenberg Mental Hospital, wrote numerous letters to authorities claiming that medical staff, nurses, and his fellow patients abused him and in one instance, broke his rib.[20] Similarly, Kristian Johansen talked about patients and staff members physically abusing him:

> I was recently back at the Montagu police for a few days when I told the police that the patients and the male nurses push me around, strangle and stamp stamp on my left and right hips and my stomach.[21]

In a later letter, Johansen requested protection for himself and his family against the male nurses in the institution:

> Dear Dr, I will be happy if Dr out of mercy and sympathy send 10 [*illegible*] police officers to take me away, in every case the male nurses will mistreat my brothers and will mistreat worse than pigs but just as well they said that they will mistreat me, my brothers and sisters worse than pigs. [22]

The official record supports these patients' accusations. In 1958, Dr. Fisher presented a petition on behalf of approximately 1,000 friends and family members of patients in the Valkenberg Hospital about the "type of person" who was hired by the institution due to the poor working conditions.[23] In the early years of apartheid when effective psychopharmacological drugs had yet to become available and staff relied more on physical strength and restraints to contain their patients, the work of the psychiatric nurse was physically demanding. Between the 1940s and 1960s, the majority of nurses hired to work within psychiatric hospitals were white men, many of whom were former soldiers and were trained in discipline and conflict, not therapy. Moreover, it was always difficult for the Department of Health to find sufficient staff willing to work in such poor conditions, or even trained to deal with difficult patients. The overcrowding and unpleasant conditions meant that few were willing to work within these remote and dilapidated institutions. In 1944, the government established a Commission of Enquiry to investigate the poor working conditions within mental institutions. Staff members, particularly male staff nurses and clerks submitted a list of grievances about their conditions. They requested the expedition of promotions for male staff, that all male wards be placed under male nurse supervision, that salaries be increased, shifts shortened, that pension schemes and disability benefits be increased, and that family members be allowed free medical coverage as nursing staff at general hospitals were given.[24] They also equated their working conditions with slave labor. "Never so much done, by so few, for so little" they argued, and requested better pay and understanding of the difficulties of the profession. In addition, they asked for more nursing support staff, particularly white men:

> We consider 12 hrs shifts as slave labour: in no other Profession, Trade, or even among labourers anywhere in the world do we find similar conditions, can any man or woman be expected to give their best for 12 hours a day, let along 12 hours a night; without a five minute break . . . With regard to remuneration the nature of our work should also be borne in mind. Firstly the personal danger attached no nurse at any time is ever quite safe, especially with those patients harbouring persecutory delusions against the staff it is only due to the tact and wit of a nurse, that many an ugly situation has been saved "ours is an extraordinary profession" very distinct from general nursing there is no understanding and no appreciation abuse [*sic*] and threatens any nurse to six months imprisonment should he forget himself.[25]

Their complaints of their personal safety issues were certainly understandable. When taking me on a tour of the former Tower Hospital in Fort Beaufort, Joseph Nqaba Gqomfa, a nurse, told me the story of when he was taken hostage by one of the state president's patients in the hospital. While one incident in the many years in which he had worked in the hospital, he noted that the job could potentially be a very dangerous and overwhelming one.

But the staff's comment in the letter to the commission that they could possibly be imprisoned for up to six months for "forgetting" oneself, undoubtedly points to the abuse that patients endured at the hands of staff within institutions and, indeed, the dismissive attitude that many staff took towards such mistreatment.

Although the Mental Disorders Act restricted the use of "mechanical restraints" unless a practitioner signed a certificate and a log was kept, these stipulations were rarely adhered to.[26] Solitary confinement was often used for far longer periods than allowed, sometimes up to a few months, and the very presence of such places meant that their use was popular.

The limited time spent by practitioners in the institutions meant that many nurses and attendants restrained patients often without practitioners' knowledge. Practitioners were often overworked and had numerous duties within the mental health system. They not only had to examine patients, but were also expected to submit reports to superintendents and magistrates, and be on call for consultation. In addition, many practitioners taught classes or held university appointments. South Africa consistently had a deficiency in the number of psychiatrists and medical practitioners interested in mental health, and even a lower number who were willing to

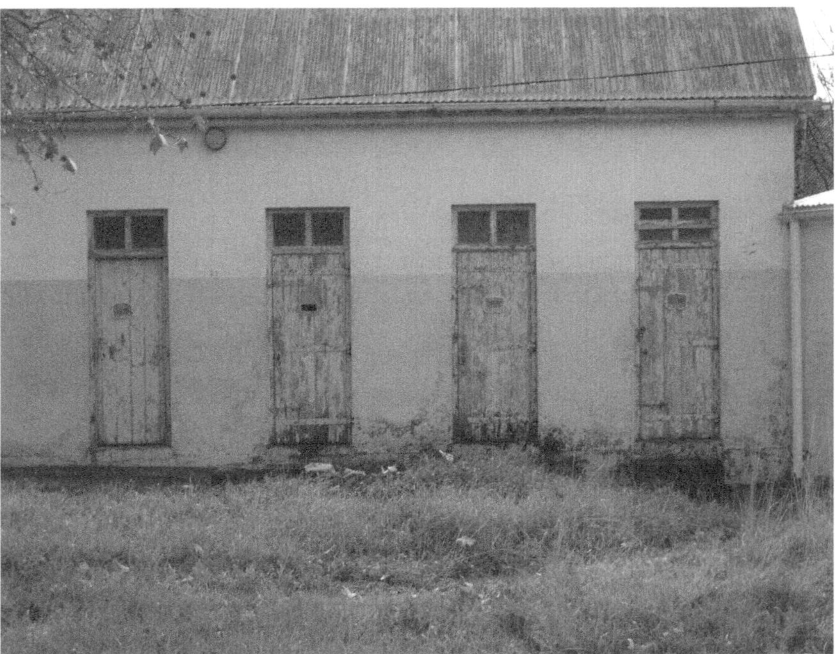

Figure 3.1 Men's solitary confinement cells at Old Tower Hospital, Fort Beaufort. Photo by author.

work in state practice. In 1950, for example, there were only forty-nine registered psychiatrists in South Africa and fifty-one medical staff members who dealt with mental health issues, not all of whom worked within South Africa's twelve mental hospitals. That year 20,631 patients were treated within the hospitals, although the actual number of individuals that practitioners examined was most likely considerably higher as not all were institutionalized.[27] While the number of registered psychiatrists, instead of general practitioners who took the role of working within mental hospitals, increased over the years, their numbers were always limited and practitioners relied heavily on nursing staff to care for and keep track of the condition of patients with little supervision.

By the late 1960s, black women and men were hired as ward "maids" to do the "rough work" so that white staff could spend more time with patients. As the National Party began to focus more on promoting and "uplifting" white men, and innovations in pharmacology meant that patients could be restrained less forcibly, in the 1970s and thereafter, black men and women gradually began to replace white men and women as nurses. In 1962, the Commissioner for Mental Hygiene, Lamont announced that "the first group of qualified non-White mental nurses satisfied the requirements of the South African Nursing Council for registration."[28] However, he also pointed out in 1967 that over a decade the number of student nurses had dropped dramatically and trained staff were being replaced by untrained assistants.[29]

Table 3.1 Number of Posts for Medical Staff Working in Mental Institutions, 1957–1970

Type of Staff	1957	1958	1959	1960	1961	1962	1963
Number of Medical Staff	67	67	68	76	79	83	93
Permanent	44	46	40	44	47	45	44
Temporary	16	16	17	21	17	22	32
Vacancies	*7*	*5*	*11*	*11*	*15*	*16*	*17*
No. of Registered Psychiatrists in South Africa				70			

Type of Staff	1964	1965	1966	1967	1968	1969	1970
Number of Medical Staff	92	91	101	104	110	113	89
Permanent	51	48	39	32	38	45	36
Temporary	27	25	35	44	49	46	36
Vacancies	*14*	*18*	*27*	*28*	*23*	*22*	*17*
No. of Registered Psychiatrists in South Africa			86				

Table 3.2 Number of Posts and Vacancies for Nursing Staff in State Mental Hospitals from 1957–1970

Type of Staff	**1957**	**1958**	**1959**	**1960**	**1961**	**1962**	**1963**
Nurses							
Number of Posts for White Male Nurses	880	895	915	933	959	1,038	1,066
Total Vacancies	96	103	93	104	66	84	76
Number of Posts for White Female Nurses	983	919	990	1,066	17	22	32
Total Vacancies	197	77	91	110	68	90	135
Number of Posts for Non-White Male Nurses	812	856	1,135	1,169	1,173	1,271	1,198
Total Vacancies	51	35	61	49	20	34	10
Number of Posts for Non-White Female Nurses	76	178	246	328	408	495	357
Total Vacancies	1	16	23	61	16	26	23

Type of Staff	**1964**	**1965**	**1966**	**1967**	**1968**	**1969**	**1970**
Nurses							
Number of Posts for White Male Nurses	1,072	1,027	1,038	1,039	1,029	1,033	833
Total Vacancies	78	97	95	107	134	127	146
Number of Posts for White Female Nurses	1,289	1,311	1,355	1,354	1,338	1,338	1,202
Total Vacancies	134	164	152	150	172	163	246
Number of Posts for Non-White Male Nurses	1,201	1,235	1,439	1,584	1,410	1,482	1,357
Total Vacancies	5	21	115	77	122	136	131
Number of Posts for Non-White Female Nurses	375	457	587	724	766	830	897
Total Vacancies	19	51	158	169	183	45	116

The high rate of staff turnover and the limited therapeutic training of those working with patients meant that relationships between nursing staff and patients mostly were strained. Staff were extremely overworked and had little time to deal with patients individually. The institution was a harsh place. In an interview, Wilhelm Bodemer, a psychiatrist, pointed out that patients were not always abused by staff, but there were incidences where staff members also "instigated other patients to subdue a patient."[30] The prevalence of staff using patients as a means to restrain and abuse other patients is unknown, yet it is likely that it occurred often as it enabled staff to maintain dominance in a space where they were a minority and to punish patients without getting into trouble themselves.

The dehumanized and arbitrary nature of the system, along with the very violent nature of staff and even some of the treatments, like ECT, perpetuated a tense and often violent atmosphere within the institution.[31] Jan Robbertze, a psychiatrist, who worked at Sterkfontein for a few months in the 1963 explained some of the abuses that occurred:

> There were no services at all. They were housed in unbelievably bad conditions. I had a lot of problems there actually about the situation. I complained about the fact that they were trying to force me to give electroconvulsive therapy to patients without fully examining them, without deciding what their psychiatric condition was. So they suspended me as a psychiatrist and I had to do all the medical work at the hospital. And then I went through the wards and I examined them all physically and found that more than thirty patients suffered from Pellagra because they were mal fed at that time. So, with the superintendent we reported the whole situation to head office in Pretoria and they eventually found out that there was a group of people stealing the meat, fruit and vegetables of all the patients and that was the main reason why they developed the lack. At that time, also they hired out psychiatric patients to the staff to work in their gardens and so on at one and six a day. I said well that was terrible, they should at least pay them two and six a day. I had such a lot of trouble about that, it was unbelievable. But eventually I was sent away when I completed the time there at Sterkfontein hospital, never to return again. I'm not allowed to be admitted to the hospital any more. And the superintendent of the hospital was eventually suspended because he had a farm near the hospital and he had more than 500 psychiatric patients working as slaves on that farm, making money out of madness, you can say. So that was my introduction to psychiatry.[32]

Whereas Robbertze in this statement tends to blame staff and the superintendent for the poor treatment of patients, practitioners also offered little in the way of treatment for patients. Patients who ended up in mental institutions could remain in custody anywhere from ten days to the rest of their lives. Even with the movement towards drug therapies that grew in popularity in the 1950s onwards, remedies were lacking. Drug therapies were, and many still are, extremely experimental. Instead of offering patients a means of release, early drugs tended to supplement straight jackets and isolation cells as a means of patients' control, although physical restraining methods certainly continued. Medication failed to address the more acute diagnoses and many patients remained detained behind the closed doors of the institution. The custodial practices of the institution are reflected in a letter by de Villiers who equates his experience to imprisonment:

> when I arrived at the place of "certain freedom" I found it to the the [*sic*] worst Ward of the lunatic asylum (a Ward reserved for violent criminals) where I was locked up in a prison cell by night and in a small yard by day.[33]

Similarly, Adrien Klipton compared the hospital to the Belsen-Bergen concentration camp in Germany that received considerable publicity in South African newspapers.[34] The parallels with prisons and concentration camps are not surprising as mental hospitals mirrored these institutions with isolatory practices, restraints, daily restrictions, dilapidated conditions, and even deaths. The incessant overcrowding, rundown buildings, and lack of appropriate facilities led to patients living in highly inadequate and unsanitary conditions. Food was minimal, toilets, most of which were squat pans or buckets, were filthy, and staff did not sufficiently clean soiled clothing and bedding. Flies infested the kitchens and wards. Evidence of mice and other vermin were present in many of the hospitals. Even at the newer hospitals, there was a constant lack of bathroom facilities and washbasins, drains never worked properly, heating during the winter remained a problem, and ceilings leaked. The conditions in non-white wards and hospitals were significantly worse than those for whites, and continued to degrade while acceptable non-white wards were taken over for white patients and little money was spent upgrading the hospitals. Patients often had chronic diarrhea due to intestinal worm infections and were infested with fleas, ticks, and other parasites. The lack of sanitary practices, inadequate nutrition, overcrowding, and malfunctioning heating also led to high incidences of tuberculosis and other respiratory diseases.[35] In 1946, there was a large number of patients who suffered from dysentery, and over 200 more patients died that year than the year before. But for the most part, the majority of illnesses from which patients suffered were influenza and tuberculosis, which were also the leading cause of deaths.

Poor conditions, isolation from family, and conflicted relationships with staff meant that for most patients, the feeling of alienation loomed and life within the institution was a lonely and difficult experience. Indeed, the remote location and dilapidated structure of mental institutions was indicative of the estrangement and neglect that patients endured. The touching letter to her father that opened this chapter, written in 1944 by Anne Waterson, reveals the sense of isolation and alienation that many patients felt during their institutionalization. The letter shows her longing to see her mother and her unhappiness at the hospital, while also demonstrating her awareness of the procedures that limited her ability to communicate openly with her family. Despite Waterson's mother's intense desire to see her daughter, she had other children at home and it was difficult for her to leave Mafeking and travel to Potchefstroom to visit her daughter. Thus, she continuously wrote letters to the superintendents and Governor General to request the release of her daughter. Her mother claimed that Anne was institutionalized due to "a small misdeed birth of a child under the age of eighteen." While it is unclear as to what happened to Waterson's child, or to the man who impregnated her, for there is no mention of either in the remaining letters, in most cases, men who did not voluntarily concede to their paternity faced little consequences. Illegitimate children were often removed from their mothers, placed in children's homes, or put up for adoption. As mentioned in the last chapter, women from poor families who gave birth to an illegitimate child could be institutionalized for doing so. Underlying the admission of women such as Anne Waterson to an institution were thus patriarchal notions of control. As Sandra Burman and Margaret Naude have shown, church-run "homes" for both married and unmarried children bearing illegitimate children were set up throughout the early part of the twentieth century, but many contained racial, age, or religious restrictions and the demand for spaces within these homes far outweighed the number of women bearing illegitimate children.[36] Thus, if a social welfare officer or magistrate deemed a woman unstable in any way, they could have them placed within a mental institution. For a white woman such as Waterson, her pregnancy became the means for her exile from her family and the estrangement from her own child. Reproductive rights were, it seemed, only for married women.

Patients such as Waterson could be moved from institution to institution on a regular basis, rarely seeing their family and never feeling part of the hospital in which they lived. Over a period of eight years, Waterson was sent to five different institutions.[37] As mental institutions were inhospitable cold places, home became secure places of refuge for many patients. Waterson's thoughts, like those of many patients, were often about her family and her desire was always to be reunited with, or at least in contact with, her home. Similarly, Tiebert Botha, while in the Fort England Hospital, wrote letters that also expressed his deep need to return to or at least to hear news from home:

> Mother, I truly long for home but I must be satisfied until I can go home. I ask God day and night to help me to be merciful so that I can safely go home again. Ah mother, it is terribly dry and hot here in Grahamstown, a person can almost not sleep during the nights, it is so warm. Ah mother, I have not yet received a letter from sister and auntie anna. Ah mother is it also so dry there and how are our sheep are they still nice and fat. And how is the horse is the black horse of mine still not ridden and how goes it with the old dog does he still live. Ask

> pa that if he has not yet inoculated the calf, tell him that he must still inoculate. And ask him how is everyone there in the town. And how does the fruit look by them are there still peaches tell Nellie she must send a pair of quinces along with the pears if pa sends me the pears please. And give greetings to them and to Hester du Preez as well, if ma sees her.[38]

Another patient, Isabelle Best, for example, was reported to have spent large portions of her time writing voluminous letters to her family.[39] Unfortunately, none of these letters have survived. The sub-standard conditions in which patients were housed in mental hospitals made their stay extremely unpleasant and contact with home became immensely important. Having a family member who could send food, clean clothing, and offer some means of diversion and connection with the outside world became increasingly important for patients who spent countless hours within the stark walls of institutions. Yet for most patients, regular contact with family members was difficult or impossible.

Individuals had little say in where they were admitted and were often detained in remote hospitals far from their families. In 1941, Rian Nederboom visited the local Native Commissioner's office to send a request for the transfer of his brother to a closer mental hospital. His brother had been admitted to the Fort Beaufort Mental Hospital in the Cape, and he asked if the authorities could transfer him to the Pietermaritzburg Mental Hospital so that his wife and children could visit him. Due to overcrowding in the Pietermaritzburg Mental Hospital, his request was denied.[40] Similarly, in 1948, Martha Gowen, a black women living in Germiston, visited her local magistrate to request assistance to visit her husband in the Grahamstown Mental Hospital. Two years previously, her husband had been admitted and she and their child had not seen him since. Not being able to have her husband transferred to a mental hospital closer to Johannesburg, in desperation, Gowen requested two free rail passes from the Native Affairs office so that she and her father could visit her husband in the hospital. Her request, like that of Rian Nederboom's, was denied.[41]

Some relatives wrote numerous letters in attempts to have their family members released even if just for a visit. Janice Pretorius, a former patient herself institutionalized at Witrand, for example, wrote many letters in her quest to get her daughter released:

> I will be glad if you can let me know about my daughter, Philomena Pretorius of Witrand Institution, Potchefstroom if I can get her hom [*sic*] to me and I have got plenty room for her and I can look after her very well. She is the only one [who] is locked up. Why can't she come home even for a little holiday just to stay a few months she had plenty people in the war. Why can't she come down to see me. She did not do any murder or steel [*sic*] why must she be locked up. I would like to

> have her down for Christmas and I will be glad if you sent my daughter down to me. Please, and here is work for her and please let me know when can I go and fetch her, or what day will she be here.[42]

Her daughter had been removed from her home by a social welfare officer who considered her and her husband unable to care for her, and in a later report suggested that the "the morals of the home left much to be desired."[43] The reference to the fact that many of her relatives had fought in the war was an attempt by Janice Pretorius to promote her status within the eyes of government officials. She believed that because her family fought for the South African government during the Second World War, government officials would perhaps overlook the fact that she and her husband had both been deemed mentally disordered. Indeed, her husband had fought in the war despite being diagnosed as a moron, a feat that was not uncommon, as we will see later.[44] Nevertheless, despite the reference to the war and the fact that her daughter had not been convicted of any criminal charges and had family members who wanted her home, Pretorius's request failed. Her daughter remained in the Witrand Institution for another four years before she was allowed to be released for a six month stay with her family.

For some families, having a patient institutionalized meant a removal of financial and physical support. A few families relied on their patient relatives for their livelihood. Albert Gilomee, for example, explained that he and his wife missed his institutionalized son's assistance around the farm: "This son was always a help around the farm and my wife and I are affected by much exhaustion and miss his help a lot.[45] Similarly, Jan Grober, a Governor General's decision patient had a mother who needed his help at home. His mother wrote numerous letters to the Governor General explaining her need to have her son take care of her.[46]

Whereas most of these stories reflect the pain most families felt when their relations were institutionalized, because of the negative stigma attached to mental disorder, a few families who may have been responsible for having them institutionalized in the first place, may have simply disowned their relative. As time passed, it became easier for family members to choose not to keep in contact with their institutionalized relatives or had no means to assist them. Philip Levin, for example, was granted permission to be released if his family wanted him home, but his family declined to take him. He therefore remained housed in the Witrand Institution for the Feebleminded.[47] Jan Pretorius, a declared inebriate coloured patient, was also due to be released, but as his wife could not financially support him or stop him from purchasing alcohol, the Physician Superintendent of Valkenberg Mental Hospital decided that he too should remain institutionalized.[48] Due to limited social support offered to family members, it is not surprising that many were unwilling or unable to take care of their relatives. Once discharged from institutions, patients became the sole responsibility of family members, who not only had to financially support them, but had to be accountable for their well-being. Paul Olivier, for example, was discharged from the Pretoria Mental Hospital in 1944 into the custody of his father. Olivier had to report to the district surgeon with his father every three months for an examination. At any time, the magistrate could decide whether he would remain in the custody of his father, or be returned to a mental hospital.[49] No government support was offered to his father, although many families were reliant on charity from the churches, such as the Dutch Reformed Church, to which they belonged. However, churches had strict stipulations to which families had to abide, and not all fit the parameters of the church or were willing to conform to them in order to have their relatives home.

For patients without relatives, their discharge was uncertain and meant that they could end up staying in institutions regardless of their mental condition because they had no family members who could vouch for their care. Derrick DeBeers, for example, had been institutionalized at the Pretoria Mental Hospital when he was eighteen as a Governor General's decision patient in 1938, only to remain in the institution indefinitely because according to the superintendent he could not be released as there was "no suitable custodian to take him on conditional discharge."[50]

These are just a few of the poignant stories that depict the everyday obstacles that family members and patients faced when attempting to visit with their relatives or when wanting to be released. Wrapped up in a highly complicated bureaucratic system and having little say and money, most patients lived in a state of exile and alienation from their communities, their families, and society in general. For patients without family members or who did not have good relationships with their relatives, the isolation was all the more pervasive.

CHALLENGING EXILE

Whereas many scholars writing about alienation have suggested that individuals estranged from their communities and their role within their communities often internalize their situation and fail to recognize their own powerlessness,[51] what is apparent in the letters of patients and family members, however, is the fact that the process of institutionalization, while often brutal and painful, was not necessarily all encompassing and completely debilitating. Many patients looked for ways to challenge the restrictions or to maneuver within them. Patients were not simply complacent, but challenged institutional staff and government officials. Superintendent reports were full of accounts of individuals being noncompliant. Albert Augustus, for example, a coloured man was described as "argumentative."[52] Joseph David, an Indian man, according to a practitioner's report, showed "marked lack of inhibition—is familiar, cheeky and jaunty and says just what he likes."[53] A coloured woman, Agnes Letoi, was described as "inclined to the habit of domineering and complaining and even during the short period of her residence here her emotional instability has revealed itself by her insolence and general insubordination."[54] Whereas all of these attitudes of non-white patients could have been deliberate attempts to challenge staff's authority, as Geoffrey Reaume points out in his study of patient experiences in the Toronto Hospital for the Insane in Canada, "one should be careful not to read into *all* such examples a deliberate effort to subvert authority" for at times they may not have been intentional resistance at all. On occasion patients may have been tired, drugged, or simply unable to cooperate.[55] Moreover, the idea that patients were difficult could also have been the perceptions of white staff who insisted on the subordination of those deemed racially inferior to themselves and viewed any non-compliant behavior, especially by black patients, as a threat.

Yet, staff also saw white patients as non-complacent. The superintendent's report on George Leroux, a white male patient, for example, claimed that "he maintains that he is being illegally detained here. His attitude is supercilious and he answers in an insolent manner when questioned."[56] Victoria George, a white female patient, was also described as having "abusive" language, "her conduct on occasions aggressive and even reprehensible and her whole outlook obstructive and unco-operative."[57] Indeed, anyone challenging the authority of staff in any way or showing any form of independence were likely to be so described. Erving Goffman calls this "looping," that is, when an agency creates an atmosphere of defensiveness among patients and uses their very responses as a means to apply further punishment. Therefore, the institution provokes a "self-protective expressive response to humiliating demands" by patients that will lead staff to "directly penalize inmates for such activity, citing sullenness or insolence explicitly as grounds for further punishment."[58] Thus, patients acting out in the system rarely won. This does not mean, though, that they did not try.

For many patients, particularly those who believed themselves not to be mentally disordered, acting out against staff was unsurprising. Indeed, the number of patients described as uncooperative suggests that patients regularly and intentionally retaliated against staff. In 1943, approximately 250 black patients at Fort Beaufort Mental hospital picked up table legs, boots, and work benches and began a riot in their ward. Patients became angry when after having been given the task of dishing out their own meat rations for some time because of their good work, and often able to obtain double meat rations because of surplus, their privileges were abruptly stopped and their meat rations halved. Hospital staff also searched their bags for undesirable objects and one patient's money that he had earned by mending shoes was taken away from him. After clashing with the nursing staff, patients broke into the cupboards that held numerous garden tools with which they broke all the locked doors. They also tried to set fire to the ward using old cleaning cloths, a few sheets and two sleeping mats. Nursing staff wielded sticks to placate the patients and the police were called in to help restrain the outbreak. Patients were quickly returned back to their wards. Although during the disturbance twenty-one patients and seven black nurses were injured, and the estimated cost of the damage reached £75, these were relatively minor damages in relation to what could have happened if the police had not been called.[59] Nursing staff blamed the injuries on those that began the riot. Individuals who were implicated in initiating the riot were first isolated from other patients and then transferred to different wards. One patient, whom staff deemed the leader, was eventually sent to another institution. Patients never did receive their extra meat rations or the respect of their property that they desired. Institutional authorities simply removed any loose benches and tools from the wards and replaced the locks.

The riot that took place indicated patients' frustration with the lack of self-determination granted to them. Protesting, even though easily quashed, was a means by which they could attempt to collectively challenge their sub-standard conditions and assert their authority. Whereas patients' riots were few and far between, there were some reports of patients setting fire to wards or influencing other patients to commit havoc in the institution. A specific section was even set aside at the Bloemfontein Mental Hospital called the Fort section where troublesome patients could be housed.[60] Some patients stole money from the staff and flagrantly broke the rules. In 1959, Koebus Joubert wrote about patients stealing money and smoking in the office of Witrand Institution:

> I would like to tell Dr that some of the patients of the male nurses said that patients had nicely stole money from the male nurses and when I came to the office of the Home in which I am in they had rolled tobacco and smoked then I told this also to the Montagu police and also told the male nurses.[61]

Institutional staff often relied on some patients to help maintain their authority, and Joubert obviously was one of those that could be counted on to inform on others. Whereas stealing from staff and disobeying rules was a means to dispute the system, it could also have been a survival tactic for some patients who had little or no money with which to buy necessities or extra goods. Nevertheless, the very act of stealing from staff and smoking in the office was itself a pro-active stance by these patients to improve their sub-standard living conditions and defy the institutional rules.

Some patients even threatened to sue the government for falsely institutionalizing and costing them their employment. Joseph Stone argued that if the government did not give him his job back, he would have to make a claim against it:

> I serve notice here Sir your Highness the Hon Dr. Jansen that if the proper dept of the Union Government should disdain as usual to take my views seriously and meet me successfully I should have no

> ulturnative [*sic*] but henceforth to make it my business to endeavour by rightfull [*sic*] means to lodge via law a claim against your hon. Union Government of South Africa for my certification & definition [*sic*] of character & severe individual damaged prestage [*sic*] which I must need's suffer personally having been an inmate of the mad house close on twenty years.[62]

Carl Van der Walt also stated that he had thought about suing the government, although he recognized the futility of such a proposition:

> I had intended to sue the responsible parties for £10,000 damages to go into a trust fund controlled by an authority like the Master of the Supreme Court to make my treatment free for medically hopeless cases in the last extremity . . . but to succeed against the unindictable [*sic*] Crown is like asking it to convict itself and seel [*sic*] out to the sovereignty of the people. The fall of the Roman Empire was never as rotten as this."[63]

Most patients' challenges to the social order within the institution were more understated than those mentioned here, and instead of openly protesting and threatening staff and government officials, patients often undertook activities such as letter writing as a means of protest. Despite the fact that officials often dismissed patients' views as delusional, writing letters to the Governor General or family members was a way that they could resist their separation from society. Patients specifically used their words as a means by which to express their displeasure with government policy and convey their desire to be considered. Attempting to defy their exile, patients continued to view themselves as part of the larger political world and integral parts of society.

One of the most common means by which patients could do so was through religion. In a society that relied on Christian-nationalism to support its political ideologies, it is not surprising that patients continually invoked concepts of religion to advance their position in society or as a prescription to what they saw as problems with the political structure. Although Sigmund Freud argued that the use of religion by patients was a form of neurotic and compulsive behavior, [64] John Hull has pointed out that "religious imagery can be the inspiration for social change,"[65] and it was not uncommon for patients to see themselves as contributing to positive social transformation through religion. William Ngcobo, a black patient in Fort Beaufort Hospital, for instance, continually preached to other patients. A report purported to explain his thoughts: "He states that he has the mission to preach to the natives and bring them to the Lord. He has the delusion that he is a prophet."[66] Similarly, Moses Debert argued that he had been sent by God to deliver an important political message:

> How are you government. Have you managed to release the people from the oppression. What do you expect people to say when they talk to you whites. The whites from Magudu have visited us[67] from their place, over pongolo. They gave way to the blacks so that we should be released from this hospital at Fort Beaufort. We request you [father] doctor who is (or) black(s) at Magudu before we run out of time. Jehova has sent me for this job of his. You see whites if you want to build this land of Africa because it is not yours, yours is in England, for others it is in Holland. I am helping you because I have been sent to you, this is the ninth year that Jehova has sent me—God Almighty, the Father, the releaser[68] of those who are oppressed. I am calling you, Moses Debert, the one who is sent. If the time that God has set passes He will punish you whites severely because there is nothing that you don't know. I am stopping there.[69]

The apocalyptic images and talk of prophets contained within Debert's letter were commonly invoked by black activists as a means to obtain inspiration for their activities, particularly in times of stress. One need only think of the Xhosa cattle killings of 1856 or the rebellion by rural laborers and members of the Industrial Commercial Union in the 1920s and 1930s to recognize its significance.[70] The use of religion, however, was not limited to black patients. A white patient, John Rulling, feeling that politics was not the answer to the problems in the area, also suggested religion as the answer:

> Politics will never bring peace in this country. Preach to and with everyone and naboor [*sic*] love will be the only way for having peace for ever . . . To pray to black and also all white like Dr. Billy Graham how sooner things can settle in this country and the Union as politics will let my country down.[71]

Throughout these letters, solutions to racial struggles were sought in religious belief and expression. These letters suggest that despite their isolation, patients were well aware of the political and social differentiation that was becoming increasingly formalized, and, in turn, were attempting to instigate social change.

During the Second World War and thereafter, patients' desire to be valuable participants in society was especially apparent. Several patients wrote letters expressing their desire to join the war effort. Zabia Solomon for example claimed that she was sane and wanted to be released so that she could partake in "war work."[72] Mike Venter also argued that he would have liked to assist his country in the war on the front lines.[73] Whereas patients were never officially released to join the war effort, some former patients did manage to sign up for service by escaping. It is difficult to determine exactly how many were able to enlist, particularly as the army never kept records of such events. But surviving patient files show a few cases of individuals who managed to sign up. Jan Stoebert, for example, escaped from the Grahamstown Mental Hospital in 1943 to join the Union Defence Force where he remained for three months when he was eventually discharged and shortly thereafter readmitted to the Valkenberg Mental Hospital.[74] The number of patients who managed to escape and sign up for military service was significant enough to prompt the Secretary of the Interior, A. B. Moore, to state, "I may say that our experience is that feebleminded ex-patients who by some means have managed to join the Defence Force are a great nuisance and are usually promptly discharged by the authorities as soon as their peculiarities show up."[75]

The desire to be free from institutional control either through escape or discharge is evident in the countless of letters that patients sent to the Governor General. Some patients were able to get themselves released by presenting themselves to the hospital board or writing letters to the Governor General's office. Between nine and ten percent of all resident patients were discharged annually between 1939 and 1950, a considerably low discharge rate. Yet discharge rates steadily increased after 1950 so that by 1960, approximately thirteen percent of all patients were being released. The increase in discharges was mostly due to new open-door policies and community-orientated approaches to patients' care by practitioners, but many of the releases were also the result of appeals to the hospital board.[76] As practitioners visited the wards and reviewed patients' conditions so infrequently, it was often up to the patient themselves to make the case for release.

Because staff recorded escaped patients as discharges, it is difficult to determine the number of patients that were officially discharged or the exact number of patients that escaped from institutions. Yet from the many reports of patients who had run away, it is probable that the rate of escape was quite high. For the most part, mental hospitals took a lax attitude towards patients who ran away, most likely because the procedure to readmit an escaped patient was the same as that for involuntary patients and the process was somewhat tiresome. Furthermore, mental hospitals had limited resources and were reliant on the police or relatives to pick up escapees and readmit them. In 1941, R. J. P. Otto who lived close to the Pietermaritzburg Mental Hospital complained about the large number of escaped patients who turned up on his farm and the failure of the mental hospital staff to even recognize that they had escaped or to bother to pick them up.[77] The inability of hospitals to effectively keep track of their patients and to search for them once they escaped, meant that patients could break out relatively easily. Yet as these institutions were in rural areas, and patients had limited money, it is unlikely that many of those who escaped were not captured shortly thereafter.

For those few patients that managed to be discharged, their lives outside the institutional walls were not easy or free of struggle. Patients such as a Janice Dickhart, for example, felt the strain of dealing with the stigma attached to being classified as mentally disordered. During one of her periods outside of the hospital in 1948, she wrote a letter to the Governor General explaining her difficulties and her awareness of the discrimination against mental patients:

> Sir,
> Just to give you my new address. I had to go as Mrs White was getting very nasty. I can't let my letter go there as she opens the letters and no one in Cape Town knows about my troubles. I am out job hunting in the factorys [*sic*]. I can't sell any more of my clothes the Lady I am sharing a room with is very poor but respectable and one of the best.[78]

Dickhart's poverty was typical of what many patients with limited education and work experience encountered outside of the institution. For some patients, readmission was their only means of obtaining shelter, food, and employment (for patients often worked within the institutions). Ran Botha, for example, regularly escaped from hospitals, but readmitted himself when he lost a job or had problems with the family members or individuals with whom he was living.[79] The amount of time that patients spent within institutions meant that many patients became dependent and unable to live outside on their own. This institutionalization has been depicted by many scholars, such as Erving Goffman and David Vail, who illustrate the "total institutionalization" or "dehumanization" of long-term patients in isolated and controlled environments. Yet as Goffman points out, many patients did not lose their identities or their humanity, but continued to challenge, manipulate, and work the system, and at times even used the system to their advantage.[80]

CONCLUSION

An analysis from the patients' perspective emphasizes the pervasiveness in their lives of the state's custodial structures. Yet it also reveals a system that was susceptible to manipulation and protest by patients and their families. This standpoint underlines both the negative effects of government policy and the limitations of its power. Patients endured intense marginalization and exile from their families and communities throughout the process of admission and thereafter, while they also remained determined to defy this exile. Moreover, an analysis of their letters reveals that the voices of inmates are not simply incomprehensible and irrelevant. Rather, as Roy Porter has argued, if they are analyzed as "products of their situation and their times . . . their testaments plainly echo, albeit often in an unconventional or distorted idiom, the ideas, values, aspirations, hopes and fears of their contemporaries."[81] Indeed, the desire to be restored to one's community, the focus on family structures, the belief in religion, the fear of war, the concern over political, racial, and gender persecution, all these certainly reflected the concerns of many South Africans between 1939 and 1960.

Although much is revealed through an analysis of patients' and family correspondence, government reports, and superintendents' notes, great silences remain. I have based this chapter predominantly on sixty-six letters from twenty-three involuntary patients, some inside mental institutions and others released and living at home, between 1939 and 1961 that were sent to the Governor General's office or to family members. Few patients' letters after 1961 were kept in government files. There are also thirteen letters from family members on behalf of their relations requesting their release. These letters are only a small percentage of those actually received in the Governor General's office, as many more were sent but then returned to the Commissioner for Mental Hygiene's Office for disposal. The letters that have survived are certainly not representative of all patients, specifically as many mental patients either could not write or never made it into the institutions at all. Thus, it is important to keep in mind that the views expressed in the letters are those of a small, somewhat unique group. With the majority of beds in institutions reserved for male patients, most of the letters sent were from men. With the exception of one letter written in Zulu and one written in South Sotho, all letters were written in either English or Afrikaans, and most were written by the educated, predominantly white, patients, although a few black, Indian, and coloured patients wrote letters.[82] A small number of illiterate patients asked staff members or fellow patients to write letters on their behalf. Supplementing these letters are superintendents' reports on patients, some degree of court testimony[83] and correspondence between government officials. These views are by no means a substitute for the more comprehensive representation of patients' perspectives that cannot be written because of the limited testimony available.

The voices of the illiterate, the less provocative, and of voluntary patients therefore remain unheard. Their silence tells us about who had agency within the institutions; it was the literate, informed patients who had more opportunity to voice their concerns through the letters that have survived, even if some of their voices have been revealed through other means of protest. In addition, although one can glean an indication of their daily routines and interrelationships with the staff and each other, the details of their lives both within the hospitals and outside remain on the whole unrepresented in the reports and letters. Their personal histories remain obscured by government processes, institutional restrictions, and the perception of practitioners. After South Africa became a republic in 1960, patients' voices became even more marginalized and difficult to uncover. The crackdown on South Africa's dissident population in the 1960s translated into an intolerance of the mentally disordered, particularly those black, coloured, and Indian decision patients held on State President's warrants. An increasingly authoritarian and intolerant government meant that the voices of the mentally disordered became progressively suppressed. The State President never kept any of the letters sent to his office by patients. The creation of bantustans permitted the state to "endorse out" dissidents, the insane, and those no longer needed in the economy to the remote and isolated homelands. Educational services dwindled, particularly for blacks, and more patients remained illiterate, while fewer letters were written or kept. At the same time, however, as shown in the next chapter, the introduction of community psychiatric practices meant more people, especially those white patients who tended to write letters, were being released, while the majority of black patients were sent to private facilities where their fate was rarely a matter of public notice or concern.[84] Either by their increased integration into society as was the case for white patients, or by their augmented segregation, as was the case for blacks, the voices of patients became even more muted.

4 Heinous Crimes

Community and Cross-Cultural Psychiatry, and State Mental Health Services for Non-Whites, 1948–1990

On September 6, 1966, just five years after South Africa had become a republic, at around 2:14 p.m., the parliamentary bells began summoning the Members of Parliament of South Africa into the chamber. As Prime Minister H. F. Verwoerd sat down at his bench, Demetrio Tsafendas, dressed in his parliamentary messenger's uniform, hurried up to the Prime Minister, pulled a large knife out of his uniform and stabbed him four times in the chest and neck. As Verwoerd slumped over, several members of parliament rushed to his aid, while others restrained his assassin. The Prime Minister was taken to Groote Schuur hospital where doctors declared him dead on arrival. The police took Tsafendas to the Caledon Square police station. That evening, police sent Tsafendas to Groote Schuur Hospital for x-rays. He had a fractured nose and jaw, which had occurred in the scuffle to restrain him. Isaac Sakinofsky, acting head of the Department of Psychiatry

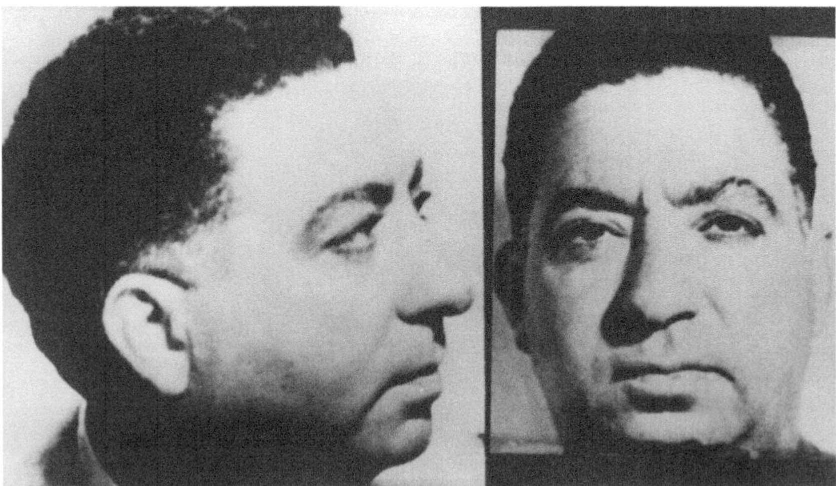

Figure 4.1 Demetrio Tsafendas, the assassin of Verwoerd, 1966. Keystone, Hulton Archive. Reprinted by permission of Getty Images.

at the hospital, examined him for about an hour and a half. When he asked Tsafendas why he had killed Verwoerd, Tsafendas vaguely stated that Verwoerd was against the "English way of life," was against a "Cape-to-Cairo movement" and supported what he saw as an unjust Immorality Act, the act that banned inter-racial sexual relations. After this examination at the hospital, the police then returned him to his police cell to await his trial.

The case of Tsafendas and Verwoed's assassination would once again bring the issue of madness to the forefront of the minds of the South African public. Directly after Verwoerd's death, politicians and journalists alike grappled with explanations for this seemingly "mindless killing"—words they used that explicitly suggested the insane nature of the act.[1] "A heinous crime," the liberal English-language newspaper, the *Rand Daily Mail,* concurred in its coverage of Verwoerd's death the day after the assassination. With little knowledge of the reasons for Tsafendas' actions, the editor of the *Rand Daily Mail* argued that it was obvious that the act was "the impulse of a crank."[2] The depiction of Tsafendas as a peculiar madman became increasingly prevalent as newspapers sought out more information about him in the days following Verwoerd's death.

Public demands for information fuelled the zeal with which newspapers sought information. The demand for stories about the death of the Prime Minister was so high that the *Rand Daily Mail* had to reprint a special edition, which they made available the following day. Tsafendas' face donned the front pages of newspapers throughout South Africa and around the world. "Face of the Assassin" blared the *Rand Daily Mail* with Tsafendas' huge eyes staring out from the page. However, few knew what type of man Tsafendas was and virtually no one knew anything about his past.

Deborah Posel argues that although the assassination of Verwoerd had "intense symbolic significance" for the South African government, the ways in which it was explained was often inconsistent and confused, partly because officials grappled with the fact that Tsafendas himself was often incoherent and viewed as mentally instable.[3] Indeed, the ways in which the government described Tsafendas's actions were not always uniform and highlighted the very confused manner in which the government approached those deemed mad. Moreover, the impact of Verwoerd's assassination on perceptions of madness could have had serious ramifications on the treatment of patients. Certainly the views of practitioners, most of whom were employees of the state, did not extend too far beyond those of the government. Psychiatric practice and theories were, as we have seen, pervaded by underlying racist and patriarchal views. All psychiatrists in the country were white until the late 1970s and early 1980s when a few coloured, Indian, and black men became certified.

Yet new trends of deinstitutionalization and the increased professionalization of the psychiatric field as a whole after the Second World War tended to negate some of the zealous public demands for increased control of the mad that emerged after the assassination of the Prime Minister. The

Society of Psychiatrists and Neurologists of South Africa (SPNSA, later the Society of Psychiatrists of South Africa or SPSA), a sub-group of the Medical Association of South Africa,[4] and more prominently, the South African National Council of Mental Health (SANCMH), to which most psychiatrists belonged, were able to assert a more critical stance that did not always support the government's or public's desire for custodial practices. In particular, the majority of practitioners continued to promote new ideas of community and cross-cultural psychiatry that advocated for more deinstitutionalized and cultural sensitive attitudes to treatment. In so doing, they were able to voice their opposition to inefficiencies of apartheid policies as applied in the mental health system and express their frustration at the low standard of mental health services in general.

Their adoption of deinstitutionalized and cross-cultural practices was a genuine attempt to benefit all patients, regardless of race or gender, by introducing less repressive forms of treatment. However, in the 1970s and 1980s the apartheid government adopted and skewed these views as a means to advance its grand apartheid strategies. Thus, practitioners, often inadvertently, facilitated the inequality of service provision on a racial basis. Nevertheless, it is still important to recognize that some practitioners did at least attempt to address the deficiencies.

BACKGROUND OF A MADMAN, RACE, AND MADNESS

Demetrio Tsafendas was born in Lourenço Marques in Mozambique sometime between 1918 and 1921. He was the son of a Greek father, Miguel Tsafandakis, who originated from Egypt, and a Mozambican mother by the name of Amelia. At the age of one his father sent him to live with his grandmother in Egypt, but after five years he returned to Mozambique to live with his father and his new stepmother, a Greek woman who took an instant dislike to him. His father worked either as an engineer or as a mechanic and moved to the Transvaal when Demetrio was ten. Demetrio attended the Middleburg Primary School in the Transvaal for two years beginning in January 1928. A fellow schoolmate remembered Tsafendas as "a popular boy who was not at all introverted."[5] However, he also described him as "not very bright" and "very dark even for a Greek."[6] Because of his "dark" skin and "fuzzy" hair, Tsafendas was nicknamed, "Blackie," which seemingly gave him an inferiority complex.[7] When Tsafendas was fourteen, he returned to Mozambique and enrolled in a church school for two more years. At the age of sixteen, he dropped out of school and took up work as a shop assistant. In 1936, he returned to South Africa and worked temporarily at a munitions factory. During World War II, Tsafendas joined a United States naval convoy, which began his extensive travels. Throughout Tsafendas' travels between the 1940s and 1960s, he picked up odd jobs. He did not keep these for very long, for he often ended up in psychiatric institutions. After he journeyed from Canada to the United States, for example, he was institutionalized as a schizophrenic for six months on Ellis Island in New York. According to his psychiatric records, he heard voices and had bouts of smearing his own feces on the walls. His racial classification seemed to cause him anxiety, for the records also reported him being in love with a white girl in South Africa but afraid to marry her in case they spawned a black child.[8] Tsafendas also spent time in Germany, Portugal, and England. By the end of his travels, Tsafendas knew eight languages, which enabled him to get a job as a translator at the immorality trials of Portuguese and Greek seamen in Durban when he returned to South Africa in 1965. These trials, which mostly dealt with interracial sexual activities, increased his concerns about his own racial categorization. Having been estranged from his mother at an early age, Tsafendas returned to Lourenço Marques that same year, in search for his mother. It is unknown whether he ever found her, but in 1966 after Verwoerd's assassination, she was reported to be still alive.[9]

Tsafendas's international wanderings and his multicultural background caused unease among those who tried to explain the assassination of Verwoerd. In the context of apartheid South Africa, where racial categorization played an important role in determining one's fate, it is not surprising that newspapers began questioning Tsafendas's racial classification. Although Tsafendas was legally white, many newspapers began arguing that Tsafendas was of "mixed" origin. Even the *Rand Daily Mail*, South Africa's more liberal newspaper, argued that Tsafendas's mother was a coloured Mozambican and stressed any connections that Tsafendas had with the non-white community. It described Tsafendas having lunch at facilities frequented by non-whites, his connections with coloured individuals and his dark complexion. Indeed, Tsafendas had spent most of his life not fully accepted by the white community and he often insisted that he preferred spending time with coloureds. His confusion over his racial classification became central to his own inner conflict and his contradictory statements to friends and associates. Just weeks before Verwoerd's assassination, newspapers reported that he had mentioned to an acquaintance that he considered changing his racial status to coloured.[10] At the same time, however, they reported that he had also commented to co-workers at the parliamentary buildings that he was angry at the low status of the poor whites in South Africa, and was upset that the government "was doing too much for, and spending too much money on the coloured people."[11] Implicit in these reports, was the idea that Tsafendas's actions were attached in some way to the rejection of apartheid, while also being the actions of a madman who thought he was the martyr of the South African republic.

The difficulty in understanding Tsafendas's behavior was due mainly to the idea that Tsafendas seemingly had little political motivation for stabbing Verwoerd. Indeed, this was increasingly emphasized by the Nationalist government, especially as rumors circulated about him being a possible Soviet spy, or someone hired by those opposed to Verwoerd policies. In the context of the Cold War, fears about the spread of communism were growing, particularly as the Soviet Union was supporting many African independence movements throughout the continent. The Justice Minister, John Vorster, who would become Prime Minister shortly thereafter, reassured the public that Verwoerd's death was the work of a sole killer and was definitely not part of a larger political conspiracy. South African embassies worldwide claimed that Verwoerd's assassination was "perpetrated by an unbalanced individual" and was, therefore, "devoid of political significance."[12] Moreover, some non-white opposition leaders were quick to disassociate themselves from Tsafendas. Rev. Benjamin Rajuill, Chief Whip of the Opposition Transkeian Democratic Party stated: "If his [Verwoerd's] murderer believed this would help the African people, he must be a misguided madman. I think I speak for all Africans in condemning this terrible act."[13]

This quick projection of Tsafendas as a "madman" and "crank" reflected the need to maintain a sense of order and control in a period where South Africa had gained the complicit support of the international community. Throughout the 1960s foreign investments in South Africa had increased, the white community as a whole had voted in the National Party with a majority and Verwoerd had stood as the symbol of the "architect of apartheid." He had endured numerous crises without retracting apartheid policies. Just six years earlier, David Pratt, a white farmer who was later deemed mentally disordered, had attempted to assassinate Verwoerd by shooting him in the head at the Rand Show, an annual amusement and exhibition event. Verwoerd had remarkably survived the gunshot wound; he seemed invincible. With his death, however, many domestic and international politicians believed that there was a chance that South Africa's political power had died with him. Stock markets initially plunged when the government released the news about Verwoerd's death, and as South Africa had recently become a republic, it was seen as increasingly vulnerable. Thus, for both the government and the public, the image of Tsafendas as a "lone killer" whose actions were mainly due to his mental imbalance was important.

Throughout Tsafendas's trial, it was not only Tsafendas who was on trial, but psychiatry as well. Government officials and the white public alike wanted to know just how someone like Tsafendas, who had a history of mental illness and had been housed in psychiatric hospitals during his travels, was no longer under treatment and even managed to obtain a job in parliament. Harold Cooper, who had spent a total of six hours with Tsafendas and testified on behalf of the defence, argued that Tsafendas was a "chronic schizophrenic" who was unable to fully understand the nature of his crime. He brought up Tsafendas' obsession with a supposed tapeworm in his stomach—a tapeworm that Tsafendas claimed had enabled him to kill Verwoerd. In cross-examination, the Attorney General of the Cape, W. M. van den Berg, asked Cooper whether Tsafendas had deliberately planned to kill Verwoerd. Cooper admitted that Tsafendas had intentionally killed the Prime Minister. However, he also pointed out that Tsafendas did not have an escape plan, therefore his act was not one of a rational clear-thinking individual. The presiding Judge, Justice Beyers, assisted by two assessors, an advocate, and a medical superintendent of a mental hospital, was somewhat skeptical of the validity of the plea for mental observation.[14] The judge's skepticism reflected the cynicism of the public against psychiatrists. To support their case, the defense attorneys obtained records from all the mental hospitals in which Tsafendas had spent time and called numerous psychiatrists to support Cooper's testimony. On the second day of the hearing, the defense called Ralph Kossew as another psychiatric witness. Kossew testified that three months before Verwoerd's assassination he had examined Tsafendas' mental state because Tsafendas had applied for a disability grant from the Department of Social Welfare. At that time, he too had classified Tsafendas as schizophrenic with a persecutive complex and hypochondria. In addition, Isaac Sakinofsky, who had examined Tsafendas the day of the assassination at Groote Schuur Hospital and two times thereafter, verified both Kossew and Cooper's findings. He argued that he had found Tsafendas mentally disordered in terms of the Mental Disorders Act and had classified him as schizophrenic.

Recognizing that skepticism against psychiatric testimony existed, on the third day of the evidentiary hearing, the defense called yet another psychiatrist, Abraham Zabow, to testify that Tsafendas was schizophrenic with paranoid tendencies. He maintained that Tsafendas suffered from delusions and thought-disorder and had lost contact with reality. James McGregor, a specialist psychiatrist and head of the Department of Neurology at the University of Cape Town, had testified earlier that he had also examined Tsafendas and found him suffering from schizophrenia of the paranoid type. He too had noticed that Tsafendas obsessed excessively about an illusory tapeworm in his stomach and found that Tsafendas had no other aspiration in life but to get rid of it. He argued, like all the psychiatrists before him, that Tsafendas had no hope for recovery. Basing his view on Tsafendas's previous escapes from mental institutions in Germany and Portugal, McGregor argued that he did not think "any ordinary asylum would hold this man for any length of time."[15] McGregor's words would form the basis of the State President's final decision to imprison Tsafendas rather than place him in a mental hospital.

Four days after the trial had begun, after hearing similar evidence of Tsafendas' schizophrenia from prosecution witnesses, Justice Beyers stated that he had no reason to prolong the proceedings of the case further. He declared Tsafendas insane and unfit to stand trial. He acknowledged that he had not immediately accepted the diagnosis of the first psychiatrist, Harold Cooper, because a court "does not lightly sit back and allow a man who has committed a grievous crime to get away on a plea or an inquiry of this nature."[16] However, as the case proceeded, he realized that Tsafendas was "obviously deranged." He stated:

> I have before me, on the evidence, clearly a man with a diseased mind, a mind subject to delusion, a mind which is so trammelled, if not guided, by irrational forces that obviously I cannot even begin to find whether he is guilty or not guilty of a crime at law. So really I have no option in the matter. There is really nothing more for me to decide and I and my two assessors find ourselves where we cannot do otherwise than say that the person presently before us is found by us to be mentally disordered.[17]

Subsequently, he committed Tsafendas to Pretoria Central Prison, pending the decision of the State President.[18] Thirty years later Tsafendas was transferred to Zonderwater Prison, and shortly thereafter, sent to Sterkfontein Mental Hospital, where he died of pneumonia in 1999. Tsafendas's funeral reflects the confusion with which people viewed his actions. His ambiguous role in shaping the history of South Africa has never quite been clarified and although there remains much speculation over whether or not he was a hero for assassinating Verwoerd, he is still very much seen as a madman. Less than ten people, none from the former anti-apartheid movement, attended his funeral.[19]

DEFENDING THE COMMUNITY? COMMUNITY PSYCHIATRY AND SOUTH AFRICAN PRACTITIONERS

The question of whether or not Tsafendas was really insane will most likely be debated for years to come. The Tsafendas case, however, at the time had revealed the cynicism and uncertainty the public and the judicial system felt about psychiatry. Psychiatrists had to explain why Tsafendas had not been institutionalized before the assassination and it forced practitioners to defend their newfound ideals of what became known as community psychiatry. Whereas debates exist as to the origins of community psychiatry in South Africa, concepts of deinstutionalization emerged due to a combination of economic and humanitarian factors, along with international influence and the introduction of psychopharmacological drugs. The involvement of the community was becoming popular worldwide, and South African practitioners readily adopted community psychiatric practices in the late 1940s when it was becoming obvious that the existing institutions and services simply could not provide the number of beds needed. Very sick individuals were ending up in the community anyway.[20] At the same time, new psychotropic drugs meant that patients could effectively be treated in non-institutional settings. These developments enabled a shift in the profession away from custodial practices toward community psychiatry.

Notions of community psychiatry were not uniform, however, and psychiatrists often had differing views about what community psychiatry entailed. Their ideas of community psychiatry also continually changed.

For some psychiatrists in the late 1940s and 1950s, community psychiatry meant applying more "therapeutic" approaches within the institution, placing these institutions within the community, or helping patients to be more socialized so they could eventually manage outside of the hospital walls. For others it signified an integrative approach between general medicine and mental health, meaning that patients could access support through general practitioners or general hospitals and they placed less emphasis on the mental hospital in general. In the 1960s, it evolved into meaning complete deinstitutionalization, the involvement of community groups and family members, and even preventative medicine.

At the 1952 South African Medical Congress in Johannesburg, many mental health practitioners criticized the general hospitals for not offering help for the mentally disordered and suggested the building of new therapeutic hospitals that would allow them to better practice their new psychological techniques.[21] Others suggested the creation of "halfway houses" for patients or "neuropathic pavilions."[22] In 1953, Alice Cox, chief psychiatrist at Tara Hospital, took community psychiatry to mean bridging the Cartesian division between mind and body and suggested that less acute mental patients be dealt with at the general hospital level. This, she argued, would address many of the accommodation and staffing problems that existed within South African mental health services.[23] A year later, G. A. Elliott, a professor at the University of the Witwatersrand, agreed with Cox and argued that integration of psychiatry and internal medicine should be South Africa's main concern.[24] Whereas these suggestions for integration with general medicine could have been due to psychiatrists' desire to gain respect within the medical field, it was also a means to address what they saw as the custodial crisis within mental health services.

Tara Hospital, the white hospital that housed predominantly white males at the end of the Second World War, was at the forefront of innovative community-orientated approaches in psychiatry. In 1953, Tara initiated the first outpatient program for a mental hospital in South Africa.[25] Its program was still hospital-based but kept the patients out of the wards. Tara, being a white, provincially funded and university-affiliated institution, had the resources with which to implement its plans. While community psychiatry in the 1950s still focused on the institution as the sole site of treatment, in the 1960s, advocates began to call for forms of treatment in smaller clinics or non-hospital settings. They also advocated co-operation between other government services, social agencies and the community in general. Within Tara's approach to community psychiatry, the mental hospital remained central to the effective treatment of seriously ill patients, but family doctors, nurses, and smaller clinics were meant to eventually replace hospital, in-patient care particularly in less acute cases. In 1960, H. Moross, then Tara's medical superintendent, also suggested the establishment of small treatment centers and mobile psychiatric clinics for whites and non-whites living in urban centers.[26] In his view, patients did not need to be admitted to, or even treated in, mental hospitals. The next step was to advocate integration of treatment in community settings through outpatient programs, that is, programs for patients who do not reside outside the institution, home-visits, group therapy, social activities, and, when necessary, through prescription of psychotropic drugs. L. S. Gillis, Senior Psychiatrist at Tara, argued that treatment of psychiatric illness should move beyond narrow clinical practice and should take full account of the patient's social and community background. In addition, he argued that already established community services should be utilized in treatment; and he advocated training black psychiatrists whom he felt would have a better understanding of black patients. Tara Hospital staff conducted home visits of their released patients and their families. It offered domiciliary nursing services to those patients waiting for inpatient treatment, enlisted social workers to visit patients in their homes and created therapeutic social clubs in various locations outside of the hospital throughout Johannesburg. It appointed a social worker to its staff. It was the first hospital to do so.[27] Tara also expanded the scope of community psychiatry to include prevention and early detection. Moross suggested that preventative programs should be set up in schools, homes and workplaces in order to enable early detection and provide basic treatment before hospital admission became necessary.[28]

The concept of outpatient programs seemed like a good idea in general to deal with an ever increasing demand on beds in institutions. It was meant to transform the custodial practices of institutions, but it failed to do so and instead ended up reinforcing custodial practices for blacks, and perpetuating inequalities within the system. The government, having heard incessant complaints about inadequate services, recognized the potential these programs could have, not only for the problem of overcrowded wards but also to save themselves money. Psychopharmacological drugs were also becoming increasingly available for mental illnesses and government officials could use them to justify their release of patients.[29] At the same time, community psychiatry seemed to support the government's mandate to create racially separate institutions for blacks, whites, and coloureds.[30]

To promote Afrikaner nationalism and white supremacy, the government spoke the language of modernity and pushed industrial development, technological advances, and private enterprise in ways that would exclusively benefit whites. These notions that put modernism at the service of narrow ethnic nationalism certainly affected psychiatrists' views of their own practice.[31] They began to advocate for reformed psychiatric practices that they thought would promote the intellectual development of white patients. Concern for the incidence of mental disease among whites reflected fears and anxiety that their racial supremacy was at risk. For example, Louis Freed, a South African doctor, compared the incidence of mental disorders among locally born and foreign-born whites. He came up with the reassuring conclusion that foreign-born South Africans had a higher incidence of mental illness than those born in South Africa.[32] His figures were disputed shortly thereafter, but the idea of carrying out such a study indicates the extent of fears that white racial superiority might be at risk. By providing supposedly scientific evidence to the contrary, Freed hoped to calm such anxieties.

Apartheid's preoccupation with particular forms of modernity was, however, itself a subject of criticism as critics warned of the negative effects that modernist ideas would have on society. Psychiatry itself was affected by the politics of modernism. As a relatively new medical sub-discipline, it was often perceived to have a weaker claim to scientific standing than general medicine. In response, psychiatrists tried to raise the status of their profession not only in the medical community but also among the wider public. Here was a powerful incentive to abandon old-fashioned clinical practices that emphasized the custodial in favor of seemingly more modern treatment strategies that were community-oriented and more visible to the public. The same motive helps to explain why psychiatrists embraced drug-treatment programs that seemed to promise up-to-date remedies for mental disease. They claimed these drugs were as effective and scientific as those that antibiotics. Claiming the authority of Western science, many psychiatrists also felt compelled, like most of their biomedical colleagues, to distance themselves from, and in some cases to condemn, indigenous healers, who performed the only forms of psychological counseling that most black people ever received.

Whereas the quest for higher professional status and greater public respect led some psychiatrists to advocate community psychiatry, their ambitions also involved contradictions. To be successful, community programs required extensive funding at a time (through most of the 1950s) when public health and social welfare budgets were seriously constrained. They also required collaboration from social and welfare workers who were already overworked and underfunded. They even, as we will see, sometimes relied on indigenous healers in the grossly underserviced black communities, which in turn may have been perceived to diminish psychiatry's claims to exclusive professional standing.

Among psychiatrists, as in the wider community, there was an ambivalence toward modernism that included a tendency to blame modernity for a host of evils afflicting society, from drug and alcohol abuse, to the fears of racial decline among whites and a related concern about a perceived rising tide of mental illness in white society. In 1964, R. W. S. Cheetham argued that the rapid advance of science and technology contributed to the increased anxiety of individuals. This in turn created a change in "traditional" mores:

> Cultural patterns and behaviour have departed radically from traditionally sound and fundamental concepts . . . the modern neurotic need

> for haste in acquisition of more and more material gain only serves to enhance the underlying emotional insecurity. Cultural patterns have therefore altered and the individual, attempting to identify himself with a rapidly changing culture suffers emotionally.[33]

Urbanization and industrialization were seen as the main causes of mental illness, specifically among non-whites, who were perceived as abandoning their traditional values. H. Moross, for example, argued that:

> South Africa faces special mental health problems in its multi-racial and multi-cultural community. The complexity of these problems is heightened by urbanization of the non-White races in a time of changing values—especially by the effects of urbanization on tribal laws, customs and taboos.[34]

Similarly, Eugene Toker argued that he only encountered cases of mental illness in the black population among those who lived in urban areas. He maintained that because black males went to urban centers to work, "traditional" family structures were broken up. "This would suggest," he wrote, "that with the urbanization of the Bantu one would expect an increased incidence of neurosis and psychopathy."[35] These practitioners' arguments, while never overtly stating that they supported apartheid policies, did advocate that blacks be protected from the perceived harshness of urban centers—views that reinforced those of the state which was attempting to force blacks into reserves under the guise of "protecting" their cultural traditions.

Even if practitioners did not support apartheid segregationist strategies, because community psychiatry was reliant specifically on community input, and in apartheid South Africa where black, coloured, and Indian communities were being broken up, divided, relocated and starved of financial and human resources, the ability of practitioners to effectively implement their strategies was thwarted. Apartheid policies were expensive and mental health was not a priority of the government. At times poor resources even affected whites. In 1958, A. Radford argued that despite the fact that practitioners wanted to treat and discharge patients, inadequate resources restricted their efforts:

> Mental hospitals differ from all other hospitals in this respect that the inmates of mental hospitals are not there with their own consent. They are people who are deprived of their liberty by the State, and it is the duty of the State to see that they are well cared for, and as far as possible returned to the community when it is safe for them and the community that they should do so. I would like to point out that conditions in this country are in such a state that this is almost impossible. A few gallant doctors in the service of the State are doing their best, and are

> getting back some people, but on the whole they are frustrated and unable to carry out this function.[36]

In 1961, the Mental Disorders Amendment Bill enabled the extension of outpatient programs to all mental hospitals. By 1966, when Tsafendas assassinated Verwoerd, approximately 42,000 patients were treated at makeshift outpatient facilities throughout South Africa. But most state-run institutions had limited resources and were not able to implement as extensive community psychiatric programs and offer social services such as at Tara.[37] Indeed, Tsafendas himself had never been admitted to Tara Hospital and had never benefited from any social services in South Africa. The advocacy of community psychiatric programs by the state was, it seemed, nothing more than a means to save money and virtually nothing was invested in social programs for released patients. Thus, in reality, practitioners chose to retain the majority of patients in institutions, or they simply released them with little follow-up support.[38] Even those white patients who were released had practically no access to formal community services. The few outpatient services that existed for black patients were often in dilapidated buildings rented by the Department of Public Works, were crammed, crowded, and offered little form of therapy.[39] In some rural cases, community clinics were held outdoors. Wilhelm Bodemer, a psychiatrist, described the local clinic:

> I always said it was a shock for my first overseas visitor, after the community when we went to the clinic, and the clinic was the third rock under the tree on the road . . . that was the community clinic. We had no buildings at that stage.[40]

When community clinics were established, they still relied on larger institutions to oversee their development, and as beds for non-white patients in these institutions were relatively few, and resources and staff were stretched, only a small percentage had access to community-based programs. Moreover, the racialized nature of diagnoses that existed in the early twentieth century became even more apparent throughout the apartheid years. Indeed, the majority of coloured, Indian, and black patients continued to be diagnosed with the more serious mental illnesses, while white patients were diagnosed with less serious illnesses such as depression. Because nonwhites were diagnosed with more serious disorders such as schizophrenia, which one psychiatrist called South Africa's biggest "therapeutic failure," community psychiatric programs rarely prompted changes in the treatment of black patients.[41] Whereas some observers suggested community psychiatry provided a means to deal with the rising numbers of black patients, they were the least likely to be released or receive post-treatment services. Even without the racialized views of practitioners and the differential diagnoses, community psychiatric programs could not have been effective because of the overall discriminate system in which they existed.

CROSS-CULTURAL PSYCHIATRY

Some practitioners promoted an extension of community psychiatry, which they called transcultural or cross-cultural psychiatry. Cross-cultural psychiatry included an insistence that mental illness had to be understood within the social or cultural context in which it occurred. Using Western therapies and anthropological methods, these practitioners set out to offer community services to Africans and to understand what was distinctive about African mental processes.

Cross-cultural psychiatry was not a new concept; it originated in the early twentieth century when practitioners began to encounter mental illness among Africans. Wulf Sachs's *Black Hamlet,* first published in 1937, republished in 1947, and again in 1969, was a popular book that asked whether Western psychiatry could be applied across cultures. As mentioned in the first chapter of this book, Sach believed that it could, arguing that "the manifestations of insanity, in its form, content, origin and causation, are identical in both natives and Europeans." He proved this through analysis of a Manyika healer whom he called John Chavafambira.[42] Also in 1937, B. J. F. Laubscher's *Sex, Custom and Psychopathology* analyzed the psychopathology of the Tembu and Fingo of the Eastern Cape and argued that "the cultural pattern to which the native belongs, determines the nature of his mental content, but does not affect the particular form of mental disorder, namely, its structure, to the extent of making it something different from that which occurs in European culture."[43] In other words, Europeans and Africans exhibited similar mental disorders, but the way they understood and expressed them was completely different.[44]

These ethnopsychiatric works were influential precursors of cross-cultural psychiatry that became increasingly popular in the later 1960s and 1970s. The re-emergence of cultural-sensitive psychiatric approaches at this particular juncture is directly connected to the rise of community psychiatric ideas—the desire to release patients into the community led to an increased interest in patients' lives. However, it can also be attributed to the fervent resistance struggles that were taking place throughout South Africa during the late 1960s, 1970s, and 1980s. Jock McCulloch has argued that ethnopsychiatric studies in colonial Africa increased significantly during periods of violent resistance or nationalist assertions by Africans.[45] Similarly, in South Africa, the increase of organized resistance among blacks, particularly in the 1970s and 1980s, certainly had an impact on the consciousness of practitioners about how to understand the discontent that Africans expressed about their social circumstances. Many practitioners, however, disregarded the real grievances of Africans and talked instead about "understanding the African mind," as if African protests were caused by a mindset or a consciousness different from that of whites. In so doing, they absurdly thought that they could understand and perhaps even defuse black anger, without having to implement expensive strategies that would address their real grievances.

It is helpful here to have a broad understanding of what exactly cross-cultural psychiatry entailed in order to understand its limitations. In 1986, Leslie Swartz performed a cross-sectional review of cross-cultural psychiatric views in a South African context. His findings not only skillfully reflect the complexity and the diversity of practitioners' beliefs, but were also written at the time that practices were being implemented. His insights are representative of how at least one practitioner was not completely ignorant of the inherent problems of the application of cross-cultural psychiatry within the context of apartheid. Swartz points to three different, although overlapping approaches that were used in South Africa throughout the 1970s and 1980s. First, there were the proponents of an "African personality." Citing individuals such as R. W. S. Cheetham and J. A. Griffiths who argued that blacks were "closer to nature than whites," and G. G. Minnaar who argued that "Westernization" had negative effects on Africans, these practitioners promoted relativist ideas in that Africans had a different and stagnant worldview of mental health than whites.[46] These relativists suggested that there were two "radically different" and "contrasting" approaches to health—the Western systematic biomedical approach and the indigenous "traditional" approach.[47] David Hammond-Tooke's anthropological studies were often used by these proponents of the "African personality" as proof that African indigenous views had barely changed since their inception and varied little among the different groups of Africans themselves.[48] These arguments explicitly supported the notion that blacks were less evolved than whites and, in turn, needed less modern services than whites.

Second, Swartz points to scholars who placed understandings of mental illness of a specific group within a larger social context. Those who supported this view were in direct contrast to those asserting the notion of the "African personality" and were universalist in their approach. These were practitioners, who were strongly influenced by anthropological and ethnographical studies that placed African understandings of mental health within local and international contexts. Anthropologists such as A. I. Berglund, for example, examined Zulu understandings of mental illness within a more holistic and broader context of Zulu thought rather than separating it.[49] Harriet Ngubane also wrote about African understandings of mental illness through anthropological methods within broader family and social structures. Arguing against those that suggested that African ideas of illness were less evolved than Western notions of medicine, Ngubane implied that African notions of illness were just as easily understood as Western notions and deemphasized the "exoticism" of traditional practices that proponents of an "African personality" projected. Jean Comaroff and J. Mills argued that one cannot study "medical anthropology as a separate discipline separate from that of social anthropology," and both attempted to reintegrate analysis of African understandings of health within a broader socio-political and everyday context.[50] Skewing these anthropological studies somewhat, some practitioners such as M. C. O'Connell, A. G. Le Roux, and T. L. Holdstock recognized that African understandings of mental illness changed depending on the social situation in which they found themselves.[51] For example, Le Roux and Holdstock argued that social change such as technology and urbanization could negatively affect the mental health of Africans.[52] These arguments, like those of community psychiatry, perpetuated the notion that Africans needed to be "protected" from the negative effects of urbanization, modernity, and social change.

Lastly, Swartz describes the views of those few practitioners who asserted psychoanalytical approaches to black understandings of mental health.[53] These methods of cross-cultural psychiatry combined both universalist and relativist approaches to mental disorders. Proponents suggested that regardless of race, culture, or ethnicity, all human beings exhibited similar mental indicators for illness and approached them through analogous psychoanalytical processes; individuals just expressed them differently. Practitioners such as Vera Bührmann, for example, analyzed indigenous practices towards mental illness through a Jungian perspective. Bührmann essentially argued that because the Xhosa were more in tune with their true natures, they practiced Jungian psychotherapy intuitively, although with a few expressive differences. Xhosa practices, she argued, focused more on the unconscious and symbolic and "*act out* what the Western people *talk about*."[54] Her views echoed those of the "African personality" by suggesting that two opposing worlds existed, "the Western world which is primarily scientific, rational and ego-oriented, and the world of the Black healer and his people, which is primarily intuitive, non-rational or orientated towards the inner world of symbols and images of the collective unconsciousness."[55] The numbers of practitioners, however, who adopted the psychoanalytical approach were less common than for those who suggested that Africans had an "African personality," and one of the last scholars to do so was S. G. Lee who looked at spirit possession among the Zulu in 1969.[56]

Although the intentions of those promoting cross-cultural psychiatry was to encourage a deeper understanding and respect for African means of treatment, and some practitioners such as N. C. Manganyi, influenced by Franz Fanon's writings and the black consciousness movement, adopted notions of a unique "African personality" as a means to promote African self-empowerment, for the most part, all three approaches to African mental health supported discriminatory beliefs.[57] Some practitioners even used these notions in a disparaging manner, by, for example, adopting the concept of an "African personality" as a means to show that Africans were simply not as intellectually developed as whites. Furthermore, most proponents of social contextualization directly promoted the notion that African culture needed to be "protected" from westernization, while psychotherapeutic approaches also often adopted notions of "African personality," and heralded Western approaches as the marker for appropriate care. Indeed, the underlying premise of all three views of cross-cultural psychiatry was to establish whether African methods were the same or different from Western practices, and Western practices were heralded as the desired means of treating individuals. This was reflected further in the incessant concern over methodology and positivist approaches towards its application that continued to promote Western notions of mental health.[58]

A way that practitioners attempted to get around these discriminatory views was by integrating healers into their practice. Indeed, practitioners such as Jan Robbertze and C. W. Allwood promoted collaboration between practitioners and healers.[59] But indigenous ways of knowing were often overshadowed by those of western practitioners.[60] Dolly Nkosi, a healer who dealt specifically with mentally ill individuals and attempted to work with Western doctors in the 1980s found that her efforts were often disparaged:

> If you would take your patient to the doctor you would be accused of the things that you never did. For instance, the doctor would say to you: "You have given the patient herbs that you were not supposed to give him or her." I used to be very angry with that. They would tell you that you decided to send the patient to them because you couldn't manage to heal/cure him or her.[61]

Many practitioners continued to see themselves as "scientists" with more skilled and systematic treatments than healers. In 1976, the *South African Medical Journal* published an editorial entitled "Herbalists, Diviners and even Witchdoctors." Whereas it promoted the use of healers, in line with separate development initiatives, it strongly discouraged any form of partnership with them. The editorial suggested that the healers' practices were different from those of the psychiatric field and argued that healers studied a completely different field:

> The strictest member of Medical Council would not have the slightest objection to a doctor's asking the advice of an architect in connection with the design and use of facilities; in fact, such intelligent gathering of knowledge is a *sine qua non* for good medical practice and is to be encouraged. But that does not mean that the doctor may set up rooms with an architect or refer patients to him. Let those in rural practice, or wherever the problem applies, sit down with witchdoctors or diviners or herbalists, whichever term is apt, and talk and learn and try to understand more about mores and taboos, but partnership is something else.[62]

Accordingly, although psychiatrists stressed an increased understanding of African culture, in actuality they promoted difference and segregation. Science and psychiatry were not politically disaffected and, as Leslie Swartz argued, "the concept of 'cultural diversity' cannot be anything but value-laden in South Africa, as it forms the basis of justification for apartheid policies."[63] As we will see, in the 1970s and 1980s, community and cross-cultural psychiatry did serve the needs of the apartheid government, but they also, in the 1960s resulted in the dis-ease with the role of practitioners in treating patients such as Tsafendas.

COMMISSIONS OF INQUIRY INTO PSYCHIATRY, MENTAL HEALTH ASSOCIATIONS, AND THE NEW MENTAL HEALTH ACT OF 1973

The same day that the judge passed down his decision on the Tsafendas case, the Minister of Justice, Petrus Pelser, announced that a commission of inquiry headed by F. Rumpff would investigate the role of psychiatry and the existing legal statutes regulating the responsibility of mentally deranged individuals. The final report stated the reason for the committee:

> Through the tragic combination of circumstances leading to the death of Dr. Verwoerd, the problem of the violent mentally disordered person was brought pertinently to the attention of the authorities, and a shocked nation wants an answer to the question of how it could be possible for attacks to be made on two occasions on the life of the Prime Minister by mentally disordered persons and how such persons could be detected before they do serious harm.[64]

The committee made note of the lack of confidence often placed in psychiatrists by the public and the legal profession. It argued that psychiatrists frequently were viewed as defending the acts of criminals and giving these criminals an opportunity to commit further crimes. As R. W. S. Cheetham from the National Council of Mental Health stated in a memorandum to the Committee:

> (i) In the present method of conducting the criminal trial, with the onus on the defence to prove insanity "as a defence," the psychiatrist, in giving evidence to indicate the presence of a mental disorder, is in reality making a diagnosis (as in any illness), and recommending therapy to the Court. This, however, is all too commonly regarded, by the public, as an attempt to defeat the ends of justice, and the purely medical attitude, required of him by his Hippocratic oath, is overlooked in the emotionality surrounding the trial and the identification of the public with the murdered or injured individual or family.
> (ii) Thus the public concept, all too frequently is that, in certain cases, psychiatrists "get people off" criminal charges.[65]

Because of this negative view of psychiatric testimony, the committee found that judges easily rejected psychiatric views that did not fit directly into the pre-existing legal perspective. For example, one of the many cases the committee cited was *Rex v. Kennedy* (1951) wherein the court refused to accept the psychiatric evaluation of Cooper, the same psychiatrist who testified at the Tsafendas case. Cooper found the accused in this case mentally disordered, but the judge dismissed Cooper's evaluation as based on improbable evidence. He argued that Cooper's definition did not fit the legal requirement and, in turn, the judge found the accused fit to stand trial.[66]

This negation of psychiatric testimony was partly due to the difficulty of determining the definition of "criminally insane." The court mainly relied on the substance of the M'Naghten Rules—five guidelines set up in the 1843 English court case of Daniel M'Naghten who had shot Sir Robert Peel's secretary and had suffered from paranoia. Generally speaking, the basis of the M'Naghten case is as follows:

> to establish a defence on the ground of insanity it must be clearly proved that, at the time of committing the act, the accused was labouring under such a defect of reason, from disease of the mind, as not to know the nature and quality of the act he was doing, or, if he did know it, that he did not know he was doing what was wrong . . . If the accused was conscious that the act was one that he ought not to do, and if that act was at the same time contrary to the law of the land, he is punishable . . . [67]

This meant that if a psychiatrist deemed an accused mentally insane and testified that he did not know the difference between right and wrong, then the accused would no longer be punished for criminal conduct. Instead, they would be placed in a mental hospital. Consequently, psychiatrists who acted as witnesses for the defense of many criminal cases were often viewed as defenders of the criminal and this placed them in direct opposition to the judge and/or jury. Furthermore, the qualities that made an individual unable to "determine right from wrong" or having a "defect of reason" were vaguely stated and open to interpretation. With no clear regulations concerning psychopaths, courts had further discretion concerning the treatment and punishment of these individuals.[68]

Some psychiatrists perpetuated this unease by stating their own negative views of the competence of psychiatric testimony. They agreed with public and judicial perceptions that psychiatry allowed individuals to avoid responsibility for their actions. For example, in 1950, J. J. de Villiers argued that psychiatrists involved in court cases merely took part in a large "poker-game" in the court where criminals tried to convince the psychiatrists of their insanity, and they were mostly successful.[69] P. H. Henning, Medical Superintendent at Fort Napier Hospital in Pietermartizburg and Lecturer at the University of Natal, argued that Zulu patients in Natal often attempted to use mental disorder as a defense in higher rates than elsewhere in the country and his solutions to solving this problem reflected an increased skepticism towards African patients.[70] He suggested that psychiatrists become more aware of falsification and that any patient that psychiatrists admit for observation be treated as a potential fraud. He also argued that mental institutions with their new "open door" policy were no longer appropriate for suspected criminals. He suggested that the new therapeutic approach gave patients extended freedom and made mental hospitals more attractive places for criminals. Indeed, in a study published just two days after Tsafendas' verdict, Henning found that almost 40 percent of state patients in Fort Napier Hospital had escaped between 1944 and 1963. Therefore, he argued that criminals would inevitably choose a mental hospital stay over prison and would be more inclined to attempt to fool psychiatrists into thinking they were mentally disordered.[71]

Similarly, a 1951 editorial argued that psychiatrists' concern did not lie primarily with the safety of society, but with the individual. Therefore, it argued that psychiatric practices made it "extremely doubtful that a person may be held entirely responsible for his actions." Moreover, it contended that while psychiatric studies could offer further insight into the reasons behind the criminal behavior, psychiatry could not take the place of the legal system.[72] The lack of services for patients, particularly those deemed dangerous, led to demands by some practitioners for stricter policies. They claimed that psychiatry was no longer adequately equipped to deal with criminal cases because psychiatric hospitals could not satisfactorily house psychopaths. M. Ginsburg, Physician Superintendent at Fort Napier Hospital, argued that sending psychopaths to mental hospitals was "not only inadvisable but wrong for several aspects."[73] He argued that they disrupted other patients and caused considerable more work for already overworked psychiatric staff. In addition, he pointed out that mental hospitals had fewer security measures, allowing patients to escape more easily.[74] These views were in turn compounded by Verwoerd's assassination, which highlighted the inadequacy of the psychiatric field to deal with psychotic and mentally deranged individuals.

Although many individual practitioners in public institutions were discouraged by the deficient nature of their programs and were aware of the public criticisms, most wanted to continue their promotion of community and cross-cultural psychiatry. The official associations of practitioners such as the SPNSA and the SANCMH undoubtedly played a role in enforcing the racialized and heteropatriarchal structure of apartheid, for the "expert" advice offered by these associations had a profound effect on the often confused views of government officials. But practitioners and their associations were also able to challenge custodial government strategies, even if only for the benefit of white patients.[75] We see this specifically in the wake of Verwoerd's assassination when practitioners, despite being pressured to abandon their community psychiatry practices, advocated for a continuation of deinstitutionalization.

The main advocate for practitioners in mental health policy revision in the wake of Verwoerd's death was the SANCMH. Established in 1920, the SANCMH was a voluntary mental health organization with numerous affiliated societies that had the objective of cooperating with government mental health programs, while simultaneously promoting additional accommodation for the mentally disordered, conducting public education, and collecting data for advocacy. It registered as a welfare group in 1949 and formed the umbrella organization for regional mental health societies.[76] In the 1950s and 1960s, however, in accordance with the rise in popularity of community psychiatry, it began to change its mandate from advocating for more hospital accommodation to preventative and rehabilitative programs.[77] Jan H. Robbertze, who became the Chairman of the SANCMH in 1966, explained the organization's role as "to try to fight *against* the psychiatric services for patients in South Africa," not one that promoted institutionalization.[78] By the mid-1960s, the SANCMH was operating subsidized community services such as developmental programs for mentally challenged and epileptic individuals, special educational services, rehabilitation services for discharged white patients and national awareness campaigns.[79] These services fit within the community psychiatric model and involved the co-ordination of social workers, voluntary workers, and mental health societies in the prevention and treatment of patients in the community.[80]

Whereas the SANCMH and its societies operated a few community services, its primary function was to campaign for changes in mental health funding and policy. It regularly asked for inquiries into conditions for mental patients, advocated for public services in the media, and participated in various government investigations.[81] After Verwoerd's assassination, practitioners actively sought to change the negative stereotypes of mental patients in their local communities. On a national level, the SANCMH submitted recommendations to the Rumpff commission.[82] It suggested that the government change existing regulations concerning the criminally insane to reflect more modern ideas of psychiatry. In 1967, the Rumpff commission heard testimony from numerous psychiatrists from different parts of South Africa and distributed a questionnaire to the departments of sociology, psychiatry/psychology and law at the various universities and numerous psychiatric and legal organizations throughout South Africa. The questionnaire concerned the existing regulations pertaining to insanity defences and requested suggestions for revisions. Psychiatrists and psychologists were virtually unanimous in their denunciation of the M'Naghten Rules.[83]

The SACMH argued that the M'Naghten Rules were outdated and did not reflect the modern community-orientated state of psychiatry. Psychiatry, they argued, had changed since the M'Naghten case in England. The M'Naghten Rules only took into account the accused's recognition of right and wrong or the cognitive mental functions, and failed to recognize the implicit desires and affective disturbances of the individual.[84] Underlying this view was the acknowledgment of the effect that socio-economic conditions had on the mental health of individuals as suggested by community psychiatry. These psychiatrists argued that because the South African law "assumes that there are still two alternative mental conditions, distinct from each other, each of which has to be assessed separately: first, a condition which can deprive a person of his capacity to discriminate between right and wrong, and secondly, a condition in which . . . an irresistible impulse has arisen," it led to conflict with psychiatric evaluations of patients whose lines between right and wrong may not be clearly defined.[85] As a solution, the SANCMH recommended that the government modify the Criminal Procedure Act to reflect that "an accused who in respect of an alleged crime was not capable on account of mental disease or mental defect of appreciating the wrongfulness of his act, or of acting in accordance with such appreciation, shall be held not to be responsible."[86] It argued that existing legislation for mental patients was outdated and did not take the circumstances surrounding a crime into account, nor did it acknowledge the degrees of disorder that could exist among individuals.[87]

Because of the submissions of practitioners and the SANCMH to the Rumpff commission, in March 1967, the apartheid government proposed appointing another commission of inquiry into mental health services and legislation in South Africa, headed by a supreme court judge, J. T. van Wyk. The Van Wyk commission included representatives from the Department of Prisons and the Department of Labour along with two psychiatrists, two sociologists, a psychologist, a hospital administrator, and a clinical psychologist. The commission's objective was to examine the existing legal regulations concerning psychiatric services such as the Mental Disorders Act and make recommendations for updating these regulations. The Vice-President of the SANCMH, R. W. S. Cheetham, sat on this committee and actively promoted the Council's community psychiatric ideals. He argued for more integrated services between general and mental practitioners and suggested that adequate outpatient services, general hospitals, and follow-up services be established.

Significantly, the Van Wyk commission began under the pretext that the terms "mentally ill" and "mental health" should take the place of terms such as "mentally defective" and "mental disorder." Psychiatrists had slowly been adopting these terms throughout the 1950s and 1960s as community psychiatry became more popular and drugs became more readily available. Indeed, the commission adopted many of the recommendations that psychiatrists had consistently made since the 1940s. The Van Wyk commission highlighted the increasing problem of lack of accommodation, facilities, and psychiatric staff. It argued that mental health's isolation from general medicine merely compounded the negative stigma attached to psychiatry and discouraged individuals from training to be psychiatrists. It suggested that the government place public psychiatric hospitals under the administration of the provinces. This, the commission argued, would allow more flexibility and more localized training. It also suggested that adequate outpatient facilities, night hospitals, follow-up programs, and general hospital services be set up. This adoption of more therapeutic and biologically centered terms, as well as the commission's concern over the isolation of mental illness, reflected the psychiatric field's effort to promote a more integrative and holistic approach to psychiatry.

At the same time, the Van Wyk commission concentrated on individuals who were a danger to society, such as state patients and the criminally insane. It dedicated specific sections to psychopathic patients and forensic psychiatry. It argued, much like the Rumpff committee before it, that psychopaths should be kept neither in prisons nor in mental hospitals, but should be kept in hospital prisons or psychopathic hospitals.[88] In addition to the separate accommodation for psychopaths, the commission suggested that a new provision be placed within the new Mental Health Act that would ensure that all medical practitioners, including psychiatrists, clinical psychologists, general practitioners etc. would report a mentally ill individual whom they perceived as dangerous to others to the magistrate or to a policeman. Under the 1916 Mental Disorders Act, police were already able to detain mentally disordered individuals who were dangerous to themselves or others. The committee suggested that the government add a further provision to the Act that when a medical practitioner reported the existence of a dangerous individual, the police shall shortly thereafter apprehend that individual.[89] With respect to those individuals who were charged with criminal offences and subsequently detained, the commission recommended that they not be released without the authority of the State President.[90] They also argued that courts should allow the execution of psychopaths because:

> It should be borne in mind that psychopathic disorders do not arise over night, and that if a psychopath has been sentenced to death the fact that he is a psychopath would in all probability have been taken into account by the judge when deciding that the death sentence should be imposed.[91]

Psychopaths, they implied, had no hope of ever rehabilitating; therefore, the application of the death penalty was justified.

In relation to psychiatric involvement in the diagnosis of a psychopath or criminally insane individual, the Van Wyk commission suggested that psychiatry be further removed from its involvement in criminal cases. It proposed that medical schools incorporate forensic psychiatry within their curriculum. Training in forensic psychiatry would emphasize that psychiatrists merely "assist[ed] the authorities in determining the aetiology of criminal behaviour, offences and crimes which require[d] psychiatric investigation . . . and not act as 'amateur advocates'."[92] Furthermore, the commission distanced itself from the issues concerning criminal regulations for the mentally insane and argued that the sections in the previous Mental

Disorder Act dealing with such cases should be removed and dealt with purely in the Criminal Procedure Act. This distancing of the mental health field from the criminally insane would enable the psychiatric field to continue to promote community psychiatry, while also allowing the apartheid government to detain mentally ill individuals in prisons rather than mental institutions if it so desired.

In 1973, the apartheid government changed the Mental Disorders Act to a new Mental Health Act that embodied many of the recommendations made by the Rumpff and van Wyk commissions. It opened more positively with a section on voluntary patients and outpatients and embodied many of the therapeutic views that psychiatrists had promoted. On the other hand, the new legislation also reflected the increased concern over the criminally insane that existed after Verwoerd's assassination and it contained stricter rules for their confinement. The solution to many psychiatrists' problems was the "psychopathic hospital." However, the government never built psychopathic prisons that would enable psychiatrists to distance themselves from psychopathic patients. Moreover, the problem of limited beds for black patients remained, and practitioners remained frustrated at the limited options offered them by state services.

GOVERNMENT APPLICATION OF COMMUNITY AND CROSS-CULTURAL IDEAS: APARTHEID HOMELAND MENTAL HEALTH SERVICES AND THE TRICAMERAL SYSTEM, 1960S–1989

Tsafendas the "madman" gradually faded into the background of the public's memory and the new Mental Health Act of 1973 seemed to reflect the new deinstitutionalized approach of psychiatry. Nevertheless, the problem of how to deal with black patients persisted. During the 1960s, the Nationalist government had transformed its apartheid policies to include the creation of "self-governing" homelands. The underlying principle of these homelands was, as Robert Ross suggests, a "denial of any share in a common South African nationality for those who were not white. Rather, they were thought to belong to one of the following groups: Xhosa, Zulu, Swazi, Tsongo, Ndebele, Venda, North Sotho, South Sotho, Tswana, Indian and Coloured."[93] The change of direction by the apartheid government has mostly been attributed to the after-effects of the Sharpeville shooting of 1960—an anti-pass protest within Sharpeville township where police opened fire and killed sixty-nine people and injured one hundred and eighty. In the wake of this atrocity, large protests broke out throughout South Africa and overseas newspapers began to take an interest in the events within South Africa. In an attempt to control social unrest and placate international criticism (and the subsequent decline of international investment), the apartheid government adopted its grand apartheid strategy by redefining its notion of "separate development" to one that included "a new ideological discourse of 'multi-nationalism' and 'ethnic self-determination'."[94] Under the guise of protecting "ethnicity," the Department of Bantu Administration and Development began huge relocation projects of non-white individuals into their respective homelands. The homeland system was anything but independent. Rather, the majority of the homelands remained financially dependent on and administratively restrained by the apartheid government.[95] For this reason, little development occurred within them, and the terrible conditions and atrocities that had brought attention to the inequalities within South Africa continued.

The intellectual basis of cross-cultural psychiatry played an important role, albeit mostly inadvertently, in implementing the government's strategy to increase self-government in the homelands in the late 1960s and early 1970s. Cross-cultural psychiatry, like community psychiatry, was ambiguous and contradictory. On the one hand, it recognized the need for effective treatment of black patients through better understanding of the cultural idioms in which they lived their lives. It also acknowledged the socio-political impact of apartheid on individuals. However, like community psychiatry, it authenticated apartheid practices by endorsing stagnant ideas of "cultural" and "ethnic" difference. Although advocates of cross-cultural psychiatry may have wanted to help Africans to rehabilitate to their indigenous cultures, government officials often used their views to promote the ethnic identifications that were central to the homeland strategy of grand apartheid. The idea that each African "ethnic group" had unique needs, could easily be translated into the view that Africans needed to be divided and treated accordingly. This was a view that supported the National Party's policies in the 1970s that forced homeland citizenship on blacks along ethnic lines, and its imposition in the 1980s of a tricameral parliamentary system for whites, coloureds, and Indians.[96]

From the late 1960s to the 1980s, the apartheid government explicitly adopted the discourse of community and cross-cultural psychiatry to promote its separate health strategies for non-whites. For blacks, the National Party's plan was to move responsibility for their mental health, and, of health in general, away from state run institutions, which also housed white patients, to the few homeland hospitals. This strategy began in 1961 after South Africa became a republic and an interdepartmental committee was set up to investigate the possibility of constructing institutions in the homelands for black patients so that beds for white patients in existing institutions could be freed. The result was the construction of the Bophelong Hospital in Boputhutswana in circa 1966 and Madadeni Hospital in KwaZulu in circa 1967 that crowded 2,708 black patients in total in their wards. It also contracted out long-term care to a private company, Smith Mitchell & Co., as a means to deal with overcrowding (see Chapter 6), and it relied on general hospitals to temporarily care for psychiatric patients. In 1971, when the Bantu Homelands Constitution Act enabled the apartheid government to begin granting quasi-"independence" to the homelands, there were eight hospitals that dealt with psychiatric patients, three of which were run by Smith Mitchell.[97] The rest were under the administration of the Department of Bantu Administration and Development, Provincial Authorities and the Department of Health (DOH). Missionary clinics also offered minimal psychiatric services, although these were gradually taken over by the government in the 1970s when it became concerned with enforcing ethnic divisions.[98] In 1971, the government explained its objectives of initiating indirect rule over the mental health facilities, as set out in the following diagram:

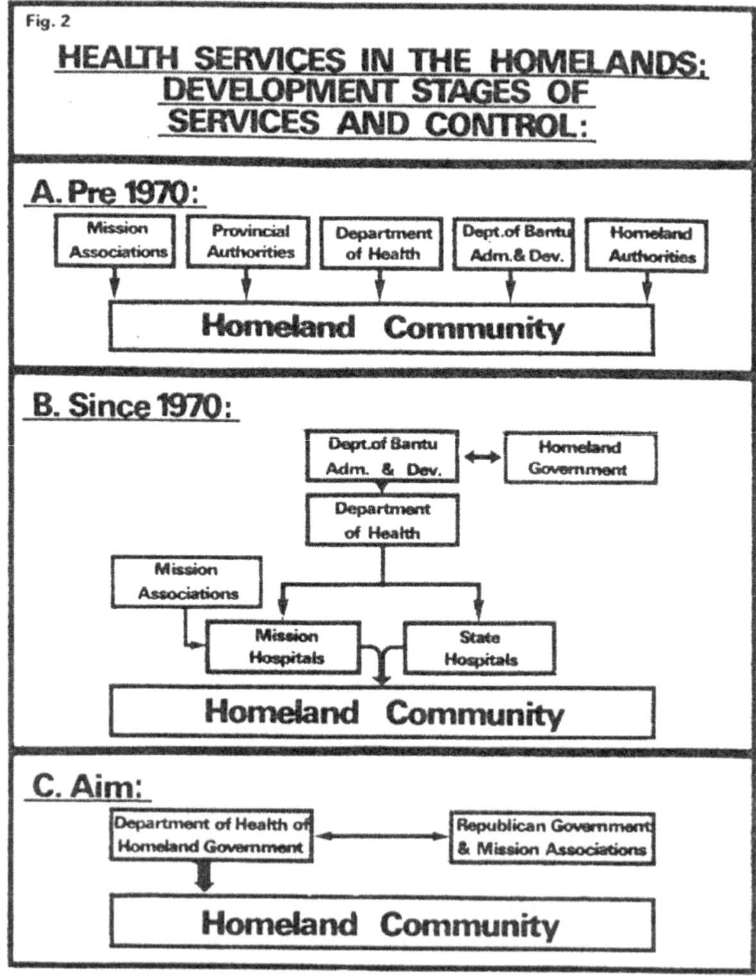

Figure 4.2 Organization of Health Services for Homeland Communities, pre-1970, since 1970, and aim, 1974. Reprinted from "Psychiatry," Bantu 21, no. 7 (July 1974), 7.

The government stated that it ultimately wanted to move the responsibility of mental health care away from itself to the homeland government, which, it argued, would implement more "appropriate" care for its population.

The South African government, instituting the language of community and cross-cultural psychiatry, suggested that mental health at first could be overseen by smaller satellite clinics administered by a central hospital in the homelands, and then ultimately could be operated on their own. These clinics would utilize black psychiatrists and staff, community members, and healers. The government's propaganda newspaper *Bantu*, which discussed issues facing Africans in the homeland system, but realistically wrote about a desired and idealized version of life during apartheid, heralded the importance of community and cross-cultural programs in the homelands:

> A good example of a homeland hospital which offers psychiatric services is the one at Groothoek . . . Here the obsolete system of isolation, by which they were more or less cut off from the community, while male and female patients were strictly segregated has been done away with. At present the organisation is modelled on the lines of the traditional way of life of the group concerned.[99]

A picture was published alongside the text meant to depict Africans partaking in "cultural activities such as traditional singing and dancing" which were to "resocialise" them back to their "traditional" culture. The underlying premise of activities such as these was that estrangement from "traditional" culture caused mental disorders in Africans in the first place.[100] Reflective of some practitioners' arguments that modernization for the African was a mentally disturbing factor, government officials argued that:

> Psychiatric problems in the Bantu homelands present a picture which often reflects the complex and difficult adaptation problems which beset a developing society when faced with the tremendous demands with which the modern technological era confronts the individual, the family and the community.[101]

The mental health of blacks therefore included removing individuals from the stressors of modern, urban life and "rehabilitating" them, that is, restoring them to their assumed original condition. In 1975, the government issued a proclamation on Rehabilitation Institutions in the Bantu Homelands that clearly set out its cultural-specific intentions. The stated purpose for these institutions was to improve individuals' "physical, mental and moral condition" by "training them in habits of industry and work" and "re-orientating them to the traditions, culture, custom and system of government of the national unit to which they belong."[102]

However, in 1982, H. C. J. van Rensburg and A. Mans showed how after the apartheid government took over control over the health services in the homelands, health care conditions were grossly inadequate.[103] Solome Malebele, a psychiatric nurse, describes the poor conditions in which she had work within a homeland psychiatric ward:

> There is no multidisciplinary team for mental health care. At Tintswalo we have no psychiatrist, no psychologist, a social worker who is overloaded and can only spend a part of her time with psychiatric patients, no minister of religion, insufficient people with therapeutic skills to deal with rehabilitation and not enough nursing staff.[104]

Homeland structures also made it extremely difficult for staff to do any follow-up community services. Because of the fragmented nature of the system, if a patient was treated in the Gazankulu homeland, for example, and thereafter crossed into Lebowa, staff could no longer offer them any more community services.[105] In 1983/1984, the total health budget for the four white-run provinces was over R1,747 ($1,215) million. The combined health budget, including pension funds, for all the homelands was only approximately R542 ($377) million.[106] As Sean O' Donoghue has pointed out, some of the hospitals and community clinics for blacks, although built, stood unused because of lack of operating funds. The Lenasia South Provincial Hospital finished in 1987 and the Mofolo South Clinic were simply abandoned.[107] Because of the chronic underfunding of psychiatry, the unequal division of budgets between the white provinces and the homelands was even worse than in the general health budget. Indeed, in 1988, ninety-three percent of the Mental Health budget remained allocated to institutions, while only seven percent was designated to community care, including preventative programs.[108] That same year, approximately forty-five percent of all patients were re-admissions, an indication of the failure of community programs in general.[109]

The apartheid government expected similar cultural-specific programs to be set up for coloured and Indian patients. Although most coloured and Indian patients remained in separate wards attached to the white hospitals throughout the 1970s and 1980s and few community psychiatric programs were ever implemented, the government did, as for blacks, promote separate administrations. Instead of setting up separate homelands for coloureds, the government's scheme was to create self-government for them in their own group areas. Mostly these were urban group areas, with a few living in rural, mainly mission settlements. In 1951, it passed the Separate Representation of Voters Bill. This meant that coloureds were placed on a separate voter's roll than whites and had a specific coloured governing body that represented coloured interests. Although rumors circulated that coloureds would be allowed equal representation in the white-dominated parliament, in 1961 Verwoerd negated this view by stating: "this would be a springboard for the integration of the races, leading to biological assimilation." The government would rather, he argued, focus on "parallel development."[110]

This meant that although the central DOH was still responsible for administering the care of coloureds and Indians, the government's aim was to have them treated in separate locations from whites, preferably in their own communities and by members of their own racial group. In 1984, President P. W. Botha initiated a tricameral parliamentary system whereby there was a Head of State, a white House of Assembly, a coloured House of Representatives, and an Indian House of Delegates.[111] This system was a means by which the government thought it could ensure that coloureds and Indians would oversee their own services and attempt to become allies with them against blacks. In the case of mental health, representatives from each group were expected to hold positions throughout the country in their corresponding areas and present their findings to the central DOH on a regular basis. This scheme was a late development in the original plan and only served to enrage blacks further, while coloureds and Indians rejected the move as the farce that it was.

Whereas the government argued that it was streamlining the administration of mental health, and creating more deinstitutionalized, culturally sensitive services, in reality, it created extensive duplication of departments, perpetuated divisions along makeshift ethnic lines and ultimately reinforced institutionalization. Services became increasingly fragmented.[112] No longer was there to be just one Department of Health, but fourteen; one central administrative department that also oversaw white care, one for coloureds, one for Indians and eleven for each of the eleven bantustans set up by the 1951 Bantu Authorities Act. Each department competed for the limited pool of staff and resources and the duplication of administration caused chaos in an already confused sector.[113] As Cliff Allwood points out, until 1984, staff working together were administered by one department. However, with the implementation of the tricameral parliamentary system, Indian staff were administered by the House of Delegates, coloureds were the domain of the House of Representatives, white staff were under the control of the DOH, and black staff were managed by the regional director of black affairs. It made it extremely difficult to implement changes in the care of patients and severely jeopardized community psychiatric programs. Clinics that had previously offered services to all races within a particular area were now expected to be divided, with very little financial support to do so. Whereas the majority of practitioners did not support the split of services, they were still reliant on funding from the government to continue these services.[114]

Moreover, those Indian and coloured representatives who were supposed to represent patients' interest were often marginalized in the decision-making process. Ashwin Valjee, who was a DOH representative for the Indian population between 1978 and 1981, describes the disinterest of the government about Indian requirements:

> I told the representative government at that meeting that I was wasting my time there, because every time I went there and told them what our

> needs were, they would say: "Have some tea and coffee," you know that kind of a thing. And I got a bit tired of that. And then a gentleman called Dr. P. H. Henning [Commissioner for Mental Health] . . . stood up in front of fifty or so people there and told me that he was sick and tired of my complaining about the various needs of the people in this area, the Kwazulu-Natal area . . . So when he finished his tirade of words, he was angry with me, I got up and told him: "Look, every time I come here, and tell you that statistics show that the highest cause of death in young Indian girls females was suicide. The number one killer of young Indian girls in the whole of South Africa was suicide, so we need more facilities for them, and I keep telling you this, and you keep ignoring it. So what's the value of me coming here, and giving you this information every three months?" . . . I tended my resignation, and told them that they would have to answer one day to a higher power than us in the country.[115]

Despite the government's arguments that posts were reserved for non-white practitioners, as there were few trained black, Indian, and coloured practitioners to fill these positions, the government ensured that it retained control. Even when an appropriate individual may have existed, the central government tended to allocate most posts to white practitioners. George Hart explains:

> There was this problem, which led to a great deal of difficulty because the white Department of Health at the time of the tricameral system had some hawks who stole all the posts which meant that there were no posts for any other groups of the tricameral system. All the people, not all the posts, were around the country, but mostly in this area and were very close to Pretoria, so Johannesburg and Pretoria were very much involved in this takeover. And hence it was that the white department paid most of the salaries to the psychiatrists because they pinched all the posts.[116]

Because of the discriminatory nature of the education system, few black, coloured or Indian psychiatrists were graduating from universities. In 1976, the government legislated that white universities could no longer admit non-white medical students. The University of Natal, which had since 1951 accepted black students into its medical program, was prohibited from doing so. This restriction would eventually be extended to include coloured and Indian students.[117] All non-white students were expected to enroll in the new Medical University of South Africa (MEDUNSA) in Pretoria, which was seriously underfunded. Those graduating from MEDUNSA were expected to work within their respective communities.[118] In 1979, there was one registered coloured, one registered Indian psychiatrist, and six Indian psychiatrists in training.[119] In 1981, there was only one black psychiatrist practicing in South Africa. The lack of sufficient psychiatric staff, along with the duplication and expense of services was causing havoc on an already overburdened system. Even less money and resources were allocated to non-white care, and with the poor administration, inadequate nursing staff, and poor treatment, the crisis in state institutions worsened.

By the mid-1980s, the homeland structure set out by the government was collapsing and the tricameral system simply was not dealing with coloured and Indian demands. Mental health services remained in crisis, and while the government was espousing notions of community and cross-cultural psychiatry in its propaganda, throughout the 1970s, it was failing to provide any effective state run services in the homelands.

5 Controlling and Challenging Sexuality

Psychiatric Struggles over Homosexuality in the 1960s–1980s

In 1973, Tom Sharpe published his satirical and comic novel, *Indecent Exposure,* which commented on the views of police about South Africa's Immorality Act, i.e., the act that controlled the sexual behavior of its population. The novel tells the story of Kommandant van Heerden, who, believing that black women were being used by South Africa's enemies to seduce his officers from their duty, decides to subject his men to a form of aversion therapy. Showing them pictures of naked black women and administering electric shocks to their genitals, he attempts to condition his men to avoid all contact with black women. However, in an unexpected twist, the therapy ends up making his officers gay.[1] Whereas Sharpe's novel is a humorous and outrageous satire of South African society, it is not that far from reality. Sharpe, who had worked as a social worker and teacher in South Africa in the 1950s, based his novels on his personal experiences, and aversion therapy was a treatment that some practitioners made use of to "retrain" white minds. Sharpe's novel is meant to highlight the ludicrousness of the fear that pervaded state official's thoughts, particularly of a black uprising, but it also highlighted the hypermasculine and homophobic nature of the society.

The issue of homosexuality came to the fore of the South African government's consciousness in the 1960s and 1970s. One of the key objectives resulting from Verwoerd's assassination and the subsequent commissions of inquiry was the government's continued focus on preserving the superiority of the white, particularly white Afrikaner male, against a foreign onslaught. When it came to discussions about sexuality, however, the ways in which the government and some practitioners attempted to preserve this purity took a perverse turn. In the 1970s, psychiatrists in the South African Defence Force (SADF) Military Hospital partook in human rights abuses by utilizing aversion therapy, hormone therapy, sex change operations, and barbiturates on young white homosexual men as a means to "cure" them from their homosexual "disease." While gay rights movements were gaining momentum worldwide, the South African government, in its homophobia, became increasingly vigilant at cracking down on any "homosexual" activities within its borders. As Glen Elder has pointed out, "discourses of sexuality in South Africa were central to the creation, support and final collapse of the apartheid state."[2] Heteropatriarchal views of sexuality supported white male power structures, promoted binary ideas of masculinity and femininity, normalized heterosexuality, and determined social roles by biological sex.[3] The state's control over the sexual activities of its population was more than just about controlling sexuality, it sought to limit the practice of inter-racial sexual intercourse and to retain white political dominance. Ideas about homosexuality threatened the Christian-nationalist procreative ideals of the apartheid government and it increased fears about the perceived moral degeneration of society. In the words of Glen Retief, the state had "the need to keep the white nation sexually and morally pure so that it had the strength to resist the black communist onslaught."[4] Psychiatric practitioners indeed played a part in supporting this objective.

Certainly in South Africa abusive psychiatric practices towards sexual "deviants" were not limited to the military. Psychiatric practitioners played their part in enforcing the heteropatriarchal structure of apartheid. Yet worldwide concepts of sexuality and gender, as well as ideas of mental illness, have always been based on changing ideas of social norms, and are thus often vaguely and confusingly defined by those attempting to understand them at a particular time. Notions of gender, sex, madness, and sexuality were often unclear and confused.[5] In South Africa, this was particularly evident in 1968 when a select government committee, initiated by the Minister of Justice P. C. Pelser and led by S. Frank, was convened to investigate the feasibility of amending the Immorality Amendment Act of 1957[6] so as to better define homosexual acts and to legislate the behavior of individuals.[7] Interestingly, while the Afrikaans newspaper, *Die Burger,* had published an article a few months earlier about homosexuality, there was little public response. It was only when the committee was established that the public reacted. Before the investigation, it seemed that homosexuality was not a primary concern for most Afrikaans-speaking South Africans, and it was the police and the Department of Justice, not the public, that brought the issue to the forefront. The Department of Justice, fearing an imagined spread of homosexual activity, and failing to fully understand the causes and manifestations of homosexuality, asked the committee to determine the best course of dealing with these "deviants." The committee turned to psychiatric practitioners for answers.

As we have seen in the previous chapters, psychiatrists' views, however, were not always clear-cut. Practitioners did not always have the definitive answers that the Department of Justice was looking for. Nor did the majority of them simply go along with the state's mandate. Indeed, the testimony and writings of practitioners of the 1960s reveal a much more complex scenario than suggested by the depiction of events that took place in the SADF in the 1970s. Their views about homosexuality, while often adhering to state ideals, at other times directly opposed them. Moreover, practitioners and psychiatrists were divided and irresolute about the origins, manifestations and treatment of homosexuality. The complex and at times noncompliant views of practitioners have yet to be acknowledged. Indeed, while many practitioners did support heteropatriarchal ideals of sexuality and normality, practitioners held disparate ideas about the etiology and treatment of homosexuality that sometimes, but not always, supported the Nationalist government's objectives.

RAIDING THE CLOSET: LEGISLATIVE ATTEMPTS AT DEFINING AND CRIMINALIZING HOMOSEXUALITY IN THE 1960S

Homosexuality in South Africa, as elsewhere in the world, had since the beginning of the colonial period been associated with criminal activity, and laws governing sodomy and "unnatural acts" had regulated "deviant" sexual behavior.[8] Legal and social ideas of homosexuality in South Africa were framed within male/female, heterosexual/homosexual, normal/abnormal, social/anti-social and lawful/criminal dichotomies. According to the Department of Justice and police authorities of the apartheid state, homosexual practices were psychological deviations that inevitably led to criminal and anti-social behavior such as rape, incest, pedophilia, bestiality, inter-racial sex, prostitution, murder, suicide, theft, public indecency, blackmail, the spread of venereal diseases, alcoholism, and exhibitionism.[9] Even traffic violations could be blamed on homosexual practices because it was suggested that homosexual hitchhiking men making advances towards innocent heterosexual drivers could cause traffic accidents.

In the 1960s, rising fears among police and government officials about an increase in public displays of homosexuality led to debate about its origins. These fears coincided with the relaxation of legislation on homosexual activity worldwide. For example, in 1957, the Wolfendon Committee in England recommended that homosexuality between men older than twenty-one years of age be decriminalized. In the United States between 1961 and 1962, the state of Illinois abandoned its sodomy laws and suggested that private sexual practices among adults were no longer legal matters of the state. A few states gradually followed suit. In 1966 legal officials in Germany argued that homosexuality among consenting adults should be legalized. Three years later Germany changed its laws so that consensual homosexual acts between men over the age of twenty-one were permitted. Shortly thereafter the minimum age changed to eighteen.[10]

Although gay rights were still far from protected in these countries, South African government and police officials were concerned that this worldwide trend of decriminalization would enable homosexual behavior to become widely accepted in South Africa. Indeed, in 1966, police raided a Johannesburg party, where approximately 300 white men were in attendance and reportedly partaking in "homosexual activities." This event prompted the police to begin discussing their concerns about the increase of homosexuality with the Department of Justice.[11] Professing to believe that homosexuality was a mental disorder that could spread to innocent white heterosexual men and women, many police and government officials wished to prohibit all homosexual activities through regulation.[12] They argued that sodomy laws, which in any event were rarely enforced, failed to allow them to investigate private sexual acts or acts that did not result in sexual penetration of a penis. These acts included the use of sexual devices, lesbianism, kissing, dancing, holding hands in public and any other sexual activity seen as abhorrent. They therefore asked that legislation be revised so that individuals who partook in any homosexual act could be convicted.

When the government's select committee commenced its inquiry into homosexuality in 1968, police testimony and submissions were somewhat confused and at times even ludicrous. To the police, homosexuals included hermaphrodites, pedophiles, bisexuals, transgendered individuals, cross dressers, or any other persons with sexual or lifestyle distinctions that varied from the heterosexual norm. In particular, police stressed the foreign, specifically English, origins of the behavior. When asked by the committee as to how he could identify a homosexual male, the representative for the South African police, Major F. A. J. van Zyl, for example, stated:

> Most people regard them as being effeminate, which most of them are not. Some of them are body-builders, and some are soccer players of repute, but they evade bodily conflict in groups. You will never find any of them playing rugby, for instance. He will be a body-builder or a fencer, or he will play squash, but when he speaks to a woman you know immediately. From his general demeanour it is very simple for me to identify them.[13]

Van Zyl's testimony is striking as he did not simply cite stereotypical notions of homosexual men as effeminate but chose rather to equate homosexuals with the type of sport they played. It is evident that his understanding of homosexuality was based on a white male heterosexual ideal. Moreover, the suggestion that homosexuals would be body-builders, soccer players, fencers, or play squash, but never rugby, the sport so closely associated with Afrikaner nationalism, reveals his perception that homosexuality was not intrinsic to Afrikaner society. Indeed, the sports that he suggested that homosexuals played are those that were associated with English-speaking South Africans. Because England a few years earlier had decriminalized homosexuality, this correlation is not surprising, and van Zyl's statements highlight the common perception among police and government offices that homosexuality was a foreign practice. Indeed, in earlier testimony, Van Zyl suggested that homosexual activities during World War II were introduced to South Africa by foreign homosexual soldiers arriving at the port of Durban. He added that immigrants, who "come mainly from countries where homosexuality is rife," brought with them pornographic material.[14] In this sense, he conceptualized homosexuality as an alien threat to the Afrikaner domain of masculinity.

What is noticeably lacking in the discussions of the committee is reference to African, coloured or Indian homosexual practices. If homosexuality originated abroad, what influence, if any, did it have on black men and women? Discussions about black homosexual activity in the 1960s and 1970s were generally rare among apartheid planners, except when such a discussion included interracial acts between blacks and whites.[15] Economic incentives may have played a role in the failure of the select committee and practitioners in general to discuss homosexuality among black men and women, particularly the absence of views on what were often wrongly perceived as homosexual activities among black men living in compounds in the gold mines. As T. Dunbar Moodie points out, mine managers often turned a blind eye to homosexual acts among black workers. In some cases, these acts were encouraged so that black sexuality could be contained within the walls of the compounds and managers could in turn retain control over their workers.[16] It is possible that the committee was instructed or felt it best not to deal with these issues as it would interfere with the mining companies' mandates.

But the government's concentration on white sexuality during apartheid was not limited to discussions about homosexuality. As Meaghan Campbell has shown, other illegal sexual activities during apartheid, such as the rape of black women in townships, were largely ignored by the state and public. It was only when it affected white society directly that the government and the white public took notice. She suggests that because the government was more concerned with the encroachment of Africans on white urban spaces, concerns regarding interracial activities outweighed any intraracial conduct. Even in the 1970s only the most scandalous activities were noted and then only in the context of the increase in township crime and African population growth.[17]

There is another absence in much of the testimony to the committee, namely, homosexual women. Whereas the committee's mandate did include a brief discussion of lesbianism—a first in South Africa's history—the discussion remained limited and almost an afterthought. Any mention of women's sexuality was couched within ideals about reproduction and procreation. Lesbian behavior threatened male dominance and the procreative ideals of the National Party, and any form of social pleasure derived from sexual interactions was seen as deviant and sinful. In the midst of discussion about homosexuality, one of the committee members asked J. A. Grobler, the Deputy Secretary of the Department of Social Welfare and Pensions: "Do you think girls in puberty should be supplied with the pill?" Such a question in the midst of an inquiry into homosexuality reveals the committee's perception that their investigation was more than just a question of homosexuality, but entailed all concepts of sexual "deviance." Grobler's response, reiterated the view that conceptions of sexual deviance were seen as foreign or alien forces from which South Africa needed to be protected:

> Well you get people who are liberal, like the Swedes, who think it must be done; but they are quite liberal. The point I want to stress is that we South Africans—thank God for it—are still conservative in many ways. We should not be influenced by the attitude of other countries on homosexuality. We have our own way of life, we have our own convictions, and I think we should lay down our policy according to our way of life.[18]

In general, having sex for pleasure, rather than reproduction, was a foreign threat against the ideals of the government. The failure of men and women who did not sexually reproduce endangered white domination, especially in light of the government's pronatalist initiatives.[19] The committee's discussions revealed another obscure fear, i.e., the importation and use of dildos. If women could have sexual relations without men, sometimes using *imported* instruments that were much *bigger* than the average male penis, then what did that say about the overall gender roles, and in turn, the sexual roles, of women and men? Nevertheless, for the most part, the discussions (and the absence of discussion) among committee members thus reflected the main concerns of the state, that is, regulating and maintaining white heteropatriarchal power and purity.

PRACTITIONERS' REPRESENTATIONS AND TREATMENT OF HOMOSEXUALITY

What is apparent in the previous discussion was that police and government officials were attempting to define homosexuality within specific gender and racial structures that fit within the confines of apartheid policy. Yet, as we have seen so far, apartheid policies themselves were ill-defined and had no set monolithic plan. Rather, definitions changed, borders moved, and ideas became increasingly layered. Although there was a desire to explicitly define homosexual acts, because of the contradictory nature of apartheid, ideas of homosexuality in South Africa were similarly ambiguous and fluid. Nevertheless, in its quest for definitive answers, the Department of Justice turned to mental health practitioners whom it hoped would provide the means of defining and "treating" such individuals. Three medical doctors were appointed as members of the committee: E. L. Fisher, a psychiatrist and a United Party Member of Parliament (MP) for Rosettenville, W. L. D. M. Venter, National Party MP for Kimberley South, and A. Radford, MP for Durban-Central. Although Fisher was the only accredited psychiatrist, Venter and Radford also worked with psychiatric patients. Because of the limited number of psychiatrists in South Africa, it was not uncommon for general medical practitioners to be appointed in psychiatric institutions or focus their work on psychiatric health. Venter and Radford had been strong critics of government policy with regard to mental institutions and had continually advocated for more beds for white men.

Debates, however, ironically existed among practitioners as to how to prevent and "cure" homosexuality. Their discussions reveal a complex interplay between two understandings of the etiology of homosexuality: one suggesting that homosexuality was a biologically inherent affliction, and a second purporting that homosexuality was brought on by social and environmental factors. Debates as to the "cause" of homosexuality continue today. The notion of homosexuality as having a biological etiology has, however, begun to be increasingly accepted in recent years.[20] In the 1960s, South African practitioners were certainly investigating biomedical reasons for homosexuality. Upon admission to a mental hospital, patients were usually put through thorough physical examinations. Blood count and protein analyses, plasma and electrolytes tests, radiological examinations of the skull and chest, bone-age estimations, urine analysis, and examinations of genitalia were conducted. In most cases, however, practitioners found little to support physical explanations. Thus, when practitioners came to define the etiology of homosexuality, psycho-sociological explanations, couched in ideas of biological difference, tended to dominate.[21]

One of the earliest and most outspoken practitioners promoting a psycho-sociological approach to homosexuality was Louis F. Freed, who had an almost zealous interest in deviant behavior within the white population. In 1954, Freed, writing one of the first articles dedicated entirely to homosexuality for the *South African Medical Journal,* stated that "homosexuality, along with alcoholism, crime, insanity, illegitimacy, homicide, suicide, infanticide, prostitution, divorce, etc., must be regarded as one of the indices of social disorganization." Homosexuality, he argued, was "largely a sociological problem."[22] Therefore, in order to effectively treat it, medical, judicial, and social welfare agencies needed to pay more attention to "ameliorating the evil human environment in which affected individuals have been projected, and from which they have to escape by the process of regressional sex behavior, be it homosexualism or any other form of sexual perversion."[23] Freed's arguments reveal his belief that it was a poor, perhaps even unchristian, upbringing that was at the root of homosexual behavior. Six years earlier, he had conducted an investigation in to white prostitution. He argued that because prostitutes came from the poorest part of society, and homosexual prostitutes came from the poorest of the poor, it was necessary to address this poverty. Katie Moodie has also demonstrated in her study of the 1950s sub-cultural masculinities in the form of "ducktail" gang members that Freed also showed increasing concern with the behavior of these "deviants." Freed's standpoint on homosexuality was indicative of his general interest in the total degeneration of white social values.[24]

Other practitioners speculated that sexual deviance was caused by "adverse childhood conditions . . . such as parental rejection of the child because of its unwanted sex,"[25] absentee fathers, overbearing mothers,[26] "abnormal environmental circumstances"[27] or a traumatic event of some sort during childhood. These ideas were founded on Freudian notions of sexuality that suggested that one's sexual identity was determined by one's childhood. It also suggested that homosexuality was a normal stage of sexual development through which all children progressed, but out of which they ultimately emerged. Thus, according to psychoanalysts, homosexuals over the age of twenty-one were individuals who were less psychologically "developed" than their heterosexual counterparts, and had either not yet emerged from this stage of homosexual experimentation stage, or would fail to do so on their own. Whereas South African practitioners for the most part steered clear of Freudian psychoanalysis in the treatment of other mental disorders, when it came to homosexuality, there were few alternatives.

These ideas of lesser psychological development substantiated apartheid ideologies, which, in an effort to ensure white (Afrikaner) supremacy, drew strongly from Christian-nationalism and social evolutionism.[28] They also further explain the lack of acknowledgement of any African homosexual practices among state officials and practitioners. Psychoanalysis itself was steeped in racialized ideals. As Sander Gilman has shown in his analysis of the treatment of Jews at the beginning of the twentieth century, because Jews were seen as less evolved than the white race, and more likely to experience mental difficulties once exposed to "modern life," homosexuality, which was seen to be brought about by trauma, was thought to be prominent. Thus, the "assumption of sexologists . . . was that the Jews, too, were fixated at an earlier stage of sexual development."[29] Similar arguments can be applied to debates about African sexuality. If Africans were inherently or culturally less "sexually developed," their predilection for homosexuality was more "natural" than that for white men, and in turn, concern about its occurrence or spread was not as necessary as for whites. In 1943, John F. Ritchie argued that male Africans who tended to suckle at their mother's breast for too long never resolved their Oedipal complex and in turn made them unable "to investigate the later interests" of heterosexuality.[30] Twenty years later, Alexander Don, a neuropsychiatrist at Tara Hospital, argued that "cultural factors play an important role in the extent to which this condition [transvestism] comes within the surveillance of the physician." Using the anthropologist Margaret Mead as evidence, he argued that many indigenous peoples embraced the idea of transvestism, while in Western culture such examples were supposedly rare.[31] Similarly, in 1968, when asked by the Select Committee if homosexuality occurred in African societies, Stephanus P. Cilliers, Professor of Sociology at the University of Stellenbosch, answered briefly: "Ethnographical material suggests that homosexualism occurs in most African societies."[32]

These arguments were not shared by all practitioners, however. In 1937, B. J. B. Laubscher, a psychiatrist who worked for the Juvenile, Criminal, and Supreme courts, published the results of a brief survey of sexual offences among magistrates in rural areas. His work was highly regarded among practitioners for many years thereafter. He specifically asked questions regarding homosexuality, transvestism, cross-dressing, rape, sodomy, and pedophilia. His findings suggested that homosexual acts, transvestism, and pedophilia were extremely rare among individuals living in the reserves, while bestiality did occur more frequently. Where transgressions did occur, he argued that it was caused by "some insecure and immature individuals, as well as those suffering from brain changes involving impairment of judgement and self-control."[33] Thus, homosexuality was not "natural" to Africans, as suggested by other practitioners. Almost thirty years later, in 1965, the Commissioner for Mental Health, Alistair Lamont, presented a paper at the forty-fifth South African Medical Congress that cross-listed diagnosis, race, and crime of State Decision patients, i.e., patients held under State President warrants, usually for criminal charges. Echoing the sentiments of Laubscher, Lamont argued that sexual crimes were most commonly associated with defective mental development, a diagnosis mostly applied to white patients, while murder was more associated with schizophrenia, a diagnosis predominantly applied to black patients.[34] What Laubscher and Lamont were suggesting was that sexual deviance was the monopoly of the white population, and Africans, while predisposed to more serious crimes, rarely partook in homosexual activities.

Because many psychiatrists based their ideas of African sexuality on ethnological studies, and indeed some practitioners such as Laubscher saw themselves as ethnopsychiatrists, this debate as to whether homosexual practices existed in Africans is not surprising, for as Marc Epprecht has pointed out, the portrayal of African homosexuality by anthropologists and social scientists from the late eighteenth century on was multifarious and often contradictory. Some dismissed or interpreted same-sex relations among Africans in such a way as to help them define a dialectic between traditional/African/heterosexual/uncivilized and modern/European/homosexual/civilized, while others acknowledged homosexuality in African culture, but often presented it as "primitive" and "natural."[35]

Because no consensus existed about the prevalence or etiology of homosexuality, treatment was correspondingly varied. Aubrey Levin, who would eventually head up the SADF's aversion therapy program in the 1970s and 1980s, actively used aversion therapy.[36] Other practitioners, such as Don, also used aversion therapy in their practice.[37] Aversion therapy could take the form of inducing vomiting or shocking individuals while they looked at naked pictures of men. Don performed sex change operations as well, but only for cases that he deemed necessary.[38] Hormonal treatment was also popular among some practitioners. G. P. Fourie, a gynecologist and obstetrician, in testimony to the 1968 select committee, argued that he "had miraculous successes with hormonal treatment in all cases where hormones are important."[39] Psychoanalysis, however, became the main choice among practitioners to treat their patients.[40]

Because homosexuality was predominately seen as a white problem that needed to be addressed, and most practitioners believed that it had to be dealt with at the psychosociological level, it is not surprising that in 1968, when the government initiated the inquiry into homosexuality, that practitioners were opposed to its criminalization. The main representative body of psychiatrists, the Society of Psychiatrists and Neurologists of South Africa (SPNSA) played a particularly prominent role in opposing the legislation. The SPNSA was officially established in 1966 when neurologists left the Society of Neurologists, Psychiatrists and Neurosurgeons, a body established in the early 1950s as a sub-group of the Medical Association of South Africa (MASA). The society was eventually renamed the Society of Psychiatrists of South Africa (SPSA).[41] Whereas the MASA had a membership of over 10,000 doctors, the SPNSA's membership averaged from only one hundred to 150 psychiatrists, about half of whom worked in the private sector.

The SPNSA argued that homosexuality was a mental disease, not a criminal activity and it campaigned against what it perceived as harsh policies towards mentally ill individuals. It was concerned that the imprisonment of white homosexuals would set a precedent for the imprisonment of other white mentally ill individuals and that consenting adults would be unfairly imprisoned. Representatives thus testified against the proposed legislation. Not having a definitive stance on whether homosexuality was caused by genetics or social circumstances, the SPNSA argued that homosexuality should not be criminalized. From a biological standpoint, they argued that it was impossible to change the genetic makeup of homosexuals and that it was therefore of no use to attempt to punish them for behavior that was essentially non-violent and unalterable. They contended that because homosexual experimentation was a normal stage of sexual development through which all children progressed, the law would ultimately require all young (white) boys to be imprisoned. Independent of the SPNSA testimony, individual practitioners also argued against criminalization. Freed published an article in the *South African Medical Journal* arguing that criminalization would do little to alleviate what he saw as the main cause of homosexuality, namely, poverty, and improper socialization.[42] Even Levin argued that criminalization would not be an effective course of action.[43]

When asked about alternatives to imprisonment, the SPNSA argued that practitioners could essentially prevent homosexuality "through a system of public education [that would] help people to bring up their children with sound attitudes towards sexual behaviour." This, they suggested, would be "far better than any immorality legislation."[44] But they were less clear about whether or not they could cure homosexuality. The SPNSA officially rejected the validity of aversion and hormone therapies. Yet they also admitted that some of their members believed they could effectively cure individuals of homosexuality through such treatments.[45] The SPNSA argued that it was more important to offer some psychological assistance to homosexuals to enable them to adapt or contain their sexual impulses, and if young enough, help them live "normal" heterosexual lives.[46] Whereas psychoanalysis in the 1960s was problematic in that it was based on a heterosexual norm, and, as Barbara Tholfsen points out, it emphasized binary and rigid stereotypes of men and women, its practice was at least physically less harmful.[47]

In large part due to the SPNSA's testimony, the legislation that ensued, although not fully in accordance with the association's stance, was less severe than initially proposed by police and government officials. Whereas homosexual activities between men at parties were banned and the legal age for consent of homosexual acts was raised from sixteen to nineteen, private homosexual activities between consenting adults remained the domain of psychiatrists.[48] It must be noted that the relaxation of policies was also partly due to pressures by anti-criminalization gay rights activists who ensured that witnesses made representations against the proposed legislation.[49] Nevertheless, most practitioners played a central part in shaping the outcome of the investigation and they did hold more unautocratic views towards homosexuality than their police and military counterparts.

THE SADF AND SHOCKING ACTIONS AGAINST HOMOSEXUALITY IN THE 1970S

Despite the SPNSA's interception in government sanctioning of homosexuality in the public domain at least, in the 1970s and 1980s, the government managed to pursue its interests in controlling white male homosexuality. After 1967, most white males were conscripted into the SADF as soon as they graduated from high school. Thus, the military served as a convenient means for the government to ensure the reproductive purity of the white race and the preservation of their Christian nationalist morality, particularly control over sexual behavior. A few practitioners actively partook in the abuses that were to take place in the military hospitals.

Ironically, while community psychiatry originated in the wake of the First and Second World Wars, the internal resistance struggles and border wars in southern Africa now facilitated a new round of abuses of white men in military hospitals, albeit under the guise of "treatment." Stories of sexual control in the military had always existed, but with threats of homosexuality seemingly on the rise, young men were caught up in a frighteningly coercive system. Militaries worldwide were renowned for being intolerant of homosexuality and most western countries disallowed individuals who engaged in homosexual activities to serve in their armies. South Africa, was not one of those countries, however, and there was a seemingly contradictory view towards homosexuality, partly because the need for conscripts was so dire, but also because they did not want individuals to escape conscription simply by claiming they were gay. While there was an overall disapproval of any form of deviant sexual activity in general, they continued to admit homosexuals in to the National Service and ultimately tried to cure them.[50] Despite the fact that the *American Diagnostic Statistical Manual of*

Mental Disorders had removed homosexuality as a psychiatric disorder in 1973, this change never was acknowledged by those in the SADF. Whereas one could not serve in the Permanent Force if deemed homosexual, this did not negate a person's conscripted status in the National Service. In 1982, a policy directive signed by General C. L. Viljoen, the head of the army, set out the policy towards homosexuality in the service:

> All possible steps must be taken to combat the phenomenon of homosexuality/or lesbianism in the Army. During the recruitment process care must be taken that persons with such behavioural disorders are not admitted to the Permanent Force.[51]

Just as police in the 1960s turned to practitioners to "cure" homosexuality, the SADF also expected medical practitioners to deal with these "behavior disorders." A separate ward, Ward 22 (later Ward 24) at 1 Military Hospital in Voortrekkerhoogte, Pretoria was set up for homosexual men. A few lesbian women were also sent there in later years. Most of these individuals were arbitrarily housed with other "deviants" such as drug users, conscientious objectors, and other mentally ill individuals.

In 1997, the South African Truth and Reconciliation Commission, received submissions from a few conscripts who alleged they had been submitted to "treatment" of homosexuality in the 1970s against their will. The Medical

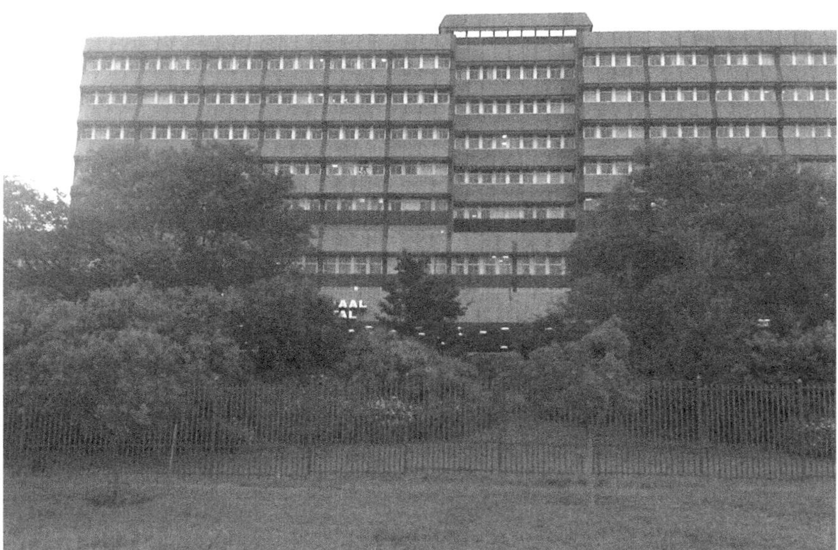

Figure 5.1 1 Military Hospital, Voortrekkerhoogte, Pretoria. Photograph courtesy of Ron Knowles.

Research Council, Gay and Lesbian Archives, the Health and Human Rights Project, and the National Coalition for Gay and Lesbian Equality, thereafter jointly conducted a study called "The Aversion Project," into gay and lesbian experiences of abuse in the military.[52] What they found was far more widespread than initially suspected. Psychiatric units were used as punitive places in order to ensure conformity. Not only did practitioners give men and women aversion therapy in attempt to "retrain" them to be heterosexual, they also administered hormonal treatment.[53] Within the psychiatric wards, practitioners arbitrarily made use of electro-convulsive therapy, sedatives, and isolation techniques, and contributed to torture manuals used by military personnel. Later reports revealed that over 900 individuals were also given gender reassignment surgery.[54] These stories of abuse were substantiated by Gerald Kraak's documentary, *Property of the State: Gay Men in the Apartheid Military*, and articles by Robert Kaplan, all of which have brought this ill-treatment of dissident and homosexual SADF conscripts by military psychiatrists to the public domain.[55]

The SADF's overarching view about homosexuality was that it was a discipline failure and made individuals more susceptible to extortion and security risks.[56] The 1970s was a period of increasing militancy in the black resistance movement, and aggressive tactics were being encouraged by the South African government as a means to restore law and order in the country along its borders and in frontline states. In the context of decolonization and the Cold War, the South African government saw threats emanating from the bordering countries of Mozambique, Zimbabwe, Namibia, Zambia, and Angola. The militarization of South Africa increased dramatically in the 1970s, and the SADF was called on more frequently by the National Party leaders to partake in missions.

The South African Medical Services, which oversaw all medical treatment in the SADF was under the jurisdiction of the Department of Defence, but most practitioners were also registered with South African Medical and Dental Council (SAMDC). The SAMDC mostly ignored the medical practices in the military and those working within the structures of the SADF rarely abided by medical ethics. As Allison D. Newton points out, those practitioners working as military psychiatrists or psychologists were first and foremost allegiant to the military, rather than the wellbeing of the patient. Their goal was to "effectively and quickly" treat the patient and "to return him to his unit as a fully functioning member."[57] Thus, quick treatments were often deemed the most valuable.

Levin was an obvious choice for overseeing the military's psychiatric rehabilitation program unit. He had been a Chairman of the Point Branch of the National Party, and Vice-Chairman of the Houghton divisional committee of the National Party of Transvaal, educated at the University of Pretoria and the University of Witwatersrand and registered as a medical practitioner in 1964 and a specialist psychiatrist with the South African Medical and Dental Council since 1969.[58] In a submission to the 1968 select committee, Levin had made it known that he had had some success in treating homosexuals using aversion therapy. He wrote: "I have in the course of my work both in General Practice and in the Psychiatric Department of the General Hospital Johannesburg, as well as Sterkfontein Hospital, treated many Homosexuals and Lesbians, and enjoyed some measure of success in therapy."[59] He joined 1 Military Hospital of the SADF in 1969.

Levin's research mostly focused on drug dependency and rehabilitation, which was a main concern to the military. He oversaw the Drug Rehabilitation Program from 1971–1974. Those found or admitting to using drugs were often sent to *Greefswald,* the drug and rehabilitation center located in a remote, dry area of present-day Limpopo Province that was renowned as a brutal labor and punishment center.[60] For Levin, the common connection between drug abuse and homosexuality was evident in that both were "deviant" conditions that could be cured. For homosexuals, however, his therapy took the form of aversion tactics. One interviewee of the "Aversion Project" explained the process as follows:

> Electrodes were strapped to the arms of the subject, and wires leading from these were in turn connected to a machine operated by a dial calibrated from one to ten. The subject was then shown black and white pictures of a naked man and encouraged to fantasise.
>
> The increase in the current would cause the muscles of the forearm to contract—an intensely painful sensation. When the subject was either screaming with pain or verbally requested that the dial be turned off, the current would be stopped and a colour *Playboy* centrefold substituted for the previous pictures . . . [The doctor] would then verbally describe the woman portrayed in glowing and positive terms. This process would be repeated three times in a single session. Sessions were held twice daily for three to four days. People subjected to this therapy experienced long periods of disorientation afterwards.[61]

Levin, a practicing psychiatrist associated with the forensic department of the University of Calgary in Canada from the mid-1990s to 2010 was ironically later charged with 21 counts of sexual assault against male patients under his care in August 2010.[62] No longer using aversion therapy in his practice in Canada, he still admitted to using it in South Africa, claiming that all patients were voluntary, although it is doubtful just how much concurrence on the part of young conscripts was due to Levin's status as Colonel.[63] Few were given adequate information about the aversion or hormonal therapy and one conscript, Clive, was told that the shocks would be benign:

> That you're going to get hooked up to something that resembles a massage device or something like that, whether it short circuited . . . I don't know, it was a peculiar thing. And he said that he'd used it on himself because he had a predilection for chocolate bon-bons and this was a

> way of getting rid of a desire for bon-bons. So well, I thought, what the hell, try it. So we tried it. I found the therapy itself terribly painful, very disorientating. . . . [64]

Other forms of treatment, specifically pharmacological, were also administered.[65] Like the limited information given about aversion therapy, few were told what drugs they were given, but most assume it was hormonal therapy. Called before a board to investigate whether or not he could be admitted to the SADF, one individual, Neil, describes being offered pills to "dampen my sexual drive, which I presumed would have been hormonal tampering with me . . . Dr Reynolds prescribed tablets that were supplied to me in an unmarked container by the pharmacist. I assumed that they would do tests on me later, and if I wasn't a co-operative patient, that they would not help me to get army exemption."[66]

Once in 1 Military Hospital, any form of viable therapy, according to Trudie Grobler, an intern psychologist, "consisted of the matron of psychiatry, the psychiatrists and psychologists sitting around a table discussing patients' cases. Each patient was brought in individually and asked a couple of disinterested questions about his medication. The patient would simply answer and leave. There was no diagnosis."[67] The very way in which individuals were sent to the military hospital for psychiatric evaluation undermined confidentiality and effective care. Rather than being treated by individual psychologists close to the base, patients were sent far from their bases for treatment. It often became common knowledge where an individual had been sent and the sense of confidentiality was frequently breached. Moreover, contrary to privacy ethic rules of the psychiatric profession, those who admitted to being homosexual were often forced by Levin to tell their parents about their homosexual behavior.[68] Although the SADF suggested that any information that a national serviceman was gay should be treated as confidential, at least to their platoons, there were numerous stories of Levin calling parents and telling them that their children were gay.[69] In the end, most of those who came in contact with practitioners associated with the SADF were left with psychological and physical scars. Many reported recurring headaches, photosensitivity, epilepsy, increased suicide rates, addiction, poor self-esteem, hormonal imbalances, depression, and impotency.[70]

At 1 Military Hospital, Barry Fowler, a former clinical psychologist in the 1980s, explains how each case was evaluated:

> The Clinical Psychology department was based within the Department of Psychiatry, which was situated in the north east side of the old 1 Military Hospital building. The Department of Clinical Psychology tended to have referred to them people who had some psychiatric diagnosis; depression, anxiety, suicide attempts, and of course, psychosis. (There was some overlap with the Counselling psychology service, and where a

> particular patient might end up often depended on who referred them.) All patients brought into casualty with mental problems were referred to psychiatry, and then often sub-referred to clinical psychology.[71]

Because of these numerous sub-divisions, a consensus did not exist among all those that worked in the psychiatric unit. Clinical psychologists tended to disagree with the psychiatrists and those working in the various bases around southern Africa could manipulate the treatment of individuals. Interviewees for "the Aversion Project" describe various individuals who attempted to make the patients' stay more pleasant. Grobler was described as "sympathetic," and nurses such as sister Snyman was also described as "sweet." Grobler had disagreed with the way that Levin conducted aversion therapy and was ultimately banned from the wards.[72]

Moreover, as Rebecca Sinclair points out, not "every white, gay soldier in the SADF in the 1970s and 1980s suffered to the degree, or suffered at all, that those mentioned in 'The Aversion Project' did."[73] Indeed, stories of fun drag parties, stealing ambulances from the hospitals to attend gatherings, and other positive experiences amongst inmates prevailed despite rampant homophobia. Sinclair suggests that because homosexuals were a minority within the military that they were not always seen as a threat, and views towards homosexuality, particularly in the 1980s relaxed somewhat, so that many were left alone. Whereas this may have been true, it also was more likely due to the fact that Levin was no longer a head psychiatrist at 1 Military Hospital after 1974.

After Levin left, throughout the 1980s, confusion still existed about the etiology of homosexuality and staff in the SADF must have realized that Levin's so-called "treatments" were outdated and ineffectual. According to Fowler, Levin became an embarrassment in military psychiatry circles and his name was used mostly in negative terms.[74] The electroshock machine was simply housed in a storage room and only brought out by practitioners to play practical jokes on each other, such as linking it up to the door handle so they could give each other low-voltage surprise shocks.[75] Instead, psychotherapy, while not vastly popular among general mental hospitals throughout South Africa, usurped hormonal and aversion therapy. The type of psychotherapy in the military, however, was somewhat different from that in the civilian sector. Partly this is because military psychiatry developed differently from civilian psychiatry in that it was always meant to serve the military first and foremost. As Newton explains in her examination of military psychotherapy in the early 1980s, "Voluntary referrals are rare. All too often it is the patient's officer or medical officer, who picking up abnormal behaviour, bundles him off to the psychiatric department with the expectancy that the soldier/patient be restored as a functioning member of his unit." [76] There was little freedom of choice of treatment and the hierarchy set up in the military undermined the open communication required for the therapy to be effective. Thus, while psychotherapy was popular in the treatment of homosexuality in the SADF, it was vastly ineffective. Much of the "therapy" took the form of short-term re-orientating or "adjusting" them to cope within the armed forces and society in general. In a letter to a friend in 1986, Fowler wrote:

> I run a group for gay "queens," teaching them more appropriate behaviour for certain conditions—i.e., when they are about to be beaten up by a group of straights. I'm not sure if its working, and it seems almost as if its becoming something of a Lonely Hearts Club for gays during the waiting time before and after sessions. I'm not happy about this, but we can't stop them talking while waiting for their transport.

For the most part throughout the 1980s, many staff at 1 Military Hospital made light fun of homosexuals and treatment was mostly inane. Concerns still existed about them being a threat to the discipline of the SADF. In an adapted lecture given on homosexuality to various units, Fowler, who was not necessarily homophobic, but felt he had to adhere to the common military doctrine, stated that:

> Gay National Servicemen often form cliques, as a "birds of a feather flock together" reaction to being in a predominantly heterosexual environment.
>
> Such groups should not be allowed to form "Power Lobbies," or to antagonise other elements of the platoon or bungalow.

And in later comments about the SADF's policy regarding Homosexuality in the SADF, Fowler declares:

> GENERAL PRINCIPALS OF MANAGEMENT
>
> Treat a homosexual person as a normal person who just happens to have a different sexual preference to heterosexual person:
>
> This is easier said than done! The majority of Gay people who create problems in the SADF threaten or challenge other people with the fact that they are Gay. ["I'm Gay—what are you going to do about it?!"] [77]

For Fowler, the concern for the SADF was no longer a matter of an individual being a security risk because of susceptibility to extortion, but instead, because now most were openly gay, it was the collective strength that these individuals posed on challenging the heterosexual norm of discipline tactics.

Although negative views towards homosexuality among practitioners certainly continued throughout the 1980s, there was an increased tolerance of homosexual behavior in general, and electroshocks and experimental hormonal therapies were less commonly used. Clive Wells, who worked as a practitioner in various bases around southern Africa and in the psychiatric ward at 1 Military hospital in 1986 argues that the psychiatric ward was actually a better place than the border posts:

> I was very bitter about the fact that people could create or have some psychological or psychiatric deviation and end up wasting thousands of hours and rands worth of taxpayers money in so called "therapy" when really they were just malingering. If you had done what you were told, and reported for duty, gritted your teeth when you didn't like it, run when they told you to, done what they told you, what did they do? They put you on a plane and send you to the border and give you the really lousy stuff to do. So the reward for good behaviour was going to hell. That seemed crazy. The reward for bad behaviour was lying on a bed trying to outwit the medical people, and that to me was a total farce! I never came to terms with that.[78]

One intake psychologist posted to 5 SAI, Ladysmith tells the story of a gay recruit whom he and a social worker agreed to transfer to a much "softer unit" where he could utilize administrative skills. They never were able to do so, however, as the individual did so well in basic training that the infantry instructors felt they had "made a man of him" and wanted him to remain an infantry officer.[79] In 1986 and 1987, Fowler recounts that many senior personnel in the department, including the head of the Department of Psychiatry and one of the three military psychiatrists were gay. Indeed, there "were a great number of gay medical staff, probably concentrated in the more humanitarian fields of psychology and psychiatry, but it wasn't a very homophobic department." One doctor working in psychiatry was openly gay, and although it initially delayed his security clearance, he was eventually deemed safe enough to be allowed to complete two border tours.[80] Thus, despite the attempts to re-orient individuals through limited forms of psychotherapy, by the end of the 1980s, homosexuality was tolerated a little more and the use of aversion and hormonal therapy, at least, had waned significantly.

CONCLUSION

Psychiatry both within and outside of the military throughout the 1970s and 1980s certainly did play a part in promoting the procreative heterosexual ideals of the apartheid state. But most practitioners' views were somewhat indefinite. They held differing opinions as to the etiology and treatment of mental disorder, and at times, their ideas may have both supported and challenged apartheid ideologies. Whereas some genuinely attempted to offer better treatment through less physically invasive practices, their endeavors were also constrained by their own heteropatriarchalism and even their desires for higher professional status. The SPNSA's mandate was to promote and protect the standing of the psychiatric discipline within South Africa and its intention may have been to ensure that the domain of psychiatry over the illness of homosexuality remained unchallenged. Even in the SADF during the 1970s and 1980s, practitioners continued to promote the notion that homosexuality was a disease. The fluidity and vague nature of practitioners' understandings of homosexuality, along with their arguments against criminalization did diffuse state authority somewhat.

When the state faced increasing resistance from African youth in the 1970s and 1980s, and its own borders were being threatened by the "onslaught" of black independence, the importance of controlling young white male sexuality became even more important—the military became the means by which to do so. But even within the military, disagreement existed as to how to treat those young white men diagnosed with disorders. Protection, rather than abuse, became the more likely intention of many of those working within the constraints of apartheid ideologies, especially in the 1980s.

6 "Monopoly on Madness?"
Private Long-Term Mental Institutions in South Africa, 1963–1989

The government and those in its employ continued to focus on protecting white men from the "evils" of black insurgence and international maladies. One means of ensuring this was to disallow most Africans permanent settlement status within white cities by creating African "homelands" and the tricameral system. Yet despite the government's intentions to move health care responsibility for blacks to homelands, it was never successful. It still needed to deal with potentially "dangerous" black individuals. In 1962, the South African government contracted long-term mental health care—particularly care of long-term black patients—to the private company Smith, Mitchell & Co. Because of the discriminate application of community psychiatric programs, the numbers of patients placed in Smith Mitchell's mainly rural institutions increased significantly so that by the mid-1980s, Smith Mitchell provided over forty percent of all mental health care beds in the country. Only about six percent of the beds were reserved for whites.[1] Charges of the government's misuse of these institutions to detain political detainees and mistreat black patients were widespread in the 1970s. Investigations by the Church of Scientology's Citizens Commission of Human Rights (CCHR), the International Committee of the Red Cross (ICRC), the World Health Organization (WHO), the Royal College of Psychiatrists, the American Psychiatric Association (APA), and an American psychiatrist, Dr. Stanley Platman and his nurse-practitioner wife Vera Thomas, substantiated these claims.

The movement of long-term black patients to contracted private institutions certainly fit with the Nationalist government's separate development initiatives. It enabled urban-based state institutions in white areas to adhere to the Group Areas Act by transferring their black patients, while they concentrated on their white patients. However, despite critics' suggestions that these were specifically warehouses where the apartheid government could house its political dissidents, the position of these institutions and those working within them was more complicated than that.

On the one hand, Smith Mitchell's position was inextricable from that of the national government. The state appointed most of the company's medical, psychiatric, and nursing staff and controlled the admission of all patients. Smith Mitchell profited from apartheid policies that produced poor conditions for Africans and benefited from the state's indifference to the welfare of black patients. Indeed, the company made most of its money by minimizing its expenditures on housing, clothing, feeding, and treating its patients. On the other hand, even though Smith Mitchell institutions remained strictly under the control of the apartheid government, it was not simply the instrument of the state. Indeed, the relationship between Smith Mitchell and the Department of Health was not always clear, and because Smith Mitchell was meant to be a temporary solution to the government's overcrowding problems, a formal relationship was never set up. Moreover, although constrained by apartheid policies, those working within the institutions expressed their frustrations to various international investigators and in turn were able to shape practices, albeit to a limited extent, within the institutions. Even the owner of the company, David Tabatznik, attempted to initiate change, although it must be said, not at the expense of profit.[2]

What is interesting about this movement of long-term patients to contracted institutions was the involvement of private and international individuals in the shaping of South Africa's mental health practices. Because of the extensive investigations into these institutions, we are able to obtain a unique comprehensive view not only into the effect of mental health policies during apartheid on patients, a view that remains more indistinct in state institutions, but we are also able to address some of the larger questions dealt with in this book through a microcosmic lens. What were the effects of apartheid policies on black patients? To what extent did socio-political forces constrain practitioners' practices? How much of a role did institutions, and in this case, private institutions and their staff play in supporting apartheid ideologies? In this chapter, we can see that these state-contracted hospitals were, to use Anne McClintock's expression, "anachronistic spaces," that is spaces in which blacks were readily perceived to exist in more "primitive" spaces within the modern world. Human rights abuses certainly took place within them, but we can also see that those who worked within these facilities were not simply placid actors in a well-structured plan. Indeed, government policy towards Smith Mitchell institutions, like that in its state-run mental health structures, was ad hoc and contradictory. Moreover, in the late 1970s, international pressures were also changing the way government officials, staff and practitioners dealt with their patients.

BACKGROUND

A wealthy entrepreneur, David Tabatznik, established Smith Mitchell in 1948 just after the *Herenigde* (Reunited) National Party won its election. It had begun as a company that provided beds first for white then black tuberculosis (TB) patients.[3] Smith Mitchell later adjoined or converted these TB hospitals to mental sanatoria. In 1962, when Alistair Lamont, the Commissioner for Mental Hygiene, faced extensive overcrowding in state-run mental hospitals, he approached Tabatznik to temporarily provide psychiatric beds until the government could create more beds or build new state hospitals. In April 1963, Smith Mitchell opened its first mental institution. As the Department of Health (DOH) never built enough state mental institutions for black patients, Smith Mitchell gradually became a permanent fixture in the mental health sector. By the mid-1980s, it had opened about twenty hospitals throughout South Africa that provided over 12,000 mental care beds for patients, three of which were in homelands.[4]

At first agreements between the DOH and Smith Mitchell were informal and the earliest written contract was only in 1975, almost twelve years after the first institution opened. Despite the large number of beds that Smith Mitchell provided and its continued expansion, the company never

Table 6.1 Smith Mitchell Institutions and Number of Beds after 1973

Name	No. of Beds after 1973
Black	
Allanridge, Welkom, OFS (1974-85)	400
Kirkwood, Port Elizabeth, Cape (1979) A – Section	700
Kirkwood B- Section (1985)	
Randfontein South Complex, Randfontein, TVL (1963)	
i) Homelake (1964)	280
ii) Millsite (1968)	175
iii) Randfontein (1964)	760
iv) Randmore	380
v) Randaf (1963)	1575
vi) Randwest (1963)	1130
vii) Randwest (children)	400
Waverley Sanatorium, Germiston, TVL (1972)	520
Waverley (children)	200
Homeland	
Ekuhlengeni, KwaZulu Natal (1975)	1300
Ekuhlengeni (children)	
Poloko, Thaba 'Nchu, Bophuthatswana (1973)	1200
Poloko (children)	
Thabamoopo (1972)	1000
Thabamoopo (children)	
White	
Hillbrow Lodge Halfway House, Jhb, TVL (1974)	60
Majestic Hotel, Kalk Bay, Cape (1974-82)	170
Simmer, Germiston, TVL (1969-78)	255
Struisbult, Daggafontein, TVL (1961-1987)	100
Turrets, Johannesburg, TVL (1974-1978)	131
Witpoort, Brakpan, TVL (1978)	386
Indian and Coloured	
East Rand, Benoni, TVL (1975)	450
East Rand (children)	50
Springfield, Durban, Natal (1964)	250

signed a long-term agreement with the national or homeland governments. Rather, the Nationalist government, insisting that the contracting out of long-term patients to Smith Mitchell was only temporary, renewed the contracts on an annual basis.[5] Terms for most hospitals were the same, except for the patients' daily tariffs that varied between hospitals. Tariffs in the homeland institutions were particularly low and the company negotiated them annually with the Department of Bantu Administration and Development (BAD), while the DOH formed the overriding contract.[6] The company charged a *per diem* rate per patient that was almost half of the patient cost in state hospitals. For example, from 1974 to 1975, state hospital daily costs ranged from R2.13 ($1.45) to R15.04 ($10.23) per patient per day depending on the race of patient (black patients were designated lower rates). The daily rate paid to private mental institutions by the Nationalist government the same year ranged from as little as R1.22½ ($0.83) to R4.31 ($2.94) per patient per day.[7]

The "temporary" status of Smith Mitchell institutions was somewhat conducive to all parties, allowing Smith Mitchell the flexibility to increase *per diem* rates on an annual basis, while the state was able to retain control over the mental health care of patients. The temporary status also meant, however, that Smith Mitchell remained vulnerable to the policies of the DOH. The number of patients accommodated in Smith Mitchell facilities, most of whom were transferred from state or local general hospitals, with the exception of a few children directly admitted from the community, was controlled by the DOH.[8] The DOH also appointed most of the employees working within Smith Mitchell facilities. State appointed or seconded staff, which included psychiatrists, general practitioners, qualified nurses, and nursing assistants were paid by the government and were a way that the government could retain some control over the treatment of patients, while also ensuring that Smith Mitchell would not poach the state hospitals' most capable staff. The complex role of seconded staff within the institutions will be discussed, but suffice to say that their presence did enable the DOH to exert further influence over company procedures.

Tabatznik was able to maintain command over his company by recruiting ministers of the National Party into the various boards of directors of each institution. Smith Mitchell had approximately eighty-nine subsidiaries in South Africa, many of which were mental sanatoria, each with its own board of directors.[9] In the 1970s, Connie Mulder, the MP for Randfontein and Vorster's Minister of the Interior and of Information who later had his career ended by the "Muldergate" information scandal of the late 1970s, was accused of profiteering from his holdings of shares and his directorship of one of Smith Mitchell's largest institutions, Randwest.[10] Mulder resigned from Randwest but apparently kept the shares.[11] Although Tabatznik denied Mulder's financial interest in the company, he did confirm that other

Table 6.2 Smith Mitchell & Co. Per Diem Rate Per Patient, 1973–1988

Name	No. of Beds after 1973	*Per diem* rate 1973-74	*Per diem* rate 1974-75	*Per diem* rate 1975-76	*Per diem* rate 1976-77	*Per diem* rate 1977-78	*Per diem* rate 1978-79	*Per diem* rate 1979-80	*Per diem* rate 1980-81	*Per diem* rate 1981-82	*Per diem* rate 1982-83	*Per diem* rate 1983-84	*Per diem* rate 1984-85	*Per diem* rate 1985-86	*Per diem* rate 1986-87	*Per diem* rate 1987-88
Black																
Allanridge, Welkom, OFS (1974-85)	400	-	R 1.375	R 1.45	R 1.48	R 1.938	R 2.145	R 2.45	R 3.135	R 3.92	R 5.34	R 6.32	R 7.14	-	-	-
Kirkwood, Port Elizabeth, E. Cape (1979) A - Section	700		-	-	-	-	-	-	R 3.55	R 4.43	R 6.31	R 7.46	R 8.43	R 9.66	R 11.09	R 15.22
Kirkwood B- Section (1985)		-	-	-	-	-	-	-	-	-	-	-	R 10.00	R 11.72	R 15.39	R 20.16
Randfontein South Complex, Randfontein (1963)																
i) Homelake (1964)	280	R 1.065	R 1.225	R 1.30	R 1.41	R 1.605	R 1.78	R 2.045	R 2.60	R 3.26	R 4.45	R 5.28	R 5.97	-	-	-
ii) Millsite (1968)	175	R 1.065	R 1.225	R 1.30	R 1.35	R 1.54	R 1.705	R 1.96	R 2.49	R 3.12	R 4.27	R 5.07	R 5.73	R 6.61	-	-
iii) Randfontein (Non-White) (1964)	760	R 1.10	R 1.26	R 1.335	R 1.445	R 1.645	R 1.825	R 2.095	R 2.665	R 3.33	R 4.55	R 5.39	R 6.09	R 6.95	R 8.04	R 10.89
iv) Randmore	380	R 1.08	R 1.24	R 1.315	R 1.425	R 1.625	R 1.80	R 2.065	R 2.63	R 3.29	R 4.50	R 5.34	R 6.03	-	-	-
v) Randaf (1963)	1575	R 1.08	R 1.24	R 1.315	R 1.365	R 1.555	R 1.72	R 1.975	R 2.51	R 3.14	R 4.29	R 5.09	R 5.75	-	-	-
vi) Randwest (1963)	1130	R 1.08	R 1.24	R 1.30	R 1.365	R 1.555	R 1.72	R 1.975	R 2.51	R 3.14	R 4.29	R 5.09	R 5.75	R 6.61	R 7.65	R 10.73
vii) Randwest (children)	400	-	-	-	R 1.54	R 1.755	R 1.945	R 2.23	R 2.85	R 3.57	R 4.87	R 5.77	R 6.52	R 7.82	R 10.53	R 14.83
Waverley Sanatorium, Germiston, TVL (1972)	520		R 1.225	R 1.50	R 1.47	R 1.675	R 1.855	R 2.13	R 2.71	R 3.39	R 4.63	R 5.49	R 6.20	R 7.17	R 8.27	R 11.46
Waverley (children)	200	-	-	-	-	-	-	-	R 3.25	R 4.05	R 5.52	R 6.54	R 7.39	R 8.89	R 11.89	R 16.29
AVERAGE RATES:		R 1.08	R 1.25	R 1.35	R 1.43	R 1.65	R 1.83	R 2.10	R 2.81	R 3.51	R 4.82	R 5.71	R 6.75	R 8.18	R 10.41	R 14.23
Homeland*																
Ekuhlengeni, Umbogintwina, KwaZulu Natal (1975)	1300	-	-	-	R 1.34	R 1.50	R 1.635			R2.86~						
Ekuhlengeni (children)		-	-	-	R 1.45	R 1.625	R 1.765									
Poloko, Thaba 'Nchu, Bophuthatswana (1973)	1050	?	?	?	R 1.35	R 1.51	R 1.645			R2.86~						
Poloko (children)	150	?	?	?	R 1.37	R 1.535	R 1.675									
Thabamoopo (1972)	1000	-	-	-	R 1.155	R 1.295	R 1.41									
Thabamoopo (children)	200	-	-	-	R 1.37	R 1.535	R 1.675									
AVERAGE RATES:					R 1.34	R 1.50	R 1.63			R 2.86						
White																
Hillbrow Lodge Halfway House, Jhb, TVL (1974)	60	-	R 4.50	R 5.18	R 5.18	R 5.905	R 6.540	R 7.325	R 9.555	R11.13~	-	-	-			
Majestic Hotel, Kalk Bay, Cape (1974-1982)	170	R 3.85	R 4.31	R 4.46	R 5.13	R 5.85	R 7.475	R 8.37	R 11.30	-	-	-	-			
Simmer, Germiston, TVL (1969-78)	255	R 3.00	R 3.60	R 3.73	R 4.29	R 4.89	R 5.33	R 5.415	-	-	-	-	-			
Struisbult, Daggafontein, TVL (1961-1987)	100	R 3.85	R 4.31	R 4.46	R 5.13	R 5.85	R 6.475	R 7.25	R 9.46	R 11.70	R 15.85	R 18.67	R 21.10			
Turrets, Jhb, TVL (1974-1978)	131	-	R 4.31	R 4.46	R 5.13	R 5.85	R 6.375	R 6.475	-	-	-	-	-			
Witpoort, Brakpan, TVL (1978)	380	-	-	-	-	-	R 5.77	R 6.46	R 8.425	R 10.43	R 14.13	R 16.66	R 18.83			
AVERAGE RATES:		R 3.57	R 4.21	R 4.46	R 4.97	R 5.67	R 6.33	R 6.88	R 9.69	R 11.07	R 14.99	R 17.67	R 19.97			
Indian and Coloured																
East Rand, Benoni, TVL (1975)	450	-	R 1.625	R 1.715	R 1.945	R 2.215	R 2.455	R 2.80	R 3.585	R 4.47	R 6.09	R 7.20	R 8.14	R 9.40	R 10.97	R 14.89
East Rand (children)	50		-	-	-	-	-	-	R 4.25	R 5.29	R 7.19	R 8.49	R 9.59	R 11.34	R 15.31	R 20.77
Springfield, Durban, Natal (1964)	250	R 1.15	R 1.75	R 1.15	R 1.875	R 2.14	R 2.37	R 2.705	R 3.73	R 4.38	-	-	-	-	-	-
AVERAGE RATES:		R 1.15	R 1.69	R 1.43	R 1.91	R 2.18	R 2.41	R 2.75	R 3.86	R 4.71	R 6.64	R 7.85	R 8.87	R 10.37	R 13.14	R 17.83

All amounts are based on letters and memos from Department of Mental Health archives, A12/2/1 vol 1-21 and 17/3/2/3 vol 1-4. Fiscal years run from 1 April to 31 March. Amounts shown are those in use at the end of the fiscal year. Because patient numbers, staff ratios, transferal fees and interest rates continuosly changed the amounts paid during the year may vary slightly.

*Homeland institutions had tarriff agreements with the Department for Bantu Administration and Development members of parliament had holdings in the company; the MP for Bloemfontein, P. L. S. Aucamp, was Director of the Smith Mitchell subsidiary, Poloko Sanatorium (Pty) Ltd., and a former Cabinet member, W.A. Maree, and MP and Johannesburg City Councillor, Alf Wideman, were also directors of the company.[12] Indeed, Smith Mitchell used its shares and directors' fees to secure political support. Jan H. Robbertze, who had chaired the National Council of Mental Health, in a 2002 interview confirmed these allegations. He argued that

> The problem with that [contract] is that the high up people in the Department of Health, they were making money out of this. They were all appointed as Directors of the Smith, Mitchell institutions. The Secretary of Health and even the Minister of Health was involved in that. Some of them are still getting cuts from that side.[13]

It was not uncommon for MPs to be associated with private business or receive gifts from businesses, and this was a way for private industry, specifically in the medical field, to ensure they retained contracts.

CONDITIONS AND TREATMENT IN SMITH MITCHELL INSTITUTIONS

Although the situation varied among Smith Mitchell institutions, in general, conditions, particularly for black patients, were appalling and these hospitals were reminiscent of pre-1930s institutions—they were mainly places of custody. As these institutions had been established at a later period, their facilities did surpass those at some state institutions in some aspects. With regards to treatment, however, the company rarely offered any form of restorative therapy. In 1969, the Commissioner for Mental Health, Alistair Lamont, stated that those occupying the beds in the institutions were "deteriorated to the extent that they can no longer benefit from intensive and specialised psychiatric treatment."[14] Thus, he felt that there was no need to attempt to implement restorative strategies.

Company institutions, similar to their state counterparts, were established in abandoned buildings. However, instead of utilizing former military camps like state institutions did, Smith Mitchell institutions were established mainly on abandoned remote mine compounds. Thus, most institutions were comprised of blocks of large square buildings with a high barbed-wire fence surrounding them. As a 1975 newspaper article described it: "The atmosphere of compound rather than hospital clings to the uniformed guard at the entrance."[15] Many historians have written about the substandard living conditions in which mineworkers lived in the compounds. In 1972 Francis Wilson, for example, described the older mine compounds as follows:

> The compounds which house . . . 99% of the labour force vary from very old pre-first World War buildings with rooms housing 50 or more men living like sardines in double-decker concrete bunks to modern hostels housing between 12 and 20 men in dormitories that compare not unfavourable with those of a white boarding school . . . In compounds built before 1939 beds are not supplied and men either sleep on the concrete bunks or they have to make, or buy from their predecessors, wooden beds specially designed to fit the short bunks . . . On the older mines there are no dining rooms and men either eat outside or in their dormitories which generally have a coal stove for heating purposes.' . . . The organisation of a compound may be described both as authoritarian and as paternalistic . . . The size of compounds varies but all are very large by any standards.[16]

Because of the so-called temporary status of these sanatoria, Smith Mitchell at first did few upgrades to the abandoned buildings other than remove the concrete tiered bunks that had served as beds for the miners. Thus, many of the poor conditions as described by Wilson in which mineworkers had lived were transferred to mental patients. Moreover, the terrible conditions that existed for black patients in state institutions were simply transferred to these new locations. Patients' buildings, particularly those accommodating black patients, remained impersonal, poorly ventilated, dilapidated, crowded, and unhygienic. Wards housed on average forty patients, with some at the larger institutions accommodating as many as 250 patients in a ward. Like black wards in state institutions, most patients in Smith Mitchell institutions did not have their own beds. Patients initially had to sleep on coir mats on the floor. In the mid-1970s, these were replaced by four-inch foam and rubber mattresses and shortly thereafter Smith Mitchell began to introduce beds.[17] However, many black patients were not provided with bedding.[18] Clothing was inadequate. Black patients, had two-piece pyjamas to wear during the day, and females wore, what the American Psychiatric Association described as "sack-type dresses."[19] Few patients had shoes and infestation of warts and athlete's foot spread among them.[20] During the winter, the hospitals failed to provide adequate clothing and patients often complained of the cold. Moreover, heaters frequently did not work and electrical problems were common. Hot water geysers did not function properly and many patients had to take cold showers in the winter.[21] Bathing facilities in general were poor and lacked privacy. At the bigger institutions, patients lined up at a central outside shower, undressed and a little liquid soap was placed on their heads before they went into the shower. Standing naked in a large crowd, staff herded patients into communal showers, where they washed themselves.[22] Jan H. Robbertze, a psychiatrist who had visited the institutions in the 1960s, described what he saw as follows:

> It was atrocious there . . . the situation there, the small rooms with a lot of people. The first time I made contact with the Smith, Mitchell was when I was working at Sterkfontein hospital and they had a hospital there and I had to go there to write monthly reports for 3 months, depending on the patient. I got there at this hospital, and they had this lot of men there that they had undressed in the courtyard and they were washing them with washing hoses like animals. It was terrible. I wrote about this, but they did not improve.[23]

Toilet facilities, like those at state institutions, were also sub-standard and frequently the cause of disease. Whereas toilets for those few whites and coloureds who were sent to Smith Mitchell institutions had doors and toilet paper, black wards often made do with buckets. In some black hospitals, toilets were outside the wards in a central yard and these were mainly rows of squat toilets with no doors or seats.[24] Flush toilets, when installed, frequently did not flush, and there was often no toilet seats or toilet paper.[25] Sewage gutters were open and patients sometimes used them as urinals, which made them sites for the spread of disease.[26] In most black hospitals, there were neither sinks nor taps near the toilets, and soap and towels were not provided for patients to wash their hands.[27] As patients often took food from pots with their hands, food was unsanitary.[28] Moreover, meals were often inadequate and worse than the food provided for black miners in the 1930s and 1940s who had at least received a "scientific diet" for the heavy manual work they performed. Many staff complained that the food given patients was inedible and they themselves refused to eat it.

Like state institutions, Smith Mitchell also had "industrial therapy" programs, although Smith Mitchell's programs were much larger than those at state hospitals. These were on-site factories assembling asbestos heaters and plugs, putting together hair accessories and watch labels, or making coat hangers, clothes and shoes for patients.[29] Patients also created crafts, such as toy animals, baskets, macramé items, or potted plants, all of which were sold to the public.[30] Moreover, like prisoners in South Africa's state-run jails at the time, most patients worked on the grounds of the facilities. Many worked in the gardens, wards, kitchens, laundry, and even in the adjoined TB sanatoria.[31] Between thirty and fifty percent of the patients worked within the hospitals, saving the company a considerable amount of money.[32] Patients were paid very little to nothing for their labour. Some were paid in tobacco, others in tokens that they had to spend at the onsite tuckshop, which charged higher prices than the shops in the closest towns. By 1984, institutions began remunerating some patients and patients could be paid between 50 cents ($0.35) and R8 ($5.56) a month, depending on the type of work they did.[33] TB patients fulfilling the same duties as mental patients in their sanatoria were paid considerably more, between R12 and

R16 ($8.34 to $11.13) a month, whereas white patients could be paid up to R30 ($20.85) a month. Labor practices therefore reinforced both racial and mental discrimination.[34]

At night, staff locked all patients in the wards in order to stop them from wandering off, often without adequate on-duty staff for the evening.[35] Some more chronic patients were locked up in wards not only in the evenings, but also for most of the day. So-called "difficult" patients were locked in seclusion rooms that had no toilet facilities, no windows through which staff could see the patients, and were dirty. Many staff who used "seclusion rooms" as a form of discipline subjected patients to physical abuse as well. Sexual abuse was also evident, both on the part of patients and by staff. The numbers of patients sexually assaulted by staff or other patients is unknown, mainly because patients' complaints received little credence and many incidences remained unreported. Patients had practically no opportunity to voice complaints as practitioners and administrators spent little time with them, and their families did not have regular access to them. Both physical and sexual abuse by staff could continue unknown for many years. Staff and superintendents seemed aware of the predominance of sexual activity, but took few steps to investigate it.[36] Instead, female patients were "sterilized" or were put on the birth-control pill, had IUDs or were given the controversial birth control injection of Depo-Provera.[37]

This denial of reproductive rights of mentally disabled women, directly contradicted the idea that these women could be pseudo-mothers. Indeed, the use of psychiatric female patients as "mothers" to children in the institutions was common. These women often worked long hours, had few breaks, and were paid very little. In 1982, in the East Rand Sanatorium for example, "mothers" were paid R3.20 ($2.95) a month. They ate and slept in the children's areas, often getting up in the middle of the night to help incontinent patients and had very little escape from their work.[38] At Poloko, ten "mothers," along with twelve staff, had been assigned to 101 physically and mentally challenged children.[39] At Randwest/Millsite, where care for children was somewhat better than that at other black institutions, forty "mothers" worked seven days a week.[40]

Medical care was poorer at Smith Mitchell institutions than at state institutions, mainly because on average, general practitioners spent very few hours a day at the hospitals treating patients, and transfer of patients to general hospitals was more difficult. Death rates were high and frequently deaths went unexplained.[41] Patients with easily treatable illnesses, even if visiting physicians would accurately diagnose them, rarely received medications such as antibiotics, and many died unnecessarily.[42]

Psychiatric care was even more deficient than general medical treatment. Psychiatrists rarely worked full-time at company facilities. They usually served several institutions, including state institutions, and held university appointments as well.[43] Like in state-run hospitals, consistent patients' reviews were rarely done and many patients retained the same diagnosis as when they were first admitted.[44] Patients were also over medicated and harmful combinations of drugs were often administered. For those psychiatrists who attempted to see patients regularly, they simply could not cope with the large workload.

Like at state institutions, to the extent that patients were treated at all, it was mostly by nurses and nursing assistants. However, a "gentleman's agreement" with the DOH involved the company's agreement not to recruit psychiatric nurses in government service."[45] Chronic shortage of nurses throughout the health system meant that Smith Mitchell had to make do with inexperienced nurses and those without psychiatric training. Although the DOH granted Smith Mitchell a higher staff/patient ratio, it was rarely met. Because of the stigma attached to psychiatric patients, many general nurses did not like to work in psychiatry. As we have seen for state institutions, the working conditions were more difficult than in general medicine.[46] The job was physically demanding and intensely stressful psychologically. Moreover, staffing problems were compounded by apartheid policies. Smith Mitchell was strongly encouraged only to hire staff members who were from the same ethnic group as the patients, or who were citizens of the designated homeland in which some of the institutions were based.[47] In the 1960s, the government also directed that white patients be solely under the care of white nurses. Because of the difficulty of finding adequate numbers of white nurses, this prohibition was dropped in the mid 1970s as long as the company made every effort to obtain white staff and that white patients indicated "in writing that they have no objection to be nursed by black staff."[48] There is no evidence of white patients granting such permission, but black staff did become more evident in white institutions.

If patients had any capacity for self-reliance, they soon lost it in the regimented world of the institutions. Although Smith Mitchell began what they called occupational therapy programs in the 1980s that taught patients the basics of "self-care, exercises, color concept training, transportation, sports, and recreation," the lack of occupational therapists and staff meant that even these cursory programs were extremely limited.[49] For example, Platman, who visited the institutions regularly in the 1980s, reported of patients that could have used some sort of occupational therapy, but due to a lack of staff and appropriate program, they remained incapable of taking care of themselves. He described the patients in one ward as follows:

> There are young late adolescent retarded girls . . . who drag themselves around and yet do not appear to have a reason for not being able to walk. There is a young hydrocephalic girl . . . who has reasonable

> intelligence and flaccid paralysed legs probably from spinal damage. Her arms are also effected [*sic*] and yet she is capable of using both arms and hands. Yet she is fed when she could be taught to feed herself. She probably could be taught to drive a suitable wheelchair and yet she is being made more dependent. This is very sad in view of her potential long life. There are many more examples like these patients and each one requires a careful individual multidisciplinary review.[50]

Patients were placed in wards according to a crudely graded system. Four categories were set up depending on the amount of effort a patient was to staff. "A" type patients were those patients who showed no signs of psychosis. These patients were well aware of their surroundings and had insight into their condition. "B" category patients were those who were not obviously psychotic, but needed help with some activities. "B" type patients could easily be promoted to the "A" category. "C" type patients were those that "looked" mentally disturbed and were not as aware of their surroundings as the previous categories. "D" category patients included patients who required special nursing such as those who were incontinent, physically disabled, or blind.[51] The indistinctness of these groups reveals the confusion that practitioners and staff had between mental acuity and psychosis, and physical and mental ability. Indeed, as we have seen in Chapter 2, individuals showing no signs of psychosis or those with physical disability could easily find themselves swept into the institutions. As social services for Africans were not a main priority of the apartheid government, and the government had means other than mental institutions to control the black majority, such as the military, police, and prisons, most who ended up in Smith Mitchell institutions were those who were difficult or inconvenient to leave loose in the streets.[52] Company institutions therefore became a place where the government and practitioners could warehouse problematic black individuals for long periods away from society.

Overseeing these custodial institutions were divisional and hospital superintendents. These men (and all of them were men) were usually former public servants sympathetic to the Nationalist government's initiatives. They had held jobs as former staff sergeants in the South African Defence Force, former prison wardens, town clerks, or BAD administrative officers.[53] Few had medical or psychiatric training. Because the company was in the business of simply warehousing people, it is not surprising that they hired former prison wardens and other types of custodial staff. Nor is it surprising that these administrators rarely challenged the sub-standard conditions for black patients or the policies forwarded by the apartheid government. Indeed, most abided by the racial, gender, and class discrimination endemic in the National Party.[54]

State appointed practitioners and nurses also seemed simply to accept government procedures that created the substandard conditions for patients.

Psychiatrists and general practitioners never took any unified overt stance in opposition to the regulations creating poor conditions for black patients, nor did they attempt to make changes through their representative body, the Medical Association of South Africa (MASA) or its sub-group, the Society of Psychiatrists of South Africa (SPSA).[55] MASA failed to investigate or concern itself with Smith Mitchell institutions. As the Health and Human Rights Project, which was initiated jointly by the Trauma Centre for Victims of Violence and the University of Cape Town, argued, MASA's main concern was "maintaining the security of the State above human rights considerations."[56] MASA itself recently acknowledged that it was "a part of the white establishment . . . and for the most part and in most contexts, shared the worldview and political beliefs of that establishment."[57]

Complaints and suggestions for improvement from MASA members working in Smith Mitchell institutions, all of whom, with the exception of one Indian doctor, were white, were also sporadic and rarely challenged the policies of the government or the company. Psychiatrists and general practitioners worked part-time and rarely spent enough time within the institutions to form any working coalition. Tensions also existed between psychiatrists and general practitioners who were often confused about their responsibilities and their working relationships with each other. One psychiatrist at Waverley complained that no communication existed between general practitioners and psychiatrists at all. No group meetings were held, and often differences of opinions existed over the treatment of patients, particularly epileptic patients whom most general practitioners felt were their jurisdiction.[58] When both psychiatrists and general practitioners worked at the same institutions, psychiatrists were held responsible for patients' well-being, but with little interaction between the two, often they became critical of one another's treatment of patients.[59] The fact that the company sometimes hired its own practitioners to work within the institutions also caused further conflict. As Platman relates, one nursing staff manager for various institutions described the tenuous relationship between a state-paid psychiatrist and a company-paid general practitioner:

> She stated it was not a good relationship and they had many fights over the new medical record. She found herself caught between the wishes of psychiatrist and the health department and those of Dr. Sachs. Unfortunately Dr. Sachs is anti-state. However as a nurse she has the state and nursing council to please.[60]

This description is an example of the multifaceted and somewhat tenuous relationships between the various levels of state-paid and company staff that existed within the mental institutions, particularly between psychiatrists and general practitioners, but also between nurses and psychiatrists.

As can be seen from the organizational chart, head nurses and nursing staff, the majority of whom were black women, held the most difficult position of all within Smith Mitchell institutions, having to deal with the often conflicting and contradictory pronouncements of the state, company, superintendents, general practitioners, and psychiatrists, while trying at the same time to cope with the demands of their patients.[61] Nurses performed most of the labor within the institutions and constituted the majority of the employees, but had the least say in the overall policies. As Shula Marks points out, nurses throughout South Africa were "subject to highly contradictory political and social pressures" and these pressures were just as prominent in the semi-private world of contracted psychiatric institutions.[62] In the 1960s, with the government's 1950s onslaught against political dissent and the banning of the ANC and PAC, the complaints of nurses went largely unheard. Up until the mid 1980s, black nurses had little official influence on government policies except through the South African Nursing Council (SANC) and its associative body, the South African Nursing Association (SANA), which the DOH established in accordance to the Nursing Act, No. 45 of 1944. The SANC and SANA's leadership was white and its mandate was to control nursing standards and education on behalf of the government, not deal with labor issues or concerns of its black workers. Indeed, the SANC and SANA staunchly penalized any nurses who did not adhere to its policies or who showed any form of political dissent.[63] Those working in Smith Mitchell institutions had even less say about government and company policies and had to conform if they wanted to keep their jobs. No organized labor union existed for Smith Mitchell nursing staff and even in the 1980s, when more organized forms of protest and strikes were erupting around the country, nurses working within Smith Mitchell institutions were never represented. Without an organized union, there were limited opportunities for Smith Mitchell nursing staff to voice their concerns without trepidation. The remote areas in which Smith Mitchell institutions were located meant that it was difficult for individuals to organize with staff from other institutions. Moreover, the mixture of state-paid and company-paid staff meant that they did not have a shared employer to which they could voice their complaints; nor did they necessarily have the same concerns. Company and seconded employees had different salaries, work guidelines and benefits, and they even lived in separate areas.[64] Without collective representation, many staff members were apprehensive of communicating their individual complaints and they believed that if they did give suggestions, they would not be implemented.[65] The lack of a coalition among Smith Mitchell nursing staff also was affected by the fact that many nurses and assistant nurses became institutionalized themselves and over time failed to recognize the sub-standard conditions in which they and patients worked and lived. Sometimes the line between staff member and patient

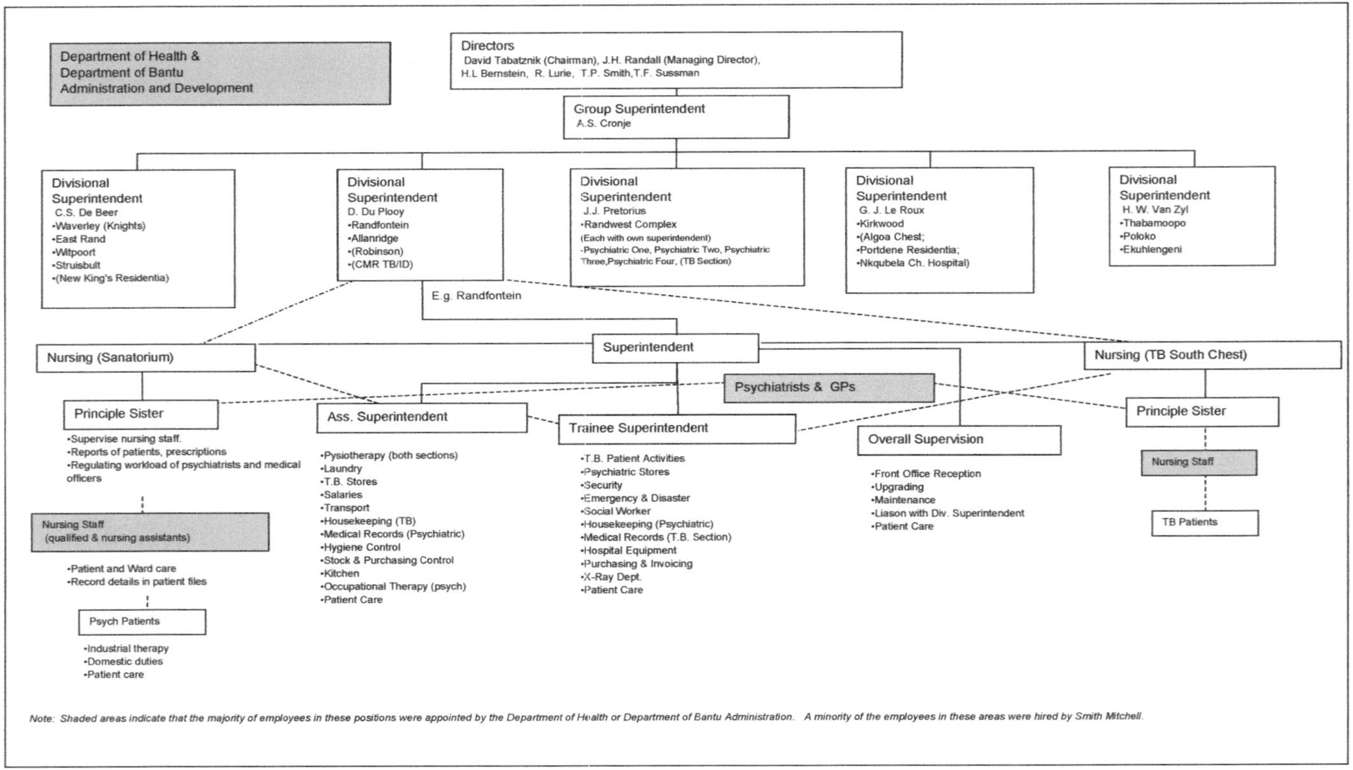

Department of Health &
Department of Bantu
Administration and Development

Directors
David Tabatznik (Chairman), J.H. Randall (Managing Director),
H.L Bernstein, R. Lurie, T.P. Smith,T.F. Sussman

Group Superintendent
A.S. Cronje

Divisional
Superintendent
C.S. De Beer
•Waverley (Knights)
•East Rand
•Witpoort
•Struisbult
•(New King's Residentia)

Divisional
Superintendent
D. Du Plooy
•Randfontein
•Allanridge
•(Robinson)
•(CMR TB/ID)

Divisional
Superintendent
J.J. Pretorius
•Randwest Complex
(Each with own superintendent)
-Psychiatric One, Psychiatric Two, Psychiatric Three,Psychiatric Four, (TB Section)

Divisional
Superintendent
G. J. Le Roux
•Kirkwood
•(Algoa Chest;
•Portdene Residentia;
•Nkqubela Ch. Hospital)

Divisional
Superintendent
H. W. Van Zyl
•Thabamoopo
•Poloko
•Ekuhlengeni

E.g. Randfontein

Superintendent

Nursing (Sanatorium)

Nursing (TB South Chest)

Psychiatrists & GPs

Principle Sister
•Supervise nursing staff.
•Reports of patients, prescriptions
•Regulating workload of psychiatrists and medical officers

Nursing Staff
(qualified & nursing assistants)
•Patient and Ward care
•Record details in patient files

Psych Patients
•Industrial therapy
•Domestic duties
•Patient care

Ass. Superintendent
•Pysiotherapy (both sections)
•Laundry
•T.B. Stores
•Salaries
•Transport
•Housekeeping (TB)
•Medical Records (Psychiatric)
•Hygiene Control
•Stock & Purchasing Control
•Kitchen
•Occupational Therapy (psych)
•Patient Care

Trainee Superintendent
•T.B. Patient Activities
•Psychiatric Stores
•Security
•Emergency & Disaster
•Social Worker
•Housekeeping (Psychiatric)
•Medical Records (T.B. Section)
•Hospital Equipment
•Purchasing & Invoicing
•X-Ray Dept.
•Patient Care

Overall Supervision
•Front Office Reception
•Upgrading
•Maintenance
•Liason with Div. Superintendent
•Patient Care

Principle Sister

Nursing Staff

TB Patients

Note: Shaded areas indicate that the majority of employees in these positions were appointed by the Department of Health or Department of Bantu Administration. A minority of the employees in these areas were hired by Smith Mitchell.

Figure 6.1 Smith Mitchell TB/Psychiatric Institutions Organizational Chart (c1982)—example of Randfontein.[66]

blurred, particularly as many patients worked side-by-side with nurses and domestic staff, and staff lives revolved around the institutions.[67]

Yet, not all of those working in the institutions remained mute about their views or were completely powerless to generate change. Rather, some took advantage of various surveys to express their discontent against the company, psychiatrists, general practitioners, administrators, and to some degree, the state. From the late 1970s, investigations by the Church of Scientology's Citizens Commission of Human Rights, the American Psychiatric Association, and especially Dr. Stanley Platman became the principle means by which staff members could convey their dissatisfaction of government and company policies. It is to these investigations that we now turn.

ENABLING CONTESTATION: INTERNATIONAL INVESTIGATIONS

> The company that runs [these institutions] provides accommodation—if little else—for South Africa's Black chronic insane. But all indications are that what once might have been excused as a temporary measure to relieve the pressure on State mental hospitals is today a permanent, expanding and unhealthy feature of mental health care in South Africa—a "growing malignancy." The number of these human warehouses where care is reduced to a minimum and cure a forgotten word is growing year by year—as are the profits of the company which now has such a monopoly on madness that as one authority told me, "it can virtually dictate mental health care in South Africa."[68]

In 1975, thirteen years after Smith Mitchell opened its first mental health facility, the *Sunday Times* published the article that highlighted the appalling conditions within the Smith Mitchell hospitals and accused the company of profiting from psychiatric "illness."[69] A month later, the *Rand Daily Mail* published a series of articles describing the sub-standard conditions and treatment within both public and private mental hospitals in South Africa.[70] In 1976, *Scope* magazine published a series of articles about an ex-psychiatric patient's experiences within mental institutions in South Africa that eventually caused debate within parliament.[71] Internationally, newspapers such as *The Observer* in London, *Dagens Nyheter* of Sweden, the New York *Voice* also described the atrocious conditions within South African mental institutions.[72]

These articles originated from investigations and articles written by the Church of Scientology's Citizens Commission of Human Rights (CCHR), established in 1969, that staunchly opposed psychiatry and psychiatric drugs in general. The role of the CCHR will be discussed further in the next chapter, but the organization's reports, which described Smith Mitchell facilities as "human warehouses" and "labour camps" had an immediate impact.[73]

In the years after the publication of the articles, the government responded in a contradictory manner. First it attempted to seriously thwart the ability of individuals to express their concerns about the mental institutions. In 1976, it enacted the Mental Health Amendment Act, similar to the interdictions in the Prisons Act of 1959, that prohibited the publication of any photographs, sketches, or information regarding mental patients or institutions, and declared violators "guilty of an offence and liable on conviction to a fine not exceeding one thousand rand or to imprisonment for a period not exceeding one year," or given both a fine and imprisonment.[74] Whereas the act was promoted as a means to protect patients' privacy and curb false accusations, it was really about shielding both the government and the company from public scrutiny.[75] To ensure that individuals adhered to the act, the Bureau of State Security (BOSS) consistently placed pressure on journalists and CCHR members threatening to publish material.[76]

Secondly, however, in an attempt to show that the allegations were unfounded, in June of 1976, the Minister of Health, Schalk van der Merwe, invited the International Committee of the Red Cross (ICRC) and the World Health Organization (WHO) to inspect South Africa's mental institutions.[77] The ICRC, whose main concern at the time was the treatment of convicted and political prisoners, conducted a preliminary investigation into whether any political detainees were held in state and private institutions. As the ICRC found no evidence to suggest that political prisoners were detained in psychiatric institutions, it conducted no formal investigation.[78]

The WHO, which the United Nations Special Committee Against Apartheid had also requested to conduct a review of Smith Mitchell institutions, decided against visiting South Africa, stating that the 1976 Amendment Act would taint inquiries and distort any investigation. Instead, it wrote a report based on House of Assembly debates, government reports, and medical publications. Its scathing report discussed the atrocious conditions in the hospitals. It condemned the custodial nature of the institutions and stated that in general, the institutions were "open to abuse" and were manifestations of apartheid.[79] Soon after the release of the WHO investigation, the Nationalist government began publicly talking about the phasing out of the use of private mental institutions. In 1977, the government released a press statement to local press stating that it would allocate sixty million rand to the building and expansion of state-run black institutions that would replace private institutions and gradually phase out the use of beds in private hospitals.[80] This plan was never implemented and no state expansion program for black patients was ever undertaken. Thus, criticisms of South Africa's use of private facilities for black patients persisted, particularly in the international press.

In 1978, in an attempt to quell allegations of human rights abuse raised in the WHO report, Smith Mitchell & Co. invited the American Psychiatric Association to visit their institutions. Soon thereafter, the DOH backed up this invite with an official invitation to visit all mental health facilities in the country. Unlike the WHO that rejected the invitation, the APA accepted under the condition that they would not be charged under the 1976 Amendment Act. In September 1978, a committee made up of four members arrived in South Africa prepared to investigate all types of South Africa's mental health institutions. Once in South Africa, however, the DOH told the committee that they could not conduct detailed inspections of state institutions. The APA therefore based its report on their visits to nine Smith Mitchell institutions and a few guided tours of state and general hospitals. Its findings echoed many of those of the WHO. They found evidence of unnecessarily high death rates in the hospitals, unsatisfactory care, abusive practices, deficiency of professional staff, improper use of drugs, and general exploitation of patients' labour. But they found no evidence of the improper institutionalization of black dissidents or abuse of ECT, accusations that had initially formed the main basis for the APA's investigation.[81]

The APA's report was the first in-depth analysis of private mental hospitals and apartheid in South Africa based on on-site visits. The APA had the opportunity to interview staff, patients, and administrators on the daily affairs of the institutions. Their report showed that staff were concerned about some policies and practices perpetuated by apartheid: "Indeed, we were heartened," wrote the committee, "to discover concern about and criticism of these abusive apartheid practices among psychiatrists, physicians, medical students and nurses within South Africa."[82] The APA's investigation was limited, however, and while it publicized the racial differentiation that existed within the hospitals and highlighted apartheid's effect on the daily workings of the institutions, it did nothing to stop the DOH's continued movement towards the use of private mental health care. Privatization of long-term care was "even more enthusiastically pursued" after 1978.[83]

The WHO and APA criticisms led the Nationalist government to suggest that Smith Mitchell conduct its own surveys. Although the company conducted its own short reviews of its institutions that reported to the head office, David Tabatznik with the help of his brother, Bernard Tabatznik, a cardiologist living in Maryland, decided to recruit an American psychiatrist, Stanley Platman, to conduct comprehensive internal reviews of the facilities. Platman was then the Assistant Secretary of the Mental Health and Addictions centre for the State of Maryland. Platman agreed under the condition that he and his wife, Vera Thomas, a South African born midwife, were given full access to institutions at any time of the day or night and that they paid his expenses. In 1981, Platman and Thomas conducted their first review. Despite the unfavorable conclusions of their reports and some resistance by psychiatrists to their visits, Tabatznik invited Platman and Thomas back five more times for reviews, the last of which was in 1990.[84] As Tabatznik ensured that superintendents and staff gave Platman access to all files, free reign to drop in to any facility any time of day or night, and consent to interview any staff member, patient, and administrator, Platman's reports and subsequent superintendents' responses offer a rare glimpse into the world within the institutions. They reveal surprisingly critical and candid accounts of conditions in the facilities by some staff members, and were generally well received by Tabatznik and Andre Cronje, the group superintendent.[85]

Many staff were aware of this positive reception. In a letter to Vera Thomas, Rian Venter, a nurse working at one of Smith Mitchell institutions wrote: "Why get somebody to come and try get to the root of things? I have decided to come to a positive conclusion—that somebody up there has realized all things are not what they are dished up to be. That somebody up there has decided the patients are perhaps entitled to a better deal by the Company."[86] Tabatznik was well respected among staff and practitioners and they were aware of the changes that were implemented after the surveys. As Venter wrote, some staff felt that "now we can get more out of them because they think the Platman's will be impressed—and if they threaten to come often enough we will get all we have been asking for."[87] Therefore, Platman's reports became an effective vehicle for staff of all levels to initiate change.

Concerns voiced by the various levels of staff showed the different priorities of each group. Many nursing staff complained about the lack of patients' care. Some showed frustration at the difficulty of discharging patients; others objected to the limited medical and psychiatric coverage and noted the poor facilities and conveniences given to patients. Many also objected to their own working conditions and complained about their substandard living conditions and the lack of social activities.[88] Nurses also frequently commented on the limited number of staff in the institutions and complained about being overworked.[89] Other complaints were about general racial differentiation, such as when some black head nurses complained of having to eat lunch separately from the white staff or when superintendents did not know the names of black staff.[90] Others objected to differential pay scales. Even though the company could set its own wages and it usually paid more than the state, racial disparity in pay continued. For example, in 1978, it was estimated that black nursing assistants received half the salary of white nursing assistants.[91] In 1984, this inequality continued. The head black nurse at Randfontein earned R907 ($630.65) net annually, whereas the white head sister at Allanridge earned R1,000 ($695.31) a month.[92]

Those at the higher levels, such as practitioners and superintendents on the other hand generally complained about the daily administration of the hospital and the discord between each other. Practitioners and superintendents of the institutions described a lack of communication among practitioners and nursing staff, whereas superintendents expressed frustration that practitioners left them out of decisions concerning policies and patients' care.[93] They also complained about the DOH's regulations concerning patients' transfers, funding, and general procedures, while superintendents voiced their discontent that they had no jurisdiction to discipline or control the actions of seconded staff.[94]

Many of the concerns raised by staff led to some, albeit superficial, improvements in Smith Mitchell institutions. Improvements over the years were far from comprehensive, but they helped quell criticisms of the institutions and made the hospital environment tolerable. Television sets were introduced, pictures were put up, old cars were put in the playground for children, patients were given stationery, food, and hygiene standards improved.[95] More activities were planned and patients were given better clothing.[96] Some wards were renovated. Toilets and bathrooms were gradually decentralized, new boilers were installed, and patients had more access to hot water.[97] Ceilings were installed in the wards, floors were tiled, and drains were closed.[98] Those invited to visit the institutions in 1987 commented on overall good conditions of the institutions. Helen Suzman commenting on Smith Mitchell's biggest institution stated that "it provides excellent care of the Black patients—young and old—entrusted to it."[99] One doctor stated: "what I saw on our visit, impressed me, especially the dedication of your staff and the standard of facilities."[100] A doctor from the United States, also visited one of Smith Mitchell institutions and argued that he was surprised to find no evidence of the "'shocking conditions' reported by the 1978 American Psychiatric Association investigation."[101]

The superficial changes made to the institutions, however, did not address the custodial nature of the hospitals. In 1998, the Centre for Health Policy at the University of Witwatersrand (CHP) conducted a comprehensive comparative study of public and private institutions in South Africa and found that the contracted institutions still were mostly "institutions for 'control'" and were "producing low quality care at low costs."[102] The CHP, like many before it, called for a "strategic redesign" of these institutions.[103]

It must be noted that a quandary existed for Smith Mitchell concerning improvements within the institutions. As buildings were upgraded, the situation within the hospitals often became better than the daily living conditions for those in the rural and township areas of South Africa. Psychiatrists and staff continuously reported of cases of patients who should not have been in the hospital, but either chose to stay because their lives were better in than out, or had no other places to go, as the local community had no rehabilitation programs and had insufficient living facilities for these individuals.[104] Indeed, mental diagnoses are not all-powerful, or free from manipulation from "below." Whereas conditions within mental institutions paralleled those within prisons and it is unlikely that many individuals chose to feign mental illness whereby they could be committed indefinitely, it is possible that some manipulated the system in order to stay within the institutions. For example, Platman reports of one patient from the Transkei who refused to leave as he felt he was better off in the hospital than at home. He stated that he was at least fed, clothed, given a roof over his head, and was allowed to go into town whenever he wanted.[105] Many nursing staff also stated that patients "were better off then [*sic*] being cared for at home."[106] Platman himself believed that there were many patients who had "learned [*sic*] to 'play the game' and spend their time gambling and even apparently are able to satisfy their sexual needs."[107] Whereas Platman and the staff's views should not be viewed without some scrutiny, it is possible that some patients ironically used these private sanatoria as an escape from the hardships of everyday life, especially as conditions in surrounding areas deteriorated.

CONCLUSION

Smith Mitchell institutions were essentially subsidiaries of the apartheid state and were controlled through contractual oversight provisions, directorships, and control of appointments. Black patients were warehoused in poor facilities in mostly rural areas with little effective treatment. These private sanatoria certainly met the mandate of the apartheid government. Yet, Smith Mitchell hospitals, like state institutions, were more than a disciplinary tool of the apartheid government. They held paradoxical positions within the structure of the apartheid. If they operated as sub-standard places of custody for the DOH, they also became places of refuge as conditions for the average black person outside the hospitals worsened. Smith Mitchell sanatoria were closed places of confinement in purposefully remote locations, yet their doors remained surprisingly open to inquiries and investigations originating in South Africa and elsewhere. The contradictions inherent in the Smith Mitchell setup were aggravated by the nature of its staffing and administration, which created a confused web of state and company controls and appointments. Like state-run mental health facilities, the company harbored both apologists and critics of the system. Superintendents, practitioners, and staff tended to conform to the values of the white establishment. Initially opportunities to dissent were mostly stifled by the confused yet authoritarian system. However, they often found their institutional role frustrating and unsatisfactory. With the onset of external review and investigations, their voices of reform within the institution began to be heard at decision-making levels in the company and the government. Living conditions gradually improved until they surpassed those in surrounding black rural areas and townships. Ironically, these belated and cursory improvements simply underlined the extent of the immiseration of living conditions for blacks that were the legacy of apartheid.

7 Critics of the System?

The Church of Scientology and the International Vilification of Psychiatry in South Africa

In 1976, reports emerged that members of the South African division of the Scientology organization broke into the Minister of Health and Smith Mitchell offices and stole files in order to substantiate claims of the mistreatment of black patients within South African mental institutions, particularly in the government contracted private institutions of Smith, Mitchell & Co.[1] Shortly thereafter, they sent press releases to the international media reiterating their accusations. This began an influx of international investigations into psychiatric institutions in South Africa.

Apartheid and mental health policy in South Africa did not exist in an isolated bubble on the edge of the African continent. The Cold War, decolonization, and changes in international psychiatric trends very much played a role in the ways in which the apartheid government, and those housed and released from mental institutions, were viewed. Whereas the government was concerned with foreign encroachment, it also saw foreign enemies within its own borders. One of these was the international organization of the Church of Scientology and its subsidiary, the Citizens Commission of Human Rights (CCHR). The CCHR alleged that South African psychiatrists were using state-contracted mental institutions to confine political detainees, exploit patients for their cheap labor, and control individuals with electroshock and excessive use of drugs. These accusations were picked up by the international press and published worldwide.

However, Scientology had not always positioned itself against the apartheid state. Since its inception, the organization attempted to ally itself with the National Party, arguing that psychiatrists were the true enemies of the country. The CCHR had self-promoting reasons for attacking the psychiatric field. Scientology dismisses psychiatry as a valid science and promotes its own doctrine as a means to obtain mental clarity. However, the organization was never successful in allying with the National Party. Instead, they played an important role in publicizing the overall substandard conditions in the hospitals and began a succession of investigations that would ultimately end with the international community ostracizing South African psychiatrists. From the late 1970s onwards, international governments and organizations vehemently criticized the practices of the apartheid government and those working within its constraints. These attacks on apartheid affected South African psychiatrists, who were working within both local and international mandates and ultimately resulted in a transformation in the way that South African psychiatrists saw themselves.

Through an examination of Scientology's role in South Africa, we not only see the complexity and changing nature of international relationships with the South African government, we also indirectly see the multifaceted relationship between psychiatric practitioners, the government and various other international players during apartheid South Africa. Although psychiatrists were not merely collaborators or agents of the apartheid state, and at times they actively advocated against apartheid legislation, there were times when they were also intrinsically ingrained with the government and supportive of apartheid practices. Scientology's anti-psychiatric actions in South Africa reveal an instance where the relationship between psychiatrists and the government was close enough to warrant the government to become concerned about Scientology, so much so that it set up a commission of inquiry into the organization in 1969.

SCIENTOLOGY VERSUS PSYCHIATRY

Scholars have generally examined the Church of Scientology as a sect, a cult, and a religion. Yet since its inception, disputes have arisen as to whether Scientology is a bona fide religion. In the late 1960s, the British, Australian, and South African governments initiated their own investigations into the matter and more recently, debates have continued within Germany and the United States as to whether Scientology constitutes a religion or not. Because Scientology was initially registered as an international organization in South Africa before it claimed non-profit church status, and because the CCHR, while affiliated with Scientology, was meant to be an "independent body" that was set up to "investigate and expose psychiatric violations of human rights and to clean up the field of mental healing,"[2] it makes sense to address it as a transnational organization, influenced at least in part by religious beliefs. This is not to deny that Scientology may be a bona fide religion, as some scholars such as Bryan R. Wilson have suggested,[3] but we can not ignore that it was first and foremost an international organization or that the CCHR sometimes operated as an independent commission without a specific religious mandate.[4]

In 1957, the Hubbard Association of Scientologists International (HASI) opened offices in Johannesburg and Durban, and another office opened in Cape Town in 1961 and in Port Elizabeth in 1962, the same year that Ron L. Hubbard sent a letter to all branches stating that Scientology was to slowly convert from business to church status.[5] Scientology's head office was located in England, with city offices or branches also in Australia, New Zealand, and the United States.[6] It has since opened offices in many countries including Russia, Germany, Austria, Portugal, Greece, Israel, Hungary, Netherlands, Japan, Italy, Denmark, Sweden, Norway, France, Belgium, Switzerland, Argentina, Colombia, Spain, Mexico, Venezuela, Zimbabwe, and more recently Botswana.

On 31 August 1965, HASI incorporated its South African branches under the name of the Hubbard Scientology Organisation in South Africa (Proprietary) Limited, with L. Ron Hubbard, his wife, Mary Sue Hubbard, and Marilyn Routsong as directors.[7] The full name change occurred in 1967. One of the main objectives of the South African city offices was to "conduct and carry on any and all kinds of scientific research especially with reference to the human mind, spirit and soul in mental psychosomatic and allied fields and the grounds and processes of human knowledge, and to apply that knowledge."[8] This mandate ironically reads as if the organization wanted to partake in psychological research, much like registered practitioners. Indeed, Stephen Kent, a critic of Scientology, argues that one of the objectives of the organization was to partake in a type of pseudo-psychiatry, that I would add had a goal to ultimately eclipse the work of psychiatrists.[9] The organization argues that it does not practice psychiatry of any kind, especially after it moved from being an incorporated organization to a church, but many of its practices did utilize a form of psychotherapy where individuals talked about themselves and their lives as a means to move to a higher mental level. In 1968, the Church of Scientology in South Africa (Proprietary) Ltd was incorporated under the Companies Act No 46. of 1926 to usurp the Hubbard Scientology Organisation in South Africa. From then on, it began promoting itself as a church in South Africa.[10]

Whereas specifics about South African members are difficult to obtain, from its publications and interactions with the South African government it is clear that the organization's membership was made up mostly of white South Africans. In 1971, the organization claimed that it had 25,000 members in South Africa. This, however, was the number of names on its mailing list. As many members repeatedly requested to be removed and were not, it is unclear how accurate this number is.[11]

From its inception in South Africa, the Church of Scientology tried to align itself with the apartheid state. The public relations committee, led by Joy Ollemans, directly targeted local municipality and government members in order to gain support for the organization's mandate. In 1966, the "Director of Success," P. Dallas, invited the Minister of Justice, B. J. Vorster, to a Scientology CLEAR congress in Johannesburg. The Minister declined.[12] The organization also employed the services of Jan Hendrik du Plessis, a former captain in the South African Police Force, who was to obtain them a meeting with Vorster and other members of parliament of South Africa, while simultaneously working on their behalf in Rhodesia. Throughout the 1960s, there are numerous examples where the organization expressed its direct support of the apartheid government. For example in a 1967 letter to the Minister of Justice and Prisons, P. C. Pelser, Joy Ollemans, on behalf of the organization, wrote:

> The Hubbard Scientology Organisation, by it's [sic] Code of Honour is loyal to the Government in power. It upholds and supports, inter alia, any and all measures taken by the Governemtn [sic] to handle those forces which seek to cause internal unrest and plan any form of overthrow of our fatherland."[13]

In a memorandum to the Minister of the Interior, S. L. Muller, the organization's public relations chief for Africa stated that the church "fully support[ed] the laws of the Government of South Africa" and in turn, did "not offer services to Africans."[14]

Scientology seemingly fit well with the National Party's objectives at the time. The theory of Dianetics, which is the foundation upon which Scientology is based, is inherently racist. Hubbard's *Dianetics: The Modern Science of Mental Health* argues that:

> Primitive societies, being subject to much mauling by the elements, have many more occasions for injury than civilized societies. Further, such primitive societies are alive with false data. Further, their practice of medicine and mental healing is on a very aberrative level [i.e., not rational] by itself. The number of engrams [i.e., mental image usually unconscious, involving pain or a threat to survival] in a Zulu would be astonishing. Moved out of his restimulative area and taught English he would escape the penalty of much of reactive data [i.e., unconscious or involuntary data]; but in his native habitat the Zulu is only outside the bars of a madhouse because there are no madhouses provided by his tribe. It is a safe estimate, and one based on better experience than is generally available to those who base conclusions on "modern man" by studying primitive races, that primitives are far more aberrated than civilized peoples. Their savageness, their unprogressiveness, their incidence of illness: all stem from their reactive patterns, not from their inherent personalities.[15]

He argued further that Africans were of too low intelligence for them to become effective members of the organization. In an auditor's bulletin he stated that:

> In South Africa they had a bit of the whip but everybody just gave up. The South African native is probably the one impossible person to train in the entire world—he is probably impossible by any human standard.[16]

Hubbard's racist rhetoric has been examined in detail by many critics of the organization and there is much to point to.[17] He specifically differentiated along color lines and argued that the "white race" is more "progressive but more frantic," while the "yellow and brown races do not understand white concern for 'bad conditions' since what are a few million dead men?"[18] We need to recognize that Hubbard's views of Africans at the time reflected common perceptions that existed about Africans in South Africa and around the world, and he certainly was not alone in his racism. Yet, despite his early racist rhetoric and the organization's continued assurance to the apartheid government that it supported its mandate, Scientologists were never able to gain the trust of government officials.

Early in 1966, the police began investigating the organization. This was mainly because of its attacks against psychiatry and prominent psychiatrists who were aligned with the state. Since opening its branches in South Africa, the Scientology organization began targeting individual practitioners who headed up the large mental health organizations or had political connections, such as T. J. Stander, the Director of the South African National Council for Mental Health, and his 1966 replacement, Jan H. Robbertze. They also targeted United Party Members, E. L. Fisher and A. Radford, both psychiatrists. All had been strong advocates for improvements to mental health care, albeit mostly for white men.

Ironically, it may also have been Hubbard's attempts to contact Prime Minister H. F. Verwoerd that made the police further suspicious of the organization. After Demetrio Tsafendas assassinated South Africa's Prime Minister, Hubbard publicly insinuated that the assassination of Verwoerd was a plot by the psychiatric profession to overthrow the government. He explains:

> In 1966 I wrote Dr Verwoerd the South African Prime Minister a letter that I had information that a dangerous situation might exist in his vicinity. He wrote back thanking me.
>
> I was suddenly made non persona grata in Southern Africa. Shortly afterwards Dr Verwoerd was assassinated by a psychiatric patient.[19]

Hubbard seems to be stretching connections between his status in southern Africa and Verwoerd's assassination somewhat. Although Hubbard claimed to be banned from southern Africa in general, he was in reality only asked to leave Rhodesia after the Ian Smith government rescinded his visa. [20] He claims to have attempted to gain admittance to South Africa, albeit with an expired passport, and ultimately rejected, but the government never had records of his application for a visa.[21] The myths surrounding Tsafendas and Verwoerd's assassination are interesting in themselves, considering that a known mental patient was able to obtain a position as parliamentary messenger. But the implication by Hubbard and his followers was that Tsafendas was a communist spy incited by psychiatrists who had their foul tentacles reaching into every part of society.

Hubbard's accusations emerged at a period of intense international skepticism of psychiatry, particularly because Soviet Russian psychiatrists were aiding the Soviet government in detaining political dissidents. Within the context of the Cold War, when the international community was already aware of the abusive practices by psychiatrists in the Soviet Union, Hubbard and Scientologists argued against what they called "Russian psychopolitics." They defined psychopolitics as "the art and science of asserting and maintaining dominion over the thoughts and loyalties of individuals, officers, bureaus, and masses and the effecting of the conquest of enemy nations through "mental healing."[22] In 1968, the organization issued a South African broadsheet arguing that "South Africa is a primary target for attack by subversive groups anxious to spread the influence and demoralization of the new Russian Imperial Empire."[23] They argued that "South Africa's vast natural wealth makes it an obvious plum for plucking" and that international financiers and an international communism cartel was financing media opposition to Scientology and more importantly, was expanding communism under the "guise of psychology." They also claimed that the World Federation of Mental Health was "an ideal tool for furthering international Communist causes and is well used for this purpose."[24] Because the National Council for Mental Health in South Africa belonged to the World Federation of Mental Health, they believed that it was part of the larger conspiracy against the South African government and Scientology.[25] Psychiatrists were the agents through which such communist psychopolitics were practiced. Hubbard, in a 1969 information letter related psychiatry as a political entity, and argued that "psychiatric treatment is actually psychiatric political treatment, nothing more, to rid the world of anyone who might disagree."[26]

With these depictions of psychiatry in mind, the South African Scientology branches launched a full front anti-psychiatric public relations campaign that played on the South African government's affront to international criticism and the public fears of internal threats of communism. In 1969, the Church of Scientology published articles and pictures in its *Total Freedom* circular that demonized psychiatrists, whom they argued were protecting "subversive interests" and were backed by international interest groups. Psychiatrists, they argued, were the enemy and perpetrators of death, destruction, and human rights abuse. One of the pictures, entitled "The Enemy Within!" is of a grim reaper straddling the Republic of South Africa and holding a scythe enscribed with the word "psychiatry." Another drawing titled, "Psychiatry's Triumph and Conquest of the world" depicts pychiatrists with devil horns and tails conducting labotomies and electric shocks on lines of waiting, straightjacketed patients. In the foreground, two small billboards read:

> Mobile Mental Health Clinic: Open in your area 24 hours a day. Electroshock, topectomy and lobotomy operations done on the spot. Fast

> helicopter service. It's your duty to inform us of anyone you think is in need of mental treatment. We'll see they get it within 24 hours! No charge to you. The government foots the bill.[27]

The article directly insinuated that there were incidents of "psychiatric patients involved in political assassination" and it once again promoted its loyalty to the South African government.[28] The Church of Scientology suggested that the government do the following:

1. That it fully supports and backs all religious groups and churches.
2. That it turn its attention to and cease to condone the seizure, torture and death carried out by psychiatry.
3. That it investigates fully, the enemy [psychiatry] within South Africa.
4. That it protects the citizens, social groups and businesses of the nation.
5. That it look into and handle possible corruption and foreign influence in the Government concerning Mental Health and Education.
6. That it provides an atmosphere and tranquility in which people can live their lives and conduct their affairs with some certainty and stability.
7. That it investigates fully the incidence of psychiatric patients involved in political assassination.
8. That it takes an active interest in establishing and guaranteeing real human rights, in that it ceases to attack groups loyal to South Africa.
9. That the government maintains its firm stand against subversive vested interests despite pressure brought to bear on it by international bankers who are also directors of psychiatric front groups.[29]

With the belief that psychiatrists were part and parcel of a communist plot to infiltrate South Africa, the organization also set about distributing bulletins defaming prominent psychiatrists. For example, in 1968, they sent out an informational letter to all the Members of Senate and the House of Assembly that contained an article claiming that E. L. Fisher, an MP and psychiatrist who was pushing for an inquiry into Scientology, was secretly a communist. Fisher responded by suing Scientology for damages for defamation. The case was settled out of court in 1969 and the organization paid "a substantial" amount in damages and attorney costs. They also issued a public apology.[30] Nevertheless, the organization continued its support of the apartheid government while attacking psychiatrists. In April 1969, it sent a telegram to S. L. Muller, Minister of Police House, stating that the organization supported the government and that the student protests that were taking place at the University of Witwatersrand were simply being organized by psychiatrists, who were trying to "destroy the security of

South Africa." The press, according to the executive council of Scientology, was part and parcel of this conspiracy against the government.[31] Because Scientology was attacking psychiatric practices worldwide, their actions were not playing out well in the media or with governments abroad. The state of Victoria in Australia had banned Scientology as "an evil influence and threat to the community," and Scientologists began to receive bad press in Europe and Australia. The English South African press also published a few negative articles about the organization. In response, in 1967, they sued the South African Associated Newspapers Limited for slander, but later withdrew their case.

This was only the first in a series of lawsuits launched by the organization. In 1969, the organization sued T. J. Stander and the South African National Council for Mental Health (SANCMH), which they only withdrew in 1977. The same year that they sued the SANCMH, the organization launched a civil action against Jan Hendrik du Plessis, the former captain in the South African Police force, whom had promised them a meeting with the Minister and other members of parliament and had never followed through.[32] The case was adjourned after an application of absolution by the organization.[33] As part of this strategy, on an international level, the Scientology organization offered rewards of $10,000 "for information leading to the arrest and conviction of the person or persons guilty of criminal libel and conspiracy which caused the government to act against [their] innocent organization in Australia, South Africa, America and England."[34] Members of the organization also wrote letters to the Minister of Health claiming that Scientology was being distorted by the public and that the organization remained "completely loyal to the country."[35]

Although the organization had intended to align itself with the apartheid government, what it had underestimated was the close relationship between some psychiatric practitioners, mental health associations, and government members. After all, Verwoerd himself had been a trained psychologist and some of the ministers of the government were mental health practitioners. Its attack on the SANCMH, for example, was ill-thought out. The SANCMH worked closely with the government shaping mental health programs, promoting additional accommodation for the mentally "disordered," conducting public education, and collecting data for advocacy. It registered as a welfare group in 1949 and formed the umbrella organization for regional mental health societies.[36] It regularly asked for inquiries into conditions for mental patients, advocated for services in the media and general public, and also participated in various government investigations, including ironically the one that the South African government established in 1969 on Scientology.[37]

Pushed by practitioners, the government set up a Commission of Enquiry into Scientology, which reported its findings in 1972. At first the Church of Scientology co-operated. But when members realized that the government intended to undermine their organization, they quickly withdrew.

Scientology received some great blows by the South African commissions' report. The committee recommended to extend legislation that would control the use of psychotherapy, which they thought Scientology was attempting to do, outlaw any security checking and intelligence actions undertaken by independent organizations such as Scientology, and suggested the prohibition of any "inaccurate, untruthful and harmful information in regard to psychiatry and the field of mental health in general."[38]

The result of the commission was that the apartheid government denied all of the allegations and argued that the Church of Scientology was simply "waging a vendetta" against the psychiatrists and the Secretary of Health.[39] It contended that many of the allegations of abuse were simply unwarranted and argued that many of the patients in private institutions chose the sub-standard conditions themselves. For example, G. De V. Morrison, a practitioner and MP, argued that "Bantu" individuals preferred to sleep on the ground, as he believed that "it was what they were used to." In addition, the government argued that the so-called "labor" that patients performed on a daily basis was simply a form of "occupational therapy" which was for their own good.[40] In order to prevent further publications regarding conditions within mental institutions, the apartheid government inserted a clause into the Mental Health Act that read:

> No person may, without the permission of the Secretary for Health— . . . publish or cause to be published in any manner whatsoever any false information concerning the detention, treatment, behaviour or experience in an institution of any patient or any person who was a patient, or concerning the administration of any institution, knowing the same to be false . . . [41]

The government also placed a ban on any photographs, sketches, or pictures depicting mental institutions or patients of any kind. Even though many opposition MPs during the House of Assembly debate on the amendment expressed concern over the loss of freedom of the press, the Nationalist government justified its actions by couching its arguments in terms of "protection of the vulnerable." H. Miller of the National Party argued that:

> the person whom it is endeavoured to protect, the person who requires [the] most protection; the person who, of all people, is the most vulnerable, viz. the mental patient, who very often has not the funds to look after himself and cannot take the step which any organization or institution could take of instituting an action of defamation against the newspaper or any other steps that may be necessary. Therefore, the objective here is to protect this most vulnerable section of the community.[42]

The banning of what the National Party considered "offensive material" was not a new concept for the apartheid government. Indeed, the control over the media was central to the apartheid government's notion of "moral purity."[43] The state had set up a Publications Control Board in 1963 to ensure that opposition to the apartheid government was controlled and liberal ideas from the international community were not imported. Therefore, the banning of any material concerning mental institutions was merely another element of the larger process of social control devised by the apartheid government.

But the Church of Scientology and CCHR did not cease its attacks on the actions of practitioners and for the most part, disillusioned by their failure to ally themselves with government officials against psychiatrists, they now began attacking the apartheid government itself. Using burgeoning international concerns about racial discrimination that existed in South Africa, they claimed that they too were victims of persecution by the apartheid government and continued their attacks on psychiatric practices in South Africa.[44] Throughout the 1970s, the organization sent press reports to various newspapers and organizations that highlighted the atrocious conditions within mental institutions. Indeed, they purposely disobeyed legislation and continued to persist in their attacks against psychiatry, sometimes even blatantly sending information to government officials. As mentioned at the beginning of this chapter, in 1976, there were reports of Church of Scientology members who broke into the offices of the Department of Health, church offices and the office of David Tabatznik, the director of Smith Mitchell institutions, in order to obtain information regarding mental health practices. In addition, the apartheid government accused the organization of forging the Secretary of Health's signature in a letter to the World Health Organization admitting to the various ill treatments that went on in private mental hospitals. Many MPs also complained about receiving copies of the "detestful little publication" of the organization's *Freedom* journal that contained information about the conditions in mental hospitals in their mailboxes whether they wanted them or not.[45]

The continued perseverance of Scientologists and their damning publications about conditions within the mental institutions sparked both domestic and international outrage at the abusive treatment of psychiatric patients. In South Africa, *Scope* magazine published a series of articles about an ex-psychiatric patient's experiences within mental institutions in South Africa. Horace Morgan, who had reportedly lost his memory in 1937 and was held in South African mental institutions for 37 years, spoke of his detainment and his attempts to escape from the abusive environment in which he had been placed. Based on interviews with Morgan and sections of his diary which he had kept during his stay in the mental hospitals, *Scope* reported physical and mental abuse that Morgan underwent during his long stay within a mental institution and argued that he had spent most of his "wasted, tragic life in a cage."[46]

Internationally, the Swedish newspaper *Dagens Nyherter* published a series of articles in 1976 depicting the terrible conditions in which patients lived and the abusive practices of psychiatrists in South African private mental institutions. That same year, the New York *Voice* published an article entitled, "New Kind of Concentration Camp Inside South Africa" that also depicted terrible conditions in South African mental hospitals. It attributed the exposure of these conditions to the Church of Scientology and included photographs taken by the *Freedom* News Service in South Africa.

In 1979, the annual Convention of Psychiatry was held at the University of Cape Town. International participants arrived to find a circular in their hotel rooms from the Church of Scientology reiterating many of its accusations of human rights abuse. At the conference, some international psychiatrists suggested using the Church of Scientology to gain further information into conditions in institutions, much to the chagrin of the Minister of Health.[47] The result of these actions on the part of Scientologists was an international awareness of the injustices of apartheid and ultimately the reproval of South African practitioners worldwide.

PHARMACEUTICAL COMPANIES AND SCIENTOLOGY'S NARCONON PROGRAM

Although psychiatric practitioners and Smith Mitchell remained the focus of Scientology's attack on South Africa, the organization also began to raise questions about the role of pharmaceutical companies in perpetuating human rights abuses. Because psychiatry was becoming more biologically orientated and pharmacological drugs more readily available, Scientologists argued that these drugs were being used as pharmaceutical straightjackets to control patients. The campaign against pharmaceutical companies, however, was never as vocal as that against Smith Mitchell institutions. Nevertheless, the CCHR claimed that drug companies were in cohort with the apartheid government. Because of the close relationship between South African mental institutions, pharmaceutical companies, private industry, and practitioners, Scientology argued that drugs were not only exploitative of individual patients' health, but also to the South African political system as well. Drugs were a means by which psychiatrists could ultimately gain control over the whole world.

Whereas pharmaceutical companies were privately owned and did much business in South Africa, most of South Africa's pharmaceuticals were bought and distributed by the state. Throughout the 1970s, scandals emerged about "collusion" between pharmaceutical companies to set prices. In 1973, three large pharmaceutical companies, Propan, S.C.S. and Lennon Laboratories met to set prices on various drugs for provincial tenders.[48] Scandals of bribery of doctors and government officials also erupted throughout the 1970s. In 1975, the Minister of Economic Affairs ordered a Commission of Inquiry into "monopolistic activities in the pharmaceutical industry." The Commission reported in 1978 that pharmaceutical companies were involved in "questionable business practices and actions." Little was done to legislate the industry, however, partly because an argument was made that steps were already taken by the industry to legislate itself and also because the largest purchaser of pharmaceutical drugs was the state.[49] Throughout the 1980s, the Pharmaceutical and Chemical Manufacturers Association of South Africa (PCMA) expressed concern at the way in which the state was limiting their ability to sell drugs in the country. Approximately two-thirds of all pharmaceutical drugs were bought and dispensed by the state. These were mostly bought at a tender price from a "restricted 'code' list of products" that reflected only a few of the drugs available, most of the prices of which had already been agreed to by the companies.[50] In order to expand their markets, pharmaceutical companies allegedly bribed individual practitioners by sending them on international trips, buying them new cars, clothes, and various other goods. Reports of "drug pushers, " "gifts to doctors" and "drug cartels" repeatedly emerged in the 1980s.[51]

It was not uncommon for medical companies to financially back or give gifts to National Party members. Admissions by doctors and ministers of receiving pay-offs from pharmaceutical companies were widespread.[52] The CCHR, however, was particularly interested in the connections between private mental institutions and the drug companies. In the 1980s, the owner of Smith Mitchell & Co, David Tabatznik, was one of the directors of South African Druggists. In 1983, its subsidiary companies, Labethica, Banstan Holdings, and Copybrook Investments were implicated in a "gift-giving" campaign that included the Registrar of the Medicines Council and the Deputy Director of Hospital Services in the Transvaal. After initial denials, the company eventually admitted to funding a six-week overseas holiday for G. Schepers, Transvaal Deputy Director of Hospital Services, and his wife.[53] Tabatznik, on the other hand, denied his involvement stating that as a non-executive member of the South African Druggists he had no knowledge of any gift giving campaigns.[54]

Similarly, in 1986, the South African Medical and Dental Council of South Africa investigated allegations that Protea Pharmaceuticals, along with RX Pharmaceuticals with which it had an agreement, was paying kickbacks to doctors for prescribing their drugs. Tabatznik had holdings in the Australian pharmaceutical drug companies of Alphapharm Pty Ltd. and Protea Pharmaceuticals (a subsidiary of Tabatznik owned Protea Holdings in South Africa). It was alleged that Alphapharm and Protea Pharmaceuticals tested drugs under investigation in Australia on Smith Mitchell patients.[55] Indeed, the pharmaceutical companies with which Tabatznik was involved did provide all the drugs for the Smith Mitchell institutions and many state hospitals. The investigation was later dropped and Tabatznik himself denied any direct connection to Alphapharm. However, he did state that his son, Anthony Tabatznik, and other family members held shares in Alphapharm. Tabatznik also admitted to having been a director of Protea Holdings, but had resigned ten years earlier.[56] Overall, David Tabatznik was reported to be a director of approximately 123 companies, some of which were general investment, multinational medical, and pharmaceutical companies, with subsidiaries in South Africa and in other countries such as Israel, Australia, and New Zealand. His private holdings were worth at least R120-million.[57] Tabatznik's substantial wealth and his likely use of "gifts" to Nationalist party members meant that he was able to gain lucrative government pharmaceutical contracts and continue to expand the Smith Mitchell conglomerate.[58]

In an attempt to counter what they saw as an increase and rise of the use of legalized psychological drugs, Scientology established its Narconon program. In 1973, Beverley van Wysel, a professor at the Microbiology and Virology department at the University of Stellenbosch, had checked herself into Scientology's Narconon program because of an addiction to painkillers and had gone through the "drugrundown" process. She was highly supportive of the program and questioned the 1969 investigation into Scientology:

> It works fantastically and the psychologists are of the same opinion. On all levels of our society today we have this problem of addicts . . . Narconon helps them all and brings them back to a place of health and happiness. Moreover, it is permanent and no follow-up treatment is needed.[59]

Narconon, a drug rehabilitation and drug avoidance organization that has three centers in South Africa today, is closely allied to the Church of Scientology and is simply an extension of their earlier practices against psychiatric drugs.[60] Whereas the battle against the pharmaceutical companies in South Africa never became as explosive as the accusations against Smith Mitchell and South African psychiatrists, it did raise questions about the way in which psychiatrists in cohort with pharmaceutical companies, were influencing policies on mental health.

THE INTERNATIONAL OSTRACIZING OF SOUTH AFRICAN PSYCHIATRISTS

When reports of human rights abuses continued to come out of South Africa, international psychiatric organizations worldwide began questioning the role of South African practitioners in the apartheid structure. In 1977, for example, in response to the article published in *Dagens Nyherter*, Jeanne-Martin Ciase, chairman of the United Nations Special Committee Against Apartheid, in conjunction with the World Health Organization (WHO) condemned the apartheid government for permitting inhumane treatment within psychiatric hospitals. He also called for an international investigation into psychiatric practices within South Africa.[61] As we have seen in the previous chapter, the World Health Organization, the International Red Cross, the American Psychiatric Association and the Royal College of Psychiatrists all conducted investigations into the allegations. One of the results of this was intense political interest in the activities in

Smith Mitchell & Co institutions. However, another debate also ensued as to whether or not South African practitioners should be sanctioned in some way. In 1982, John Dommissee invited Alan A. Stone, one of the members of the APA that investigated Smith Mitchell institutions, to partake in an international meeting to ban South African Psychiatrists from the World Psychiatric Association. Whereas Stone acknowledged the negative impact of apartheid, he replied that he did not think that psychiatrists were directly involved in human rights abuses such as torture.[62]

Nevertheless, the move to ban South Africans from international membership continued. In 1984, the World Psychiatric Association called for the exclusion of the SPSA (formerly SPNSA), which it deemed a "racist" organization that supported the apartheid government. That same year, the United Nations Centre Against Apartheid called for the expulsion of South African psychiatrists from international organizations.[63] In 1985, despite Stone's contention that South African psychiatrists were not directly involved in torture, the APA passed a resolution against apartheid. The resolution placed the burden of responsibility on the South African government, rather than individual practitioners by arguing that it

> strongly opposes the South African government's policy of apartheid as being discriminatory and damaging to the mental health of the South African people and further urges the Society of Psychiatrists of South Africa and the World Psychiatric Association to voice opposition to this policy and to launch a vigorous protest against all aspects of discrimination in that country.[64]

The World Federation of Mental Health followed up by suspending membership of South African organizations and discouraged its members from attending any events in the country. The World Medical Association also decisively moved its 1985 meeting from Cape Town to Brussels as a means to boycott South Africa.[65] In 1987, the Royal College of Psychiatrists urged its members to adhere to the Commonwealth Accord on Southern Africa of 1985, otherwise known as the Nassau Accord, that called for "discouragement of all cultural and scientific events except where these contribute towards the ending of apartheid or have no possible role in promoting it."[66]

European and North American psychiatrists also began writing condemning articles about South African psychiatric practices and pushed for further sanctions on South African practitioners. They ceased to invite South African psychiatrists to conferences, pressured their governments into not recognizing South African medical degrees, denied South African psychiatrists visitation rights to various mental institutions worldwide, and revoked South African psychiatrists' membership from international organizations. Individual psychiatrists such as S.P. Sashidharan working at the Royal Edinburgh Hospital argued that international sanctioning was not enough. Writing letters to the *Bulletin of the Royal College of Psychiatrists* and to the *Lancet* in 1985 he argued that although it was "gratifying to note that international campaigns on psychiatric abuses under apartheid are beginning to have an effect on SPSA, it will take more than self-congratulatory statements to convince us that medical institutions and psychiatrists in South Africa are not subservient to racist governmental policies in the field of health." He called for South African psychiatrists to challenge the apartheid government and accused some SPSA members of colluding with security police in detaining political opponents in psychiatric hospitals.[67] These actions on the part of the international community further isolated South African practitioners from the international psychiatric community.

Even though most South African practitioners were being pulled into the international criticisms of apartheid, most still saw themselves as removed from political mandates. Some initially defended their position, particularly those who belonged to the Medical Association of South Africa (MASA). MASA published a scathing rebuttal to the international community entitled, "Medical Journals and International Hate." MASA denied all accusations against it and argued that Western psychiatrists were ill-informed and simply wanted to "stir up international strife."[68] Other psychiatrists also responded quite vigorously to the allegations against them. For example, L. A. Hurst of the Witwatersrand Department of Psychiatry, in a letter to the *South African Medical Journal*, strongly supported Smith Mitchell. He argued that Smith Mitchell institutions had an "encouraging therapeutic atmosphere" that should be supported.[69] In addition, L. S. Gillis, on behalf of the Society of Psychiatrists of South Africa (a subsidiary of MASA) wrote a letter in rebuttal of the WHO's report to the British journal, *The Lancet*. He stated that it was "unwarranted to tie the apartheid tin to the tail of the psychiatric cat, no matter how much of a pleasing din it makes."[70] Gillis contended that the WHO report was full of inaccurate information. Rather, he argued that the WHO did not take into account the fact that "a much higher proportion of Blacks, particular those from country areas, become behaviourally disturbed (often uncontrollably) as a result of toxic, infective, or exhaustion syndromes."[71] His argument echoed those that suggested that Africans simply could not handle "modernity."

For many practitioners, the decision to criticize South Africa was an unfair one. Cliff Allwood, for example, pointed out that if the international community and Scientology really cared about abuses in institutions, they would have investigated conditions in other African countries:

> When the report came out it was a very particular report, it was particular report, because things weren't right. It was very interesting that at the time, just before that report came out, I visited mental hospitals in Kenya, in Zambia and in Zimbabwe, and I had never seen anything so terrible in all my life, in all three countries. The sad thing was that this was a time when we were being criticized, but nothing at all was being pointed at the way the human rights abuse and the disgusting way in which patients were being held in these places. I mean, Nairobi, it was absolutely awful. Never seen anything like it, never. The dilapidation

of the buildings, the dilapidation of the patients the lack of medication, it was just absolutely awful and dirty. I mean I grew up with a pig farmer, and I would never keep my pigs like that. So, one came back with a sense of disappointment and some anger and some cynicism about the integrity of the international community, that really they are about politics and not actually about the care of people.[72]

Whereas Allwood's comments reflect a resentment towards the fact that the international community was targeting South Africa when other independent African nations had seemingly worse conditions, he rightly points out that South Africa became the popular protest target. The world remained silent on other abuses on the continent. Partly this was because Scientologists were very active in exposing some of the abuses in South Africa. The accusations brought on by the Church of Scientology that psychiatrists were involved in unethical practices that supported the mandate of the apartheid government continued throughout the 1980s.

Although many practitioners initially were defensive, some practitioners re-evaluated their apolitical positions, particularly in the 1980s. A few became very vocal and active in arguing against apartheid policies. The apartheid government was to some extent pressurizing and ostracizing psychiatrists. For example, George Hart, a biological psychiatrist who worked at Tara Hospital in the 1980s and became Chair of Psychiatry in 1987, stated that:

The Department of Psychiatry at that time was in a particularly difficult position because we were already integrating our psychiatric outpatient services despite apartheid and when the so-called tricameral system came, they tried to reverse that. And so we had enormous amount of conflict with the people who paid us, which was a problem. And, you know, you took it as just part of your job really. When I went to Pretoria to see the people who actually paid me, which was an accident of history, virtually all the staff wouldn't speak to me. You know, you were sort of ostracised because you were seen as someone who wanted an integrated system and an integrated country and it created quite a lot of difficulty.[73]

Even MASA and its subsidiary, the SPSA, by the mid-1980s changed their initial defensiveness to respond to the academic boycott by declaring that it was opposed to "any discrepancies in the quality of psychiatric services for all" and acknowledged the negative effects of racism and discrimination on patients.[74] The SPSA declared its "opposition to any disparities in the quality of psychiatric services" and deplored the "potentially harmful psychological effects" of discrimination.[75] In 1980, the South African National Council of Mental Health (SANCMH) removed any racial terminology from its constitution, disobeying government orders not to do so, and in 1985, it expressed concern about the detention of young black children by police during turbulent periods.[76] Lage Vitus, the Deputy Director of the SANCMH and the Chairman of the Society of Social Workers expressed his dissatisfaction of the treatment of black patients in an article in the *Race Relations* magazine. He received a strong reaction from both H. Moross, who was then an advisor of Smith Mitchell & Co and from the Commissioner for Mental Health, P. H. Henning.[77] Whereas MASA, SPSA, and SANCMH did pass resolutions, this did not come soon enough and many practitioners left to form an alternative organization, the National Medical and Dental Association (NAMDA). NAMDA allowed practitioners to voice their concerns about apartheid policies and offer help to political detainees. The Detainees' Parents Support Committee was established in 1981/1982 by psychologists in the aftermath of a fellow physician's detention, Neil Aggett, who had helped organize mass action against apartheid policies and was detained for over seventy days without trial and died in police custody. After his death, the committee was set up to offer therapeutic services to detainee families. In conjunction with the rehabilitation Center for Torture Victims (RCT) in Copenhagen, volunteers set up detainee treatment teams of psychologists, social workers, and NAMDA doctors.[78]

Independently, some practitioners became caught up in treating prisoners or detainees and had to deal with the security police and government officials. Most felt they were protecting the individuals rather than encouraging their detention. As George Hart explains:

> We treated people in detention for many years. We saw large numbers of people who had been put into detention, not trialed for various reasons they were sent to us. Many occasions we got suicide attempts. And what the prison services really didn't want was to have a prisoner hang himself. But they were very reluctant to relinquish control over the patient, or prisoner, or detainee. So we had a very very difficult time with the security police, because they I suppose in a way controlled patients while in hospital. They had them guarded. We would see a patient, or detainee who had become depressed and wanted to commit suicide, and we would say, "one of the things this patient needs is to see his family." Of course they did not want the family to be seen because it was part of the system of interrogation to restrict visitors. It was probably wider than that. It was probably statements like, you know, "what's happening to your family, we will have them killed" or whatever, creating insecurity. So this contributed considerably towards people's moods, and could benefit people considerably if they saw their families. And this created a lot of difficulty because we felt that the social aspect, coming from a biologist, the social aspect was important. And we had frequent, I had frequent meetings with the top brass in the security and the district surgeons.[79]

Indeed, for practitioners, mental hospitals were a sanctuary for these individuals from harsher treatment. For example, in an interview with Cliff Allwood, when I asked whether the Church of Scientology's accusations about hospitals detaining political dissidents was correct, he vehemently replied: "That is rubbish; the treaty was rubbish. The only time that political dissidents came to the hospital is when we treated them. When they came then we kept them because it protected them from going back to jail."[80]

Ashwin Valjee also relates a similar experience. In the early 1980s, after leaving state employment to open up his own private practice, he was contacted by the local district surgeon and asked if he would examine some political detainees. One patient in particular stood out to him:

> I kept this chap for nine months in the hospital. You can imagine seeing him every day, on a daily basis there would be four security police guarding him. His name was Sirish Soni and they would interrogate me first before I could see him. They would want my ID book, or some reference, or what's the purpose of my visit. They would know everyday that I am coming there, but they would interrogate me on a daily basis—in the hospital. And then, once I have identified myself, then they would refuse to leave the room—you know, the bedroom hospital. Then I would say no, I've got to have privacy with my patient. They said no you cannot do this . . . they were not convinced that the guy was [mentally] sick, so they brought their own doctors from Pretoria, from the State. And you won't believe this but, I mean I could believe this, in those days the South African government was anti-Russian, the Soviet Union, you know. Do you know what they did? They brought a Russian psychiatrist . . . So he came and interrogated this patient in the hospital for four hours, and they had to stop it when the patient started screaming so loudly that the whole hospital could hear it. He cracked him. And he put in a report that said he did not agree with us.[81]

In an attempt to stop the security police from restraining and torturing the patient further, Valjee contacted other practitioners, such as Michael Simpson, Prof. Lassage and Jan Plomp and a Dr. Verster, all of whom filed an injunction in the supreme court and managed to get the patient released. Whereas we need to be careful that these recollections by practitioners were not simply selective memory in the wake of the end of apartheid, there is plenty of evidence that practitioners made a concerted effort to stop overt abuses in the system. Simpson himself was involved in numerous cases where he attempted to release dissidents who were the clear victims of "torture, and coercive and abusive interrogation."[82] Thus, although South African psychiatrists were becoming targeted internationally, there were a few that did become very active in challenging apartheid practices and redefining their roles in a more political way.

But when attempting to speak out about policies, practitioners were vulnerable to government sanction. Valjee, for example, often received threatening phone calls from the security police because he was asked to examine African National Congress members by the local district surgeon and at times deemed them in need of appropriate care outside the prisons.[83] Simpson recalled after Soni's release of being "subjected to severe professional and personal harassment, both within the University and Medical School and privately, receiving frequent death threats and other menacing calls, and what appeared to be some attempts on my life."[84] Allwood and Hart were threatened with disciplinary action and personal threats against their family members when they questioned the efficiency of the multi-tiered department system.[85] Jan H. Robbertze, who had criticized the government for its failures in mental health care and stood against apartheid policies was threatened by the government that he would lose his job. He was shut out from various committees and told to tow the party line.[86] Robbertze resigned from his job at MEDUNSA because he did not want to "perpetrate apartheid principles in psychiatry." Similarly, Jurgen Harms, left his job at the University of Free State because of discriminatory practices.[87] These are just a few examples of the challenges that practitioners faced. Critics of South Africa's psychiatrists argue that the personal risks that psychiatrists faced were small and that psychiatrists should have done more to prevent the abuse that occurred within the hospitals. Indeed, many psychiatrists today question whether they had done enough to try to change the system. As Allwood told me: "Perhaps one looks back and feels guilty that one should have been much more politically active, and we made all sorts of excuses for that I guess, but I guess we were frightened and we lived under a vicious regime."[88]

SCIENTOLOGY AFTER APARTHEID

Scientology, endorsed by celebrities and spread by dedicated members, has become a worldwide phenomenon. In 1997, the CCHR reiterated their allegations of psychiatric abuse in a written and oral submission to South Africa's Truth and Reconciliation Commission. They argued that South African psychiatrists were agents of the apartheid regime involved in human rights abuses against the majority black population. They also presented themselves as opponents of the apartheid government and what it called "psychiatric racism." We should be careful, however, not to see Scientologists and CCHR as simple opponents of the apartheid state. Indeed, Chris Owen, a vocal opponent of Scientology and who runs an anti-Scientology website, has since 1996 questioned the organization's anti-apartheid position. Owen argues that Scientology in South Africa was predominantly a pro-apartheid organization that "actively supported the forces and philosophy of apartheid."[89] His arguments have been reiterated and developed by other anti-Scientologists who argue that racism and paternalism are pervasive in

Hubbard's writings, yet remain widely accepted by his followers.[90] According to Ted Mayette and Keshet, Scientology's worldview revolves around "white privilege"' and its position in South Africa was merely one example of racist practices in Scientology that have occurred around the world.[91] Although Owen, Mayette, and Keshet's claims are generally well substantiated, their arguments with regards to South Africa focus mainly on Scientology in the 1960s and fail to recognize the fluid and changing nature of Scientology in South Africa thereafter. L. Ron Hubbard and early South African members were, as Owen suggests, fully supportive of the apartheid government in the 1960s, but he ignores the fact that the organization began to position itself against the apartheid government after 1972 and became a strong anti-apartheid voice in the 1970s and 1980s.

Scientology's change of heart from a supporter to opponent of the South African government was mainly because the organization failed to gain support from government officials. Thus, they changed tactics in order to help facilitate the spread of their beliefs. Racism was inherent in the early doctrine of Scientology and it would seem logical for the apartheid government to support, or at the very least allow them to continue to practice. Instead, the apartheid government deemed Scientology an enemy of the state. This was because of the close relationship between some psychiatrists and government officials in South Africa. Moreover, apartheid was about protection of the white community, mainly the white man. This protection of white (male) interests certainly relied on the exclusion of "non-whites," but the fact that the Scientology organization was targeting white community members and their connections with private industry, also made the government suspicious.

Despite its self-promoting reasons for positioning itself as an anti-apartheid organization and attacking the psychiatric field, we still need to acknowledge that the Church of Scientology of South Africa played an important role in publicizing the overall substandard conditions in the state-contracted hospitals and began a succession of investigations by various international organizations to investigate allegations of abuse that would lead to the boycott of South African psychiatrists in the United States and Europe.

The CCHR continues to use its past actions in South Africa to present Scientology as an anti-racist and anti-psychiatric organization in their numerous flyers and online publications in their bid to actively recruit members. This raises interesting questions about how Scientology positions itself currently now that apartheid regulations no longer exist. Chris Owen warns us that Scientology is attempting to infiltrate the business community and is trying to "win" South Africa and ultimately the continent.[92] Since the end of apartheid, there have been accusations of an alliance between the Inkatha Freedom Party (IFP) and Scientology. In 1994 the IFP called for an investigation into South Africa's mental health institutions and in 1997, the Scientology organization "bestowed a 'freedom medal' on Lawrence Anthony, KwaZulu-Natal businessman and confidant of Mangosuthu Buthelezi." [93] The Inkatha Freedom Party (IFP) denies such links.[94] Nevertheless, Scientology has continued to spread throughout the region and has stepped up its actions targeting members in malls, leading education missions into local schools and has recently purchased the 64,000 square foot Kyalami Castle as a "spiritual retreat" in Johannesburg.[95] Scientology is currently leading missions into Botswana where in 2006, they claimed to have contacted 41,300 people, begun missions in Namibia and recently opened up a new church in northern Johannesburg.[96] It has had some success in marketing itself to schools and promotion of its education programs, offering "de-stressing" courses to the South African police force and in 2000, after a 40-year battle, the church was granted the right to perform marriages. But the organization has yet to fully affiliate itself or infiltrate the present government or rid South Africa of its psychiatrists, but it is not for their failure of trying. At their grand opening of the Church of Scientology in Johannesburg in 2003, the Minister of Arts, Culture, Science and Technology thanked the church for their work in highlighting human rights abuses and offering their "Education Alive" program to youth throughout the country. He praised their ability to contribute to the "African Renaissance" of the country and to the audience he announced: "I sincerely believe that you and your church will play a vital role in realizing that renaissance, for all the citizens of Africa."[97] In a 2003 speech given by David Miscavige, Hubbard's former personal aide and the Chairman of the Board of the Religious Technology Centre, while visiting South Africa told the crowd that "you don't just represent the hopes and dreams of a continent, you represent the hopes and dreams of all civilization." He continued to perpetuate the vision of the Church of Scientology has being an anti-apartheid group, by stating in a speech to members:

> LRH [L. Ron Hubbard, Scientology's founder,] envisioned a special role for this [South African] nation as a point of safety to yet salvage man no matter the potential devastation at the hands of a madman.
>
> That's why he descended on Johannesburg, in 1960, to take the helm of a fledgling Church. But if those were his reasons for embarking to South Africa, it took on a whole new meaning when he arrived. For what he found was a land representing both all that is good in this world, and all that is bad.
>
> In terms of the bad, a single word said it all, aprtheid and the suppression of virtually every indigenous people, perpetrated by the same psychiatric ideologies that laid 6 million to rest under the banner of eugenics during the second World War.[98]

The madman in this case was supposedly communsim, but we also see how the association of South African practitioners with Nazi Germany continues to pervade the rhetoric. Scientologists, it seems, will not be relinquishing this association any time soon.

Conclusion

It has often been stated that in the nineteenth and twentieth centuries "the personnel of science and medicine replaced the churches' ministers and priests as the custodians, confessors and controllers of [deviant behaviour]."[1] In apartheid South Africa, the formation and perpetuation of racial segregation ideologies, heteropatriarchalism, and their dependence on widespread social control was indeed closely linked to the discourse and actions of social scientists and medical practitioners. The classification of individuals lay in the hands of these professionals upon whom the state relied to implement its social policy. Throughout the different stages of the apartheid project, there were practitioners who explicitly supported the government's racial segregationist mandate and, indeed, some set out to justify it. Social policy in the years leading up to and during apartheid was extremely racialised and heteropatriarchal, and mental health services reflected the discriminatory nature of the system.

South Africa's history of apartheid, and indeed psychiatry in general, at times seems like a satirical work of fiction with various characters all playing odd roles in attempts to control the actions of the population. Yet, the impact of these actions were convoluted and severe. In 1997, the South African Truth and Reconciliation Commission (TRC) held a mental health sector workshop to highlight the need to understand the trauma induced by apartheid practices. Practitioners, staff, Scientologists, former patients, and abusees submitted reports to the commission. The TRC highlighted the role of the Medical Association of South Africa, the overarching organization for the Society of South African Psychiatrists, in placidly accepting apartheid policies in all medical practices.

The TRC focused on the abuses that occurred within the medical system, and cases of abuse certainly emerged, but more research was deemed necessary to understand the true implications of practitioners' actions. Outside of the TRC, significant evidence exists that supports the notion that practitioners were implicated in human rights abuses. Some practitioners were involved in interrogations of political detainees. Aversion therapy was certainly used, unnecessary deaths occurred in mental institutions, and racism within the treatment and rhetoric of practitioners was evident.

But the pervasive diametrical oppositions of colonizer/colonized, abuser/abusee, practitioner/patient, mad/sane as forwarded by critics such as the Church of Scientology can not be clearly defined. It is suspect to suggest that all practitioners were simply instruments of the state. First, state processes were often obscure and inept. Despite its large bureaucratic presence, the apartheid government's effectiveness was, in the words of Deborah Posel, "eroded by emerging structural inefficiencies and skills shortages" that were a result, paradoxically, of its "determination to keep vast categories of the workforce white and, if possible, Afrikaner."[2] The contradictions and inefficiencies of the state naturally filtered into the mental institutions. As we have seen, in the early years of apartheid, the government's desire to relegate administrative, nursing, and medical positions within the institutions to whites and its unwillingness to invest in mental health services meant that serious staff shortages arose. In turn, it was often forced to rely on unskilled labor. When staff shortages reached a crisis in the 1960s and blacks were allowed to take on some of the lower-paid nursing positions, the government's discriminatory education system merely perpetuated the crisis.

More importantly, however, in order for apartheid to work, it relied on maintaining a dominant white male workforce. Most beds in state hospitals were allocated to those deemed more essential to the apartheid project—white men. Recognizing this distinction challenges those accusations of practitioners as simply being a contrivance of the state. Although, the government did attempt, in vain, to deal with its disordered black population through repatriation strategies, the use of the judicial and prison system, and eventually by detaining them in contracted facilities, even in these areas, policies were confusing and obscure.

Under these circumstances, it is not surprising that mental health practitioners dealt with patients in a limited and ad hoc manner, a manner that only reinforced custodial care. Nor is it surprising that staff and patients became increasingly frustrated and attempted to challenge the system. At the end of the Second World War, South African practitioners initiated a revamping of custodial practices by advancing psychobiological approaches to patients. Beginning in the 1950s, many practitioners challenged custodial practices even further by forwarding community psychiatric practices, and in the 1970s some endeavored to address racial discrepancies in the system by advancing cross-cultural psychiatric approaches and challenging government views about homosexuality. However, for the most part, their efforts were obscured by the socio-political climate in which they practiced.

This is not to suggest that practitioners simply opposed the government. Rather, like those of the government, practitioners' views were also contradictory. They held differing opinions as to the etiology and treatment of mental disorder, and at times, their ideas may have both supported and challenged apartheid ideologies. Whereas some genuinely attempted to offer better treatment within mental hospitals through ideas of deinstitutionalization and cultural-sensitive practices to patient care, their endeavors were also constrained by their own desires for higher professional status and apartheid's discriminatory social policies. Nevertheless, the fluidity and contradictory nature of practitioners' beliefs, along with the ineffective nature of the mental health system did diffuse state authority somewhat.

Those classified as mentally disordered clearly suffered the brunt of the inadequacies of the system. All patients, even whites, were adversely affected. Alienated and marginalized from society, their voices were obscured by an increasingly bureaucratic system that failed to invest in mental health services. The letters of patients and family members, and the cases of abuse, incarceration, and even death testify to the atrocious conditions that they endured. Black patients were even more marginalized through repatriation and release from the institution. But in the context of apartheid South Africa, this may not have been completely negative, especially given governments' use of mental institutions to incarcerate political opponents, practices made infamous by Soviet Russia and Nazi Germany. Moreover, even those who were institutionalized were able to contest their positions, albeit with little success.

Underlying these arguments are understandings of what constitutes madness. Some would argue that what defines psychiatric illness is clearly defined in the *Diagnostic and Statistical Manual of Mental Disorders*, the manual to which all practitioners refer in order to make a diagnosis. Others would argue that cultural and social circumstances are more important in determining the definition of madness. Not contesting either view, this book has been more concerned with the views of practitioners and patients in their particular historical context. When viewing ideas of madness through an historical lens, one sees that they were sometimes grounded in biomedical evidence, claiming the authority of scientific fact, but were also always socially conditioned. This is, of course, not unique to South Africa. Indeed, worldwide, practitioners adopted a mix of biological and social understandings of mental health. South Africa, like in many other colonial settler states, relied on racial differentiation to shape its implementation of mental health practices. But, unlike many western mental institutions and even many institutions in African countries, women, particularly black women, were the least likely to be detained within the walls of South African mental institutions during apartheid, and black men were more likely to escape being admitted. Instead, South African mental hospitals reflected the government's racial and gendered hierarchies, privileging the white male. In this, we find the contradictions of the country's mental health process. Whereas the government did use institutions to control some of those who deviated from the socio-political norm, it also paradoxically promoted their rehabilitative nature through its concern with maintaining the dominance of heterosexual white men.

The blurred line between concepts of "madness" and "normality" has meant that this book has had to have a multifaceted scope. As notions of madness touch on many aspects of society, I certainly could not cover all these areas. Thus, there are many questions that remain. For example, the views of nursing staff have only been touched on in this book. Whereas Shula Marks has conducted extensive research on nurses within the general health system, little has been written specifically about the nurses in the psychiatric sector.[3] Because of their integral role within the institutions, their views cannot be dismissed. Social workers, physiotherapists, and psychologists also played important supporting roles. More importantly, however, the number of individuals consulting healers far outweighed those in contact with white practitioners. Healers' views have mostly been obscured by Western approaches to mental health, and whereas their profession is gradually obtaining recognition today,[4] an analysis of their role during apartheid can tell us more about the views of patients and families, and their ability to resist apartheid strategies.[5]

The legacy of apartheid on individuals pervades every aspect of South African mental health today. It is easy to suggest that because apartheid has ended, that mental health services will now be effective. South Africa seemingly enshrines psychiatric rights in its constitution in Article 12.2:

> Everyone has the right to bodily and psychological integrity, which includes the right
>
> a) to make decisions concerning reproduction;
> b) to security in and control over their body; and
> c) not to be subjected to medical or scientific experiments without their informed consent.[6]

But its current Mental Health Care Act does little to deal with this issue in its discussion of psychiatric treatment. Although South Africa revamped its mental health policy in 2002, and it shows large strides in recognizing patients' rights, it fails to recognize the intrinsic inequalities of the system and little has changed. In some cases, it has become worse.[7] The current South African government's inability to address its high levels of poverty, unemployment, and social inequality has merely perpetuated the lower levels of health care. In a 1998 study, members of the Centre of Health Policy found that even after the end of apartheid, racially integrated institutions justified their better treatment of white patients over blacks through the concept of "cultural" difference.[8] In 2004, Kohn et al. conducted an investigation five years after the end of apartheid to see if psychiatric services for Africans had improved. They found that in general, psychiatric care had deteriorated for both black and white patients and racial discrimination had continued. White patients continued to be overrepresented in the hospitals.[9] A 2006 investigation by *The* [Johannesburg] *Star* revealed that there were more than 300 potentially criminally insane individuals awaiting trial who had been housed for over a year in prison before they could be observed for the legally prescribed thirty day period in an observation ward at Sterkfontein, Valkenburg, or Weskoppies mental institutions.[10] Reports of murders by released patients have increased over the past few years, and practitioners have admitted to having to release potentially "unstable state patients" prematurely because of the lack of resources."[11] Stories of released patients being tied or locked up by family members in order to prevent them from wandering off or cases of desperate grandmothers begging courts to charge their children with a crime so that they could obtain the mental health care they think is necessary have escalated.[12]

Staff shortages, lack of sufficient beds, and limited funding for mental health all have contributed to these human rights violations. My contact with those working in the mental health sector revealed an immense desperation among those who partook in the mental health system, all of whom voiced the need for further state assistance in psychiatry. From healers who remarked on the lack of support they had when dealing with those who need care, often having to house patients in their homes, to patients who called me desperate for help, hoping that as someone who lived in North America that I would be able to help them, the situation is certainly critical. Psychiatrists also talked about the dire situation that the psychiatric field was in—that the qualified were leaving the country to work elsewhere. Western countries, including the U.S., Canada, Britain, etc. have actively sought out health professionals from South Africa and encouraged them to immigrate.

The basic questions concerning defining madness, the debates about proper policies, the divergent aims of protecting the public versus deinstitutionalization, the moral and legal dilemma of psychiatry and psychology's role in the judicial system, and how to effectively offer treatment to individuals needing it, all have remained unanswered, despite significant discussion about this issue. South African psychiatrists find themselves in a similar, if not more dismal situation than during the apartheid years. More importantly, patients are worse off today than during apartheid. Practitioners are far from being agents of the state, yet like their historical counterparts, they face similar restrictions on their activities and continue to perpetuate human rights abuses and custodial practices because of limited resources. Although community psychiatry is being re-promoted practitioners are often unable to implement these practices effectively.

Private institutions are becoming increasingly popular in today's South Africa, and with multinational corporations replacing the nation-state in socio-political influence, we need to re-examine our ideas of power structures. Michel Foucault's discussion of the state as all powerful is certainly representative of the period of which he writes. But we need to understand the rise of private health care and its influence on power structures. Are private organizations agents of the state? If not, then what are their objectives? Within the context of the National Party's gradual adoption of capitalist policies, albeit with state control, it is not surprising that in the late 1970s and 1980s semi-private institutions emerged to treat black patients. But Smith Mitchell & Co, now Lifecare Special Health

Services (Pty) Ltd (a subsidiary of Afrox Healthcare), continues to provide long-term care in South Africa, more so today than during apartheid. Their involvement in South Africa raises interesting questions about the influence and impact of the international community and private industry on South Africa and vice versa. Pharmaceutical companies are also playing an increasingly important role. Merck, for example, has financed a medical ethics center in Pretoria[13] and GlaxoSmithKline sponsored South Africa's 2007 psychiatric conference at Sun City. David Robert Lewis, a member of MindFreedom International, a mental patient rights advocacy group, has argued that:

> There is a direct correlation between drug company sponsorship of psychiatric conferences and the growth of mental illness around the world in a syndrome compounded by a strategic redefinition of mental health by big pharma in terms of production and consumption, i.e., the creation of consumers and markets.[14]

We need to examine further whether or not the involvement of private industry is a productive avenue to deal with inequalities of psychiatric care in South Africa. Certainly South Africa's public health care system is sorely lacking. However, as wealthy individuals obtain their own health care through private health care companies, whereas those without coverage stand in lines for often inadequate health care, socio-economic divisions, often along racial lines, continue to be perpetuated.

Moreover, South Africans' views towards the mad have not drastically changed. When conducting research for this book, I heard a plethora of opinions about those with mental challenges, from comments such as "You know, Hitler may have been on to something" to "Shame, they really need to be fixed [sexually]." In a country where there are high levels of post-traumatic stress disorder and high levels of daily stress, one would have thought that there would have been more empathy and compassion to those with mental difficulties. Yet, worldwide, and in Africa in particular, we are a far cry from understanding the rights and needs of individuals with mental challenges.

If South Africa, and indeed the world, is to move beyond the discriminatory practices that still exist within the system, it should not only acknowledge the socio-political manifestation of psychiatry, but also needs to accept that institutions have long been constructed along convoluted and heteropatriarchal, class, and racist ideals that have been embedded into the system. Moreover, transparency in transactions with patients is vital in order for individuals to become agents in their desired treatment. Such a recognition will be the first step in creating a successful strategy in removing those deemed deviant from the margins of society.

Notes

NOTES TO THE PREFACE

1. To protect the privacy of many individuals who are still alive, names of patients have been changed.
2. Using the 1980 exchange rate.
3. See Truth and Reconciliation Commission of South Africa (TRC), *Truth and Reconciliation Commission of South Africa Report* (Basingstoke and Oxford: Macmillan Reference Limited, 1998), vol. 4; Citizens Commission on Human Rights (South Africa & International), "Submission to the South African Truth & Reconciliation Commission: The Tragedy of Psychiatry Creating Apartheid," May 1997; Peter Deeley, "Scandal of the Money-Making Mental Homes," *The Observer* (London), 3 June 1979; and Fleur de Villiers, "Millions out of Madness," *Sunday Times* (Johannesburg), 27 April 1975. See also Hansard, House of Assembly Debates (HAD), vol. 60 (18 February 1976), col. 1522 displaying international newspaper reports and an article discussing a patient's experience from *Scope* magazine.

NOTES TO THE INTRODUCTION

1. Fleur de Villiers, "Millions out of Madness," *Sunday Times*, 27 April 1975.
2. *Peace and Freedom*, vol. 3, suppl., January 1976.
3. "A New Kind of Concentration Camp in South Africa," *New York Voice*, 21 May 1976.
4. "Calgary Psychiatrist Faces 21 Sex Assault Charges Involving Patients," *The Globe and Mail* (Calgary) http://www.theglobeandmail.com/news/national/prairies/calgary-psychiatrist-faces-21-sex-assault-charges-involving-patients/article1657274/ (accessed 12 Aug 2010).
5. A few South African political dissidents were institutionalized, but these were exceptions to the rule. As Teresa Smith and Thomas Oleszczuk point out, "the Soviet experience was unique in both the size and degree of organization of nonconformist informal groups." Theresa C. Smith and Thomas A. Oleszczuk, *No Asylum: State Psychiatric Repression in the Former USSR* (New York: New York University Press, 1996), 2. For further information on psychiatry during Soviet Russia, see Paul Calloway, *Russian/Soviet and Western Psychiatry: A Contemporary Comparative Study* (New York: Wiley, 1993); Harvey Fireside, *Soviet Psychoprisons* (New York: Norton, 1979); and Sidney Bloch and Peter Reddaway, *Russia's Political Hospitals: The Abuse of Psychiatry in the Soviet Union* (London: Gollancz, 1977).

6. For most of the apartheid era, the government failed to collect viable census data for the black population. The first authoritative census was conducted in South Africa in 1996, when it revealed that the 11 percent of South Africa's population was white, 77 percent was black, 9 percent were mixed-race, and 3 percent was Indian or Asian. Statistics South Africa, "The People of South Africa Population Census, 1996" http://www.statssa.gov.za/census01/Census96/HTML/default.htm.
7. Philip Corrigan and Derek Sayer, *The Great Arch: English State Formation as Cultural Revolution* (Oxford, New York: Blackwell, 1985), 1.
8. Corrigan and Sayer, 4.
9. Linzi Manicom, "Ruling Relations: Rethinking State and Gender in South African History," *Journal of African History* 33 (1992): 456.
10. Michel Foucault, *Madness and Civilization: A History of Insanity in the Age of Reason* (New York: Random House, 1965), 243.
11. Michel Foucault, *Discipline and Punish: The Birth of the Prison* (New York: Pantheon Books, 1977).
12. Foucault's later work on power structures shows how power is a productive process rather than merely a disciplinary one. However, it is his earlier work that has influenced mental health historians the most. Michel Foucault, *The Birth of the Clinic: An Archaeology of Medical Perception* (New York: Pantheon Books, 1973), 197.
13. Michel Foucault, "Governmentality," in *The Foucault Effect: Studies in Governmentality, With Two Lectures by and an Interview with Michel Foucault,* eds. Graham Burchell, Colin Gordon, and Pete Miller (London: Harvester Wheatsheaf Press, 1991), 92.
14. Foucault, "Governmentality," 95.
15. O. Mannoni, *Prospero and Caliban: The Psychology of Colonization,* translated by Pamela Powesland (New York, Frederick A. Praeger, 1964), 26–27, 39, 89.
16. Mannoni, 80.
17. Mannoni, 97–109.
18. Frantz Fanon, *Black Skin White Masks*, translated by Charles Lam Markmann (New York: Grove Press, 1952, 1967), 9–16, 83–108.
19. Mannoni, 110.
20. Albert Memmi, *The Colonizer and the Colonized*, translated by Howard Greenfeld (Boston: Beacon Press, 1965), 20, 146–147.
21. Memmi, 150.
22. Frantz Fanon, *The Wretched of the Earth*, translated by Constance Farrington (New York: Grove Press, 1963), 249.
23. Frantz Fanon, *A Dying Colonialism*, translated by Haakon Chevalier (New York: Grove Press, 1959, 1965), 121, 131.
24. Fanon, *A Dying Colonialism*, 145.
25. Lynette Jackson, *Surfacing Up: Psychiatry and Social Order in Colonial Zimbabwe.* History of Psychiatry Series (New York: Cornell University Press, 2005).
26. Glen S. Elder, *Hostels, Sexuality, and the Apartheid Legacy: Malevolent Geographies* (Athens, Ohio: Ohio University Press, 2003).
27. Denise Russell, *Women, Madness and Medicine* (Cambridge: Polity Press, 1995), 33, 38, 155; and Phyllis Chesler, *Women and Madness* (New York: Avon, 1983).
28. Lynette Aria Jackson, "Narratives of 'Madness' and Power: A History of Ingutsheni Mental Hospital and Social Order in Colonial Zimbabwe, 1908–1959" (Ph.D. diss., Columbia University, 1977), 211.
29. Quoted in Deborah Posel, *The Making of Apartheid 1948–1961: Conflict and Compromise* (Oxford: Clarendon Press, 1991), 81.

30. Elaine Showalter, *The Female Malady: Women, Madness, and English Culture, 1830–1980* (New York, Pantheon, 1985); Genevieve Lloyd, *The Man of Reason: "Male" and "Female" in Western Philosophy* (Minneapolis: University of Minnesota Press, 1984); and Shoshana Felman, "Women and Madness: The Critical Phallacy," *Diacritics* 5 (1975): 2–10. For further information on the connections between gender and madness, see Janet M. Stoppard and Linda M. McMullen, *Situating Sadness: Women and Depression in Social Context* (New York: New York University Press, 2003); Joan Busfield, *Men, Women and Madness: Understanding Gender and Mental Disorder* (London: Macmillan, 1996); Christina Mazzoni, *Saint Hysteria: Neurosis, Mysticism, and Gender in European Culture* (Ithaca, NY: Cornell University Press, 1996); Jane M. Ussher, *Women's Madness: Misogyny or Mental Illness?* (New York: Harvester Wheatsheaf, c1991); Yannick Ripa, *Women and Madness: the Incarceration of Women in Nineteenth-Century France,* translated by Catherine du Peloux Menagé (Cambridge: Polity Press, c1990); and P. Susan Penfold and Gillian A. Walker, *Women and the Psychiatric Paradox* (Montreal: Eden Press, 1983).
31. Ronald Bayer, *Homosexuality and American Psychiatry: The Politics of Diagnosis* (New York: Basic Books, 1981), 3.
32. Russell, 61.
33. Similarly, Diana Gittins suggests that women during twentieth-century England used mental asylums as a refuge away from their expected social roles. Diana Gittins, *Madness in its Place: Narratives of Severalls Hospital, 1913–1997* (London and New York: Routledge, 1998).
34. Showalter, 4–5.
35. Showalter, 5.
36. Megan Vaughan, *Curing their Ills: Colonial Power and African Illness* (California: Stanford University Press, 1991), 101.
37. Anne McClintock, *Double Crossings: Madness, Sexuality and Imperialism: The 2000 Garnett Sedgewick Memorial Lecture* (Vancouver: Ronsdale Press, 2001), 23.
38. McClintock, 18.
39. McClintock, 23.
40. Mahmood Mamdani, *Citizen and Subject: Contemporary Africa and the Legacy of Late Colonialism* (Princeton: Princeton University Press, 1996), 27.
41. Phillip Bonner, Peter Delius, and Deborah Posel, "The Shaping of Apartheid: Contradiction, Continuity and Popular Struggle," in *Apartheid's Genesis: 1935–1962* (Johannesburg: Wits University Press, 1993), 1–2.
42. Bonner, Delius, and Posel, 2.
43. For the most part, studies of the history of mental health in southern Africa have focused on the colonial period before apartheid. See, for example, Julie Parle's *States of Mind: Searching for Mental Health in Natal and Zululand, 1868–1918* (Scottsville: University of Kwazulu Natal Press, 2007); Jackson (2005); Robert R. Edgar and Hilary Sapire, *African Apocalypse: The Story of Nontetha Nkwenkwe, a Twentieth-Century South African Prophet* (Johannesburg: Witwatersrand University Press, 1999); Sally Swartz, "Lost Lives: Gender, History and Mental Illness in the Cape, 1891–1910," *Feminism & Psychology* 9, no. 2 (1999): 152–158; Sally Swartz, "Colonizing the Insane: Causes of Insanity in the Cape, 1891–1920," *History of the Human Sciences* 8, no. 4 (1995): 39–57; Sally Swartz, "The Black Insane in the Cape, 1891–1920," *Journal of Southern African Studies* 21, no. 3 (1995): 399–415; Shula Marks, ed., *Not Either an Experimental Doll: The Separate Worlds of Three South African Women*, (London: The Women's Press, 1987); M. Minde, "History of Mental Health Services in South Africa: Part II. During

the British Occupation," *South African Medical Journal* 48, no. 38 (1974): 1629–1632; M. Minde, "The History of Mental Health Services in South Africa: Part I. In the Days of the Dutch East India Company," *South Africa Medical Journal* 48, no. 29 (1974): 1270–1272; and M. Minde, "Mental Health—Past, Present and Future," *South African Medical Journal* 29, no. 47 (1955): 1124–1127.

44. Erwin Heinz Ackerknecht, *A Short History of Psychiatry* (New York and London: Hafner, 1968), 39.
45. In this instance, non-systematic ideas are those that are commonly viewed as out of the "norm" or "irregular," and/or exist outside Western scientific systems of research or study. These are usually ideas that are *seen* to lack any systematic arrangement or proof, and are often dismissed as archaic and inexplicable, particularly by scientific psychiatrists.
46. Ackerknecht, 1.
47. Bayer, 9.
48. Russell.
49. Edward Shorter, *A History of Psychiatry From the Era of the Asylum to the Age of Prozac* (New York: John Wiley & Sons, 1997).
50. Norman Dain, "Anti-psychiatry," in *American Psychiatry After World War II (1944–1994)*, eds. Roy W. Menninger and John C. Nemiah (Washington: American Psychiatric Press, 2000), 286.
51. His italics. Roy W. Menninger, "Introduction," in *American Psychiatry After World War II*, xxiii.
52. Ran Greenstein, "The Study of South African Society: Towards A New Agenda For Comparative Historical Inquiry," *Journal of Southern African Studies* 20, no. 4 (1994): 643.
53. See Susanne Klausen, "'For the Sake of the Race': Eugenic Discourses of Feeblemindedness and Motherhood in the South African Medical Record, 1903–1926," *Journal of Southern African Studies* 23, no. 1 (1997): 28.

NOTES TO CHAPTER 1

1. Erwin H. Ackerknecht, *A Short History of Psychiatry*, 2nd revised ed. (New York: Hafner, 1968), 39.
2. See Albert Kruger, *Mental Health Law in South Africa* (Durban: Butterworth, 1980); Lewis A. Hurst and Mary B. Lucas, "South Africa," in *World History of Psychiatry*, ed. John G. Howells (New York: Brunner/Mazel, 1975); M. Minde, "History of Mental Health Services in South Africa: Part III. The Cape Province," *South African Medical Journal* 48, no. 53 (1974): 2230–2234; M. Minde, "History of Mental Health Services in South Africa: Part II. During the British Occupation," *South African Medical Journal* 48, no. 38 (1974): 1629–1632; Charlotte Searle, *The History of the Development of Nursing in South Africa, 1652–1960* (Cape Town: Struik, 1965); and M. Minde, "Mental Health—Past, Present and Future," *South African Medical Journal* 29, no. 47 (1955): 1124–1127.
3. As Hurst and Lucas point out, the Cape settlement was established as a rehabilitative centre where ships could purchase food and goods that would offer holistic help. One of the first establishments in the Cape was a hospital. Thus, from the early years, the Cape became a hospice for sick individuals. Hurst and Lucas, 600–601. For further information on pre-union mental care, see Harriet Deacon, "Racial Categories and Psychiatry in Africa: The Asylum on Robben Island in the Nineteenth Century," in *Race, Science and Medicine, 1700–1960*, eds. Waltraud Ernst and Bernard Harris (London; New York:

Routledge, 1999), 101–122; M. Minde, "History of Mental Health Services in South Africa: Part II."; M. Minde, "The History of Mental Health Services in South Africa: Part I. In the Days of the Dutch East India Company," *South African Medical Journal* 48, no. 29 (1974): 1270–1272; Percy Ward Laidler, *South Africa: Its Medical History 1652–1898: a Medical and Social Study* (Cape Town, C. Struik, 1971); Searle, 108–123; Edmund H. Burrows, *A History of Medicine in South Africa up to the End of the Nineteenth Century* (Cape Town: A. A. Balkema, 1958).

4. See Julie Parle, "Witchcraft or Madness? The Amandiki of Zululand, 1894–1914" *Journal of Southern African Studies* 29, no. 1 (2003): 105–132; Robert R. Edgar and Hilary Sapire, *African Apocalypse: The Story of Nontetha Nkwenkwe, A Twentieth-Century South African Prophet* (Johannesburg: Witwatersrand University Press, 1999); Henry Sigerist, *A History of Medicine*, 2 vols (New York: Oxford University Press, 1951 and 1961); and John Koty, *Die Behandelung der Alten und Kraken bei dun Naturvölken* (Stuttgart, C. L. Hirschfeld, 1934).
5. See Lynette Aria Jackson, "Narratives of 'Madness' and Power: A History of Ingutsheni Mental Hospital and Social Order in Colonial Zimbabwe, 1908–1959" (Ph.D. diss., Columbia University, 1997), 2; M. Vera Bührmann, *Living in Two Worlds: Communication Between a White Healer and Her Black Counterparts*, (Cape Town: Human & Rousseau, 1984); Jean Comaroff, "Healing and Cultural Transformation: The Tswana of Southern Africa," *Social Science and Medicine—Part B, Medical Anthropology* 15, no. 3 (1981): 367–378; and M. Vera Bührmann, "Western Psychiatry and the Xhosa Patient," *South African Medical Journal* 51, no. 14 (1977): 464–466.
6. Discussions concerning this question have a long history and are complex; they cannot be reiterated in detail here. Nevertheless, simply stated, opinions have tended to fall into two camps—those who believe that madness is universally experienced, and those that argue that it is culturally relative. For a more detailed discussion about the difference between universal and relativist beliefs of mental health, see Leslie Swartz, *Culture and Mental Health: A Southern African View* (Cape Town: Oxford University Press, 1998). See also Chapter 6.
7. Minde, "History of Mental Health Services in South Africa: Part II," 1629; and Minde, "The History of Mental Health Services in South Africa: Part I," 1271.
8. Andrew Scull, *The Most Solitary of Afflictions: Madness and Society in Britain, 1700–1900* (New Haven; London: Yale University Press, c1993).
9. Scull, *The Most Solitary of Afflictions.*
10. Andrew Scull, "Psychiatry and Social Control in the Nineteenth and Twentieth Centuries," *History of Psychiatry* 2, no. 2 (1991): 149–152.
11. Johann Louw and Sally Swartz, "An English Asylum in Africa: Space and Order in Valkenberg Asylum," *History of Psychology* 4, no. 1 (2001): 20.
12. M. Minde, "History of Mental Health Services in South Africa: Part XIV. Psychiatric Education," *South African Medical Journal* 51, no. 7 (1977): 213; Searle, 117 and 312; and A. Simpson Wells, "Notes on the Training of South African Doctors," *South African Medical Journal* 26, no. 4 (1952): 61.
13. Gerald Grob has similarly argued that urbanization and industrialization in nineteenth-century America changed family responsibilities towards the mad and public institutions were fashioned in order to fulfill the need. Gerald Grob, *The Mad Among Us: A History of the Care of America's Mentally Ill* (New York: The Free Press, 1994), 24.
14. In 1931, the Parliament of the United Kingdom passed the Statute of Westminister that allowed the South African government even more legislative

independence from Britain and freedom in how they chose to deal with the "native problem." In 1936, the South African government approved the Representation of Natives Bill that gradually excluded Africans from the vote. This was a blow to the African community who were feeling the effects of the Great Depression and whose previous attempts at rebellion had been mostly quashed by government forces. The poor conditions that existed in the African reserves meant that many moved to urban areas. This influx of Africans enabled a more united spirit of resistance against racial oppression, but also facilitated a rise in the popularity of right-wing racist ideas within the white community who felt increasingly threatened.

15. Sally Swartz, "The Black Insane in the Cape, 1891–1920," *Journal of Southern African Studies* 21, no. 3 (1995): 399–415.
16. M. Minde, "History of Mental Health Services in South Africa: Part VII. Services Since Union," *South African Medical Journal* 49, no. 11 (1975): 406.
17. For further information on South African mental laws, see A. Kruger, *Mental Health Law in South Africa* (Durban: Butterworth, 1980).
18. Mental Disorders Act No. 38 of 1916.
19. Wealthier citizens were usually treated in their homes. Hurst and Lucas, 606; and Searle, 108.
20. Searle, 114.
21. Minde, "History of Mental Health Services in South Africa: Part XIV," 210.
22. It was only in 1959 and 1968 that psychiatry acquired its own full-time Chair at the University of Witwatersrand and the University of Cape Town respectively.
23. Sally Swartz, "Changing Diagnoses in Valkenberg Asylum, Cape Colony, 1891–1920: A Longitudinal View." *History of Psychiatry* 6, no. 24, Pt 4 (1995): 431–451.
24. Jacalyn Duffin, *History of Medicine: A Scandalously Short Introduction* (Toronto: University of Toronto Press, 2000), 285.
25. Alex Butchart, Brandon Hamber, Martin Terre Blanche, and Mohamed Seedat, "Violence, Power and Mental Health Policy in Twentieth Century South Africa," in *Mental Health Policy Issues for South Africa,* eds. Don Foster, Melvyn Freeman and Yogan Pillay (Pinelands: Medical Association of South Africa, 1997), 238.
26. Michel Foucault, *Madness and Civilization: A History of Insanity in the Age of Reason* (New York: Random House, 1965). For debates concerning Foucauldian applications in an African context, see also Megan Vaughan, *Curing their Ills: Colonial Power and African Illness* (California: Stanford University Press, 1991); and Alex Butchart, *The Anatomy of Power: European Constructions of the African Body* (London; New York: Zed Books, 1998).
27. Although women and blacks did volunteer in the war, they were not allowed to be part of the armed services. Neil Roos, "Homes Fit for (White) Heroes: Servicemen, Social Justice and the Making of Apartheid, 1939–1948," *Journal of the Georgia Association of Historians* 20 (1999): 26.
28. Andreas Sagner, "Ageing and Social Policy in South Africa: Historical Perspectives with Particular Reference to the Eastern Cape," *Journal of Southern African Studies* 26, no. 3 (2000): 534.
29. Hansard, HAD, Vol. 47 (28 February 1944), col 2115.
30. Roos, 29.
31. Roos, 29.
32. Roos, 35.

33. Lewis A. Hurst, "Hereditary Factors in Mental Disorder and Mental Defect," *South African Medical Journal* 18, no. 23 (1944): 397.
34. Central Archives Depot (CAD), Pretoria, Supreme Court Criminal Case, Transvaal Provincial Division (TPD) 558/1958 (1954).
35. Incidentally, the word "psychiatry" originated from two Greek words meaning "soul" and "healer." The Afrikaans word is not far off from the literal translation from Greek. J. J. de Villiers, "The Aetiology of Mental Illness," *Edinburgh Medical Journal* 57 (1950): 276; and Jacalyn Duffin, *History of Medicine: A Scandalously Short Introduction* (Toronto: University of Toronto Press, 2000), 277.
36. De Villiers, 277.
37. J. J. de Villiers, "Letter to the Editor: Psycho-Analysis," *South African Medical Journal* 25, no. 36 (1951): 36.
38. His emphasis. CAD, Governor General's Records (GG) 33/2129 (1953).
39. It is not my intention to determine whether de Villiers was mentally "ill" or not, but he did have extensive support from religious groups and family members who signed numerous affidavits testifying to his mental sanity. Yet he was never able to convince authorities of his mental capacity and acquire his license to practice psychiatry again. CAD, GG 33/2129 (1953).
40. R. E. Fancher, "Freud's Attitudes towards Women: A Survey of his Writings," *Queen's Quarterly* 82, no. 3 (1975): 368–393.
41. Susan P. Penfold and Gillian A. Walker, *Women and the Psychiatric Paradox* (Montreal: Eden Press, 1983), 97. See also Joan Busfield, *Managing Madness: Changing Ideas and Practice* (London; Dover, N. H.: Hutchinson, 1996), 168; Juliet Mitchell, *Psychoanalysis and Feminism* (London: Allen Lane, 1974); and Kate Millett, *Sexual Politics*, (New York: Avon, 1971), 172–190.
42. Sigmund Freud, *Totem and Taboo: Resemblances between the Psychic Lives of Savages and Neurotics*, trans. A. A. Brill (New York: Vintage Books, 1946), 3 and 85.
43. Jock McCulloch, *Colonial Psychiatry and 'the African Mind'* (Cambridge: Cambridge University Press, 1995), 11.
44. Wulf Sachs, *Black Hamlet,* with a new introduction by Saul Dubow and Jacqueline Rose (Johannesburg: Witwatersrand University Press, 1996).
45. B. J. F. Laubscher, *Sex, Custom and Psychopathology: A Study of South African Pagan Nations* (London: George Routledge & Sons Ltd., 1937).
46. Saul Dubow, Introduction: Part I to *Black Hamlet,* by Wulf Sachs (Johannesburg: Witwatersrand University Press, 1996), 13.
47. *Sex, Custom and Psychopathology* and *Black Hamlet* were precursors to cross-cultural psychiatry, an approach that would become increasingly popular in the 1970s.
48. As Dubow has pointed out, Sachs's strong belief in psychoanalysis continuously came under criticism. Dubow, 3.
49. Lewis A. Hurst, "Heredito-Constitutional Research in Psychiatry," *South African Medical Journal* 14, no. 18 (1940): 384.
50. P. J. G. de Vos, "Some Aspects Concerning the Treatment of the Mentally Diseased," *South African Medical Journal* 19, no. 10 (1945): 180.
51. Union of South Africa, *Annual Report of the Commissioner for Mental Hygiene, Statistical Tables 1940*, U. G. No. 47 (Pretoria: Government Printer, 1941).
52. Hurst, "Heredity Factors," 397–398.
53. H. Moross, *Tara, The H. Moross Centre* (Johannesburg: Smith Mitchell Organisation, n.d.), 45.
54. Lewis A. Hurst, "Electroencephalography in Mental Hospital Practice," *South African Medical Journal* 20, no. 3 (1946): 54–55; Lewis A. Hurst,

"Electroencephalography in Mental Hospital Practice," *South African Medical Journal* 20, no 4 (1946): 87–89.

55. Mental Disorders Act No. 38 of 1916, sec. 3.
56. Susanne Klausen, "'For the Sake of Race': Eugenic Discourses in the *South African Medical Record*, 1903–1926," *Journal of Southern African Studies* 23, no. 1 (1997): 27–50.
57. Saul Dubow, *Scientific Racism in South Africa* (Cambridge: Cambridge University Press, 1995), 120.
58. de Villiers, "The Aetiology of Mental Illness," 275.
59. Morris J. Cohen, "The New Hope in Mental Disorders," *South African Medical Journal* 14, no. 21 (1941): 434.
60. "Poisoning by Arsenic in South Africa," *South African Medical Journal* 14, no 18 (1940): 383–384.
61. See J. A. Higgs, "Insulin Therapy," *South African Medical Journal* 12, no. 16 (1938): 590–593; Cohen, 434–436; P. F. Cluver, "Some Technical Problems in Electro-Convulsive Therapy," *South African Medical Journal* 16, no. 19 (1942): 350 and de Vos, 178–180. Today ECT remains a treatment administered to patients of different diagnoses in psychiatric units in general hospitals and mental institutions worldwide, although anaesthesia is now used and the volt dosage is much lower. Nevertheless, it remains a highly controversial therapy. For examples of the debate about ECT, see Timothy W. Kneeland and Carol A. B. Warren, *Pushbutton Psychiatry: A History of Electroshock in America* (Westport, CT: Praeger Publishers, 2002); Max Fink, *Electroshock: Healing Mental Illness* (New York: Oxford University Press, 1999); Peter R. Breggin, *Toxic Psychiatry: Psychiatry's Assault on the Brain with Drugs, Electroshock, Biochemical Diagnoses, and Genetic Theories* (New York: St. Martin's Press, 1991); and Graham A. Edwards and Bruce Flaherty, "Electro-Convulsive Therapy: A New Era of Controversy," *Australian & New Zealand Journal of Psychiatry* 12, no. 3 (1978): 161–164.
62. Cohen, 436.
63. J. S. du T. de Wet, "Convulsive Therapy and Analytical Psycho-therapy in a Case of Psychoneurosis," *South African Medical Journal* 18, no. 18 (1944): 317.
64. G. F. Langschmidt, "Mental Health," *South African Medical Journal* 15, no. 18 (1941): 360–361.
65. See, for example, E. H. Cluver, *Social Medicine* (South Africa: Central News Agency, 1951); W. Waddell, "Psychosomatic Aspects of Obstetrics and Gynaecology," *South African Medical Journal* 22, no. 2 (1948): 63–67; R. Schaffer, "Psychosomatic Medicine," *South African Medical Journal* 22, no. 5 (1948): 167–169; Livni, 857–863; and C. D. Brink, "Psychosomatic Disorders," *South African Medical Journal* 19, no. 1 (1945): 11–14.
66. "Mental Hospital Services in the Union: An Interview with the Minister of Health," *South African Medical Journal* 20, no. 13 (1946): 390.
67. "Mental Hospital Services in the Union".
68. Hansard, HAD, Vol. 47 (28 February 1944), col. 2104.
69. Union of South Africa, *Annual Report of the Commissioner for Mental Hygiene, Statistical Tables* 1944, U. G. 3 (Pretoria: Government Printer, 1946).
70. Union of South Africa, *Annual Report of the Commissioner of Mental Hygiene* (1946), iii.
71. David Perk, "A Psychiatrist's Experience in the 2nd World War" *South African Medical Journal* 21, no. 23 (1947): 867.
72. Perk, 890.

73. Michael Gelfand, *The Sick African: A Clinical Study*, 3rd ed. (Cape Town: Juta, 1957), 533–534.
74. H. Moross, "The Neuroses," in *Social Medicine*, ed. E. H. Cluver (South Africa: Central News Agency, 1951), 131.
75. "Extract from the 1949 Annual Report of the Johannesburg Hospital" in *Tara*, 39.
76. Moross, "The Neuroses," 121.
77. A. Schenk, *Tara, The H. Moross Centre*, <http://www.health.wits.ac.za/psychiatry/tara.htm> (accessed 20 July 2003).
78. No. 134 Military Hospital was transformed into the Witrand Institute for the Feebleminded that same year. Tara would become a state institution in 1980. Moross, *Tara*, 4; and Cliff Allwood, "Problems in Institutional and Hospital Care of Psychiatric Patients," in *Proceedings of Two Symposia: Mental Health Care for a New South Africa Held at the University of Witwatersrand, May 1990 and Rural Community Mental Health Care Held at Tintswalo Hospital, June 1990*, ed. Melvyn Freeman (Johannesburg: Centre for the Study of Health Policy, 1990), 21.
79. "Annexure 4: Negotiations Between the Transvaal Provincial Administration and the Union Government: Acquisition of the Tara Property (TH/9/38; TH411)" in Moross, *Tara*, 95.
80. "Annexure 3: Conference on Hospital Accommodation for Neuro-Psychiatric Patients and Sequelae" in Moross, *Tara*, 90. Local residents objected to the establishment of a neuropsychiatric hospital in their area. Despite the attempt to evade stigma and establish itself as a medical hospital, Tara was, and always has been, seen as a mental hospital.
81. In 1958, Moross would become a Member of the Executive Board of the World Federation of Mental Health until 1961, where he, according to Hurst, "exercised his most influential public function in cross-fertilizing South African and world trends in Mental Health." While international influences on South Africa's psychiatric practice are evident, further research into South Africa's influence on world trends in psychiatry still needs to be done. Lewis A. Hurst, "Preface" in Moross, *Tara*, xvi.
82. Moross, "The Neuroses," 125–135.
83. A. Cox and R. Geerling, "Psychic Disorganization: The Psychoses as a Problem in Social Medicine," in Cluver, 185.
84. Moross, "The Neuroses," 135–136.
85. "Annexure 16: Minutes January–March 1951, 29th November, 1949" in Moross, *Tara*, 182.
86. "Annexure 13: Occupational Therapy Department" in Moross, *Tara*, 155.
87. "Annexure 15: First Psychiatric Community Service in South Africa C/11/2" in Moross, *Tara*, 161–163.
88. "Annexure 25: Letter to Dr. H. J. Hugo, Medical Director Transvaal Provincial Hospital Services, 24th February, 1951 from H. Moross, Medical Superintendent," in Moross, *Tara*, 217–219.
89. "Annexure 10: Interim Report of Tara Staff Committee Meeting Held at Tara Hospital on Thursday 24th April, 1947 at 5 p.m.," in Moross, *Tara*, 137–144.
90. "Annexure 19: The History of the First Steps Taken to Train Clinical Psychologists in South Africa" in Moross, *Tara*, 192.
91. "Annexure 11: Creation of Full-Time Post for Professor of Psychological Medicine," in Moross, *Tara*, 153.
92. Community psychiatry was a vague heterogeneous movement that promoted integration between mental and physical medicine, deinstitutionalization, the involvement of the community, and even preventative medicine. In the

1950s and thereafter, Tara would be at the forefront of these applications of community psychiatry. In 1950, Moross was already suggesting that it was not only the job of the mental institution to care for the neurotic, but family, politicians, teachers and social workers should all be involved in the treatment and care of the neurotic. Moross, "The Neuroses."

NOTES TO CHAPTER 2

1. Central Archives Depot (CAD), Secretary of Native Affairs Records (NTS) 9306 24/377 (1948).
2. "Death After Night in Shed," *Star* (Johannesburg), 26 August 1948; "Constable's Story at Inquest on Native Mental Cases," *Rand Daily Mail* (Johannesburg), 29 August 1948; and "Open Verdict Returned in Death of Two Mental Patients," *Star*, 2 September 1948.
3. CAD, NTS 9306 24/377 (1948).
4. CAD, NTS 9306 24/377 (1948).
5. Phillip Bonner, Peter Delius, and Deborah Posel, "The Shaping of Apartheid: Contradiction, Continuity and Popular Struggle," in *Apartheid's Genesis: 1935–1962* (Johannesburg: Wits University Press, 1993), 1–2.
6. Mark Finnane observes such paradoxes in colonial Australian mental institutions where he argues that the isolation of mental institutions ironically created administrative difficulties for the state. Mark Finnane, "The Ruly and the Unruly: Isolation and Inclusion in the Management of the Insane," in *Isolation: Places and Practices of Exclusion*, eds. Carolyn Strange and Alison Bashford (London and New York: Routledge, 2003), 92. In South Africa, the Commissioner for Mental Health, A. M. Lamont, noted in 1967, "the isolated mental hospital not only hampers rehabilitation of new psychiatric cases but it poses a major economic problem in terms of expert manpower." Republic of South Africa, *Annual Report of the Commissioner for Mental Health, 2-Year Period Ended 31 December, 1967* (Pretoria: Government Printer, 1968), 6.
7. Two of these institutions were designated for white "feebleminded," while the rest were for those deemed mentally "disordered." As previously mentioned, the designation between the two was unclear.
8. Union of South Africa, *Annual Report, 1948*, 16.
9. E. Northover, "Introductory Report" in A. M. Lamont, "Report by an Inter-Departmental Study Group Regarding Accommodation Requirements at Mental Hospitals and Institutions for Mental Defectives in the Republic of South Africa" (1969), 2–3.
10. Hansard, House of Assembly Debates (HAD), Vol. 64 (9 September 1958), col. 3265.
11. Alistair Lamont became Commissioner for Mental Health in 1960. Lamont, "Report by an Inter-Departmental Study Group," 5–6.
12. E. Northover, "Report by the Architectural member of the team on conditions at Fort England Hospital, Grahamstown," in Lamont, 1.
13. Jan H. Robbertze, interview by author, tape recording, Stellenbosch, Cape, 14 May 2002.
14. George Hart, interview by author, tape recording, Johannesburg, Gauteng, 27 June 2002.
15. Hart, interview by author.
16. E. Northover, "Report by the Architectural member of the team on conditions at the Komani Hospital, Queenstown" in Lamont, 1.

17. Northover, "Report by the Architectural," 1.
18. Hansard, HAD, Vol. 98 (9 September 1958), col. 3265.
19. *Source:* Republic of South Africa, "Verslag van die Interdepartmentele Komitee van Ondersoek insake die Daarstelling van Inrigtings vir Bantoesielsiekes in Bantoegebiede" (Cape Town, 1961).
20. Verwoerd was the Minister of Native Affairs until he succeeded J. G. Strydom as Prime Minister in the late 1950s. For more detailed discussion about how the idea of ethnic pluralism emerged in the 1960s, see Saul Dubow, "Ethnic Euphemisms and Racial Echoes," *Journal of Southern African Studies* 20, no. 3 (1994): 355–370. See also Mahmood Mamdani, *Citizen and Subject: Contemporary Africa and the Legacy of Late Colonialism*, (Princeton, N. J.: Princeton University Press, 1996) who also traces the movement of the state from racial to ethnic subjectification and analyses its application.
21. The initial cost was estimated to be £120,000 plus an additional £54,000 a few years later for additional land. This does not include the amount spent on upgrading or building new structures on sight. "Annexure 4: Negotiations Between the Transvaal Provincial Administration and the Union Government," in H. Moross, *Tara: The H. Moross Centre* (Johannesburg, Smith Mitchell Organisation, n.d.), 18 and 95.
22. Republic of South Africa. "Verslag van die Interdepartmentele;" Lamont, 9.
23. CAD, NTS, 9306 24/377 (1948).
24. Hansard, HAD, Vol. 17 (20 September 1966), cols. 2482–2483.
25. In 1946, the Municipality of Cape Town took over the responsibility and ownership of Valkenburg Hospital. However, approximately ten years later, there was a persistent demand for beds within the hospital and the need for more wards. The municipality simply did not have enough money to comply. Thus, the Department of Health re-possessed it and it once again became a state-run hospital. The Groote-Schuur General Hospital, however, also provided psychiatric beds in the Cape for many white patients.
26. The Department of Public Health itself was before 1945 a sub-department of the Department of Interior. The Public Health Amendment Act No. 51 of 1946 changed the department's name to the Department of Health. Mental Disorders Amendment Act No. 7 of 1944.
27. "The Mental Disorders Amendment Act 1957," *South African Medical Journal* 31, no. 31 (1957): 785–786.
28. Parliamentary Correspondent, "The Treatment of Mentally Ill Patients," *South African Medical Journal* 35, no. 10 (1961): 216–217.
29. *Sources:* Compiled from Mental Disorders Amendment Act No. 38 of 1916 and the Mental Disorders Amendment Act No. 7 of 1944.
30. Medical certificates in these cases had to be signed by a doctor unrelated to the individual.
31. District surgeons were state-paid practitioners whose duties were to collect evidence to present in court and treat patients in state custody. They were ill-trained to provide psychiatric counsel. The Truth and Reconciliation Commission's report showed how district surgeons often failed to report abuse of political detainees that was taking place within prisons. The most famous incidence of this is the Steve Biko case. See Truth and Reconciliation Commission of South Africa (TRC), *Truth and Reconciliation Commission of South Africa Report* (Basingstoke and Oxford: Macmillan Reference Limited, 1998), vol. 4.
32. In these cases, family members who were medical practitioners could sign medical certificates.
33. Natal Archives Depot (NAD), Pietermaritzburg, Supreme Court Registrar Records (RSC) 1/27/152 85 (1950).

34. NAD, RSC 1/535 I157/59 (1959).
35. Mental Disorders Act No. 38 of 1916 s31; and A. Kruger, *Mental Health Law in South Africa* (Durban: Butterworth, 1980), 24.
36. General hospitals were another option where patients could admit themselves. However, patients could not stay in general hospitals for longer than forty-nine days. Thereafter they either had to be admitted to a mental institution or discharged.
37. See Chapters 4 and 6 for information about community psychiatry and private institutions, respectively.
38. Mental Disorders Act No. 38 of 1916, s3.
39. CAD, Governor General's Records (GG) 1258 33/2110 (1943).
40. Union of South Africa, *Annual Report, 1960*, 1.
41. Mental Disorders Act No. 38 of 1916.
42. Mental Disorders Act No. 38 of 1916. s.6.4 (f).
43. Yannick Ripa, *Women and Madness: The Incarceration of Women in Nineteenth-Century France,* translated by Catherine du Peloux Menagé (Cambridge: Polity Press, 1986); and Elaine Showalter, "Victorian Women and Insanity," in *Madhouses, Mad-Doctors and Mad-men,* ed. Andrew Scull (Philadelphia: University of Pennsylvania Press, 1981), 316–317.
44. Phyllis Chesler, *Women and Madness* (New York: Avon, 1983), 31.
45. H. Roberts, *The Patient Patients* (London: Pandora, 1985).
46. Act No. 38 of 1916, s73.
47. Timothy Keegan, "Gender, Degeneration and Sexual Danger: Imagining Race and Class in South Africa ca.1912," *Journal of Southern African Studies* 27, no. 3 (2001): 475. For more information regarding "black peril", see Gareth Cornwell, "George Webb Hardy's *The Black Peril* and the Social Meaning of 'Black Peril' in Early Twentieth Century South Africa," *Journal of Southern African Studies* 22, no. 3 (1996): 441–454.
48. Elder, 11–12
49. Elder, 5, 11.

NOTES TO CHAPTER 3

1. Central Archives Depot (CAD), Pretoria, Governor General Collection (GG) 1258 33/2121 (1944).
2. Shula Marks, ed., *Not Either an Experimental Doll: The Separate Worlds of Three South African Women*, (London: The Women's Press, 1987); and Robert R. Edgar and Hilary Sapire, *African Apocalypse: The Story of Nontetha Nkwenkwe, a Twentieth-Century South African Prophet* (Johannesburg: Witwatersrand University Press, 1999).
3. Saul Dubow, "Ethnic Euphemisms and Racial Echoes," *Journal of Southern African Studies* 20, no. 3 (1994): 368.
4. Deborah B. Fontenot, "A Vision of Anarchy: Correlate Structures of Exile and Madness in Selected Works of Doris Lessing and Her South African Contemporaries," (Ph.D. diss., University of Illinois at Urbana-Champaign, 1988), iii.
5. Diana Gittins, *Madness in its Place: Narratives of Severalls Hospital, 1913–1997* (London and New York: Routledge, 1998).
6. Edwin N. Wilmsen, Saul Dubow, and John Sharp, for example, argue this about ethnicity in "Introduction: Ethnicity, Identity and Nationalism in Southern Africa," *Journal of Southern African Studies* 20, no. 3 (1994): 347.
7. Luise White, "The Traffic in Heads: Bodies, Borders and the Articulation of Regional Histories," *Journal of Southern Africa* 23, no. 2 (1997): 327–328.

8. See, for example, Janet M. Stoppard and Linda M. McMullen, *Situating Sadness: Women and Depression in Social Context* (New York: New York University Press, 2003); Susan J. Hubert, *Questions of Power: the Politics of Women's Madness Narratives* (Newark, N.J.; London: University of Delaware Press: Associated University Press, 2002); Mindy Lewis, *Life Inside: A Memoir* (New York: Atra Books, 2002); Julia Nunes and Scott Simmie, *Beyond Crazy: Journeys through Mental Illness* (Toronto: McClelland & Stewart, 2002); Kerry Davies, "'Silent and Censured Travellers'?: Patients' Narratives and Patients' Voices: Perspectives on the History of Mental Illness Since 1948," *Social History of Medicine* 14, no. 2 (2001): 267–292; Jeffrey L. Geller and Maxine Harris, *Women of the Asylum: Voices From Behind the Walls, 1840–1945* (New York: Anchor Books, 1994); Mary Elene Wood, *The Writing on the Wall: Women's Autobiography and the Asylum* (Urbana: University of Illinois Press, 1994); John S. Hughes, *The Letters of a Victorian Madwoman* (Columbia: University of South Carolina Press, 1993); Maggie Potts and Rebecca Fido, *"A Fit Person to Be Removed:" Personal Accounts of Life in a Mental Deficiency Institution* (Plymouth: Northcote House Publishers, 1991); Barbara Sapinsley, *The Private War of Mrs. Packard* (New York: Paragon House, 1991); Roy Porter, *A Social History of Madness: Stories of the Insane* (London: Weidenfeld and Nicolson, 1987); Dale Peterson, *A Mad People's History of Madness* (Pittsburgh: University of Pittsburgh Press, 1981); and Bert Kaplan, *The Inner World of Mental Illness. A Series of First Person Accounts of What it was Like* (New York: Harper and Row, 1964).
9. Geoffrey Reaume, *Remembrance of Patients Past: Patient Life at the Toronto Hospital for the Insane, 1870–1940* (Don Mills, Ontario: Oxford University Press, 2000), 5.
10. CAD, GG 1260 33/2190 (1950).
11. CAD, GG 1259 33/2160 (1947).
12. CAD, GG 1257 33/2082 (1942).
13. CAD, GG 1260 33/2190 (1950).
14. CAD, Prime Minister Records (PM) 1/2/127 PM41/14 (1936).
15. "*Soos u weet is sy begeerte on terug te kom na my toe, hier waar ek by sy ouers vandag tuis is. Sy begeerte is om vir hom in goeie werk te kry, en dat ons twee weer saam gelukkig mag lewe en sterwe. Hy het altyd in verkeerde pad geloop, in die stilleheid sonder dat ek daar van geweet het. Later moet ek alles uitvind, en in terleurstelling kry, dat hy aan die Ossewabrandwag behoort. Ek is dit nie gewoont nie, want ek is gebore, en sal sterwe vir die Engelse. So my man het sorg, en my eie ouers nou hand, en monde belowe om ook aan ons kant te wees. Sal u tog so goed wees, en hom sy ontslag gee om uit to kom in Oktober maand, want soos u seker al gehoor het, in watter toestand ek verkeer, en ek wil hom graag dan hier he na my. Ek belowe u om agter hom te kyk, dat hy nie weer die verkeerde pad sal vat nie, en as hy dit weer doen, dan kan u hom vir altyd daar hou.*" CAD, GG 1258 33/2118 (1944).
16. CAD, GG 1260 33/2192 (1953).
17. The diagnosis "dementia praecox" was renamed "schizophrenia" in 1953.
18. CAD, GG 33/207320 (1941).
19. CAD, GG 1259 33/2140 (1946).
20. CAD, GG 1259 33/2134 (1946).
21. " *. . . ek was nou vir 'n paar dae terug by die polisie van Montagu gewees toe ek vir die polisie gese dat die pasiente en die mans nursese [sic] vir my ruk en pluk wurg en in my linker en regter heupe en op my maag vir my op stamp stamp.*" CAD, GG 1260 33/2183 (1951).

22. "*Geagte Dr ek sal bly wees as Dr van genade van medelyde 10 [illegible] polisie sal stuur om my daar vergoed vergoed weg te neem, in elk geval van die mans nursese [sic] my broers gaan mishandle en gaan mishandle laer dan varke maar ewewel [sic] hulle het dit gese dat vir my en broers en susters en my erger gaan mishandle laer dat [sic] varke.*" CAD, GG 1260 33/2183 (1952).
23. Hansard, HAD, Vol. 98 (9 September 1958), col. 3254.
24. CAD, A272 224 20/76 (1945).
25. CAD, A272 224 20/76 (1945).
26. Mental Disorders Act No. 38 of 1916, sec. 77.
27. Union of South Africa, *Annual Report of the Commissioner for Mental Hygiene, Statistical Tables, 1950*, U.G. No. 19 (Pretoria: Government Printer, 1952).
28. Republic of South Africa, *Annual Report, 1962*, 4.
29. Republic of South Africa, *Annual Report, 1967*, 4.
30. Wilhelm Bodemer, interview by author, tape recording, Pretoria, Gauteng, 29 May 2002.
31. Geoffrey Reaume has pointed out that most historians tend to rationalize the abusive behaviour of staff by pointing to the terrible conditions in which they worked, but when it comes to patients' violence, they tend to offer no understanding. Patients are therefore depicted as inherently violent and staff frustrations as often justified. However, he argues that "patients were and are as diverse as any other population group" and that "no historical or contemporary evidence supports any broad brush stroke tarring all or even a majority of psychiatric patients as abusers." Indeed, the conditions in which staff worked were even worse for patients. While patients' violence certainly existed within the institutions, not all patients partook in it. Most patients' violence was likely the product of the frustrating lack of agency given to them and the overall sub-standard conditions in which they were housed. Institutions really did more to foment disturbances among patients than offer any form of restorative therapy. Reaume, 75.
32. Jan H. Robbertze, interview by author, tape recording, Stellenbosch, Cape, 14 May 2002.
33. CAD, GG 1259 33/2129 (1945–1958).
34. CAD, GG 1259 33/2160 (1947).
35. A. M. Lamont, "Report by an Inter-Departmental Study Group Regarding Accommodation Requirements at Mental Hospitals and Institutions for Mental Defectives in the Republic of South Africa" (Cape Town, 1969).
36. Sandra Burman and Margaret Naude, "Bearing a Bastard: The Social Consequences of Illegitimacy in Cape Town, 1896–1939," *Journal of Southern African Studies* 17, no. 3 (1991): 383.
37. CAD, GG 1258 33/2121 (1944).
38. " . . . *moeder ek verlang nou regtig huis toe maar ek moed [sic] spaar te vreete wees tot ek kan huis toe gaan. Ek bid die Heër dag en nag om my te help om genadig te wees dat ek weer veillig na my huis kan gaan. Ag moeder dit is bitter droog en warm hier in Grahamstad 'n mens kan amper nie slaap in die nag so warm is dit. Ag moeder ek het nog geen briewe van suster and antie anna gekry. Ag moeder is dit daar ook so droog en hoe gaan dit met ons skaape is hulle nog mooi en vet. En hoe gaan dit nog met die perde is die swart perd van my nog nie gery nie en hoe gaan dit nog met die ou hond leef hy nog. Vra vir pa as hy nog nie die kalwer geend het nie, së vir hom hy moed hulle tog end. En vra vir hom hoe gaan dit met die mense daar op die dorp. En hoe lyk die vrugte daar by hulle is daar nog*

perskes së vir Nellie sy moed [sic] vir my 'n paar kweppers stuir [sic] saam met die perskes as pa vir my die perskes stuur asseblief haar. En së ook groetnis vir hulle en vir Hester du Preez ook, as ma haar sien." CAD, GG 1260 33/2192 (1956).
39. CAD, GG 1257 33/2058 (1940).
40. CAD, Secretary of Native Affairs Records (NTS) 9306 15/377 (1941).
41. CAD, NTS 9306 21/377 (1948).
42. CAD, GG 1259 33/2140 (1946).
43. CAD, GG 1259 33/2140 (1946).
44. CAD, GG 1259 33/2140 (1946).
45. "*Die seun was altyd my hulp op die plaas en my vrou en ek raak van al baie gedaan en mis sy hulp baie.*" CAD, GG 1260 33/2192 (1956).
46. CAD, GG 1258 33/2121 (1944).
47. CAD, GG 1258 33/2100 (1953).
48. CAD, GG 1257 33/2061 (1940).
49. CAD, GG 1258 33/2117 (1944).
50. CAD, GG 1257 33/2079 (1941).
51. Influenced by Michel Foucault and Karl Marx, Richard Schmitt, for example, argues that, "alienation is more than being deprived of the ability to develop fully; it cannot be understood unless we acknowledge forthrightly that the alienated are not themselves, because their identities, having been imposed on them are not their own. Hence they are always at odds with and strangers to themselves." Thus, individuals become "self-estranged" from themselves and often become "invisible behind the derogatory definition." Richard Schmitt, "Introduction: Why is the Concept of Alienation Important?" in *Alienation and Social Criticisms,* eds., Richard Schmitt and Thomas E. Moody (New Jersey: Humanities Press, 1994), 4–6. See also R. D. Laing, *The Divided Self: An Existential Study in Sanity and Madness* (Middlesex, England: Penguin, 1965). For a detailed description of the concept of alienation, see Felix Geyer, ed. *Alienation, Ethnicity, and Postmodernism* (Westport, Greenwood Press, 1996).
52. CAD, GG 1257 33/2072 (1941).
53. CAD, GG 1257 33/2057 (1940).
54. CAD, GG 1257 33/2071 (1941).
55. His italics. Reaume, 71.
56. Quoted in CAD, GG 1257 33/2076 (1941).
57. Quoted in CAD, GG 1259 33/2153 (1947).
58. Goffman, 36.
59. CAD, NTS 7682 170/332 (1943).
60. See, for example, CAD, GG 1259 33/2126 (1945), where a patient was transferred out of Witrand Institution to Bloemfontein institution for causing trouble within Witrand and setting fire to a ward that accommodated sixty-four patients.
61. "*Wil ek aan Dr se dat party van die pasiente van de mans nursese se het pasente van die mans nursese se geld mooi gesteel gesteel en daar twak twak ingedraai en opgerook toe kom ek by die office van die Home waar ek in is toe ek dit ook dit aan die Montagu polisie vertel van en ook aan die mane nurses vertel.*" CAD, GG 1260 33/2183 (1952).
62. CAD, GG 1260 33/2167 (1948).
63. CAD, GG 1259/2129 (1950).
64. Sigmund Freud, "Obsessive Acts and Religious Practices" first published in 1907, republished in *The Collected Papers, Vol II* (London: Hogarth Press, 1924).

65. John M. Hull, "Religion, Education and Madness: A Modern Trinity," *Educational Review* 43, no. 3 (1991): 360.
66. CAD, GG 1257 33/2081 (1942).
67. Or "have crossed over."
68. Meaning the liberation of oppressed races.
69. "*Ku njanina-Rulumeni awukayi lungi-sina leyo ndaba yokukululwa kwaba ntu emba ndeze lweni kantinizwa nxa kutiwa nina belungu usubasu silena labo belungu base-Magudu bawelele kuleyo ndawo yabo epesheya kopongola bade dela ba nsundulapo sipume kule ndawo yesi bhedhlela sa se-Bofolo. Siyakona esandhleni sawo Dokontela abam nyama e-Magudu a singa dhlulisi kate simisiwe ngu-Jehova o ngitume lelo msebenzi wake niyabona belungu ukuba niyatandu kuwaka lo-mhlaba wase-Afrika ngo bakusi wona o wenu owenu se-ngilandi. abanyu-se-worandi. ngiya nisizake mine e-ngitunywe kini ngokanayini lo nyaka e ngitumilu-jehova u-tixo umkululi wenhla-nga ezisebu ko bokeni ngiyanisizake mine-Manushe-Dube o tunyiweyo nxa sekudhlula isikati sake asimisileyo u-tixo uyakuselu la kabi isandhla sake kinina lu hlango lu mhlope ngo kuba niyizazi ayiko e-yodwa into eninga yaziyo ngiyapelalapo.*" Translated by Godfrey Dlulane. CAD, GG 1257 33/2092 (1951).
70. The 1856 "Xhosa cattle killings" took place when a young woman, Nongqawuse, living in the eastern Cape, claimed the ancestors told her that all cattle needed to be killed in order to cease their hardship caused by encroaching colonialists. Similarly, in the 1920s, members of the ICU, argued that a mass-killing of white-owned animals, especially pigs, which were associated with evil and even death, needed to take place in order for salvation to occur. See J. B. Peires, *The Dead will Arise: Nongqawuse and the Great Xhosa Cattle-Killing Movement of 1856–1857* (Johannesburg: Ravan Press, 1989) and Helen Bradford, *A Taste of Freedom: The ICU in Rural South Africa, 1924–1930* (New Haven and London: Yale University Press, 1987).
71. Billy Graham was an American evangelist who travelled to South Africa and held multi-racial religious gatherings throughout the apartheid years. CAD, GG 1259 33/2156 (1960).
72. CAD, GG 1257 33/2084 (1942).
73. CAD, GG 1257 33/2086 (1942).
74. CAD, GG 1258 33/2116 (1944).
75. CAD, GG 1257 33/2087 (1942).
76. See next chapter.
77. CAD, NTS 9306 16/377 (1941).
78. CAD, GG 1259 33/2135 (1946).
79. CAD, GG 1258 33/2113 (1948).
80. Erving Goffman, *Asylums: Essays on the Social Situation of Mental Patients and Other Inmates* (Chicago: Aldine Publishing Company, 1962) and David J. Vail, *Dehumanization and the Institutional Career* (Springfield, Illinois: Charles C. Thomas, 1966).
81. Porter, 2.
82. These were the racial classifications of the practitioners or government officials and not necessarily those of the patients themselves. Moreover, the language in which patients wrote may not have been their first language. For example, many Afrikaans-speakers wrote in English as the Governor Generals were mostly English-speakers.
83. Unfortunately court testimony is not easily accessible, mostly because the technology necessary to read the recording system used by courts is no longer readily available.

84. See Chapter 6.

NOTES TO CHAPTER 4

1. Editor-in-Chief, "How Dr. Verwoerd Died," *Rand Daily Mail* (7 September 1966), 1.
2. Editor-in-Chief, "How Dr. Verwoerd Died", 1.
3. Deborah Posel, "The Assassination of Hendrik Verwoerd: The Spectre of Apartheid's Corpse" *African Studies* 68, no. 3 (2009): 331.
4. The Society of Psychiatrists of South Africa changed its name to the South African Society of Psychiatrists (SASOP) in circa 2000.
5. Staff Reporter, "Boyhood Days of Tsafendas," *Rand Daily Mail* (8 September 1966), 3.
6. Staff Reporter, "Boyhood Days," 3.
7. Staff Reporter, "Boyhood Days," 3.
8. "A wild boy nicknamed 'Blackie'" Electronic Mail & Guardian (4 November 1997), 3 [electronic journal], http://www.mg.co.za/mg/news/97nov1/4nov-assassin2.html (accessed 13 June 2000).
9. Desmond Blow, "Tsafendas' mother still alive," *Rand Daily Mail* (9 September 1966), 1.
10. Staff Reporter, "Court hears evidence of faulty reason, delusions," *Rand Daily Mail* (19 October 1966), 5.
11. George Oliver, "I have something to do, said assassin," *Rand Daily Mail* (7 September 1966), 2.
12. "Devoid of Political Meaning," *Rand Daily Mail* (7 September 1966), 2.
13. Staff Reporter, "Act Condemned by non-White leaders," *Rand Daily Mail* (7 September 1966), 2.
14. Staff Reporter, " . . . he planned to shoot Dr. Verwoerd not stab him," *Rand Daily Mail* (18 October 1966), 4.
15. George Oliver, "Doctor says no asylum could hold Tsafendas," (20 October 1966), 1.
16. Staff Reporter, "Tsafendas is found insane: committed to prison," *Rand Daily Mail* (21 October 1966), 2.
17. Staff Reporter, "Tsafendas is found insane," 2.
18. In 1999, Liza Key, a South African filmmaker, researched Tsafendas' history and conducted interviews with the assassin before his death. In the resulting film, *A Question of Madness,* she suggests that Tsafendas was part of a wider conspiracy and argues that Tsafendas was not the "madman" that he was so often portrayed as; rather, his actions seemed very thought out and with a sense of purpose. She argues that Tsafendas was a registered member of the Communist Party of South Africa before the war, and points out that although Tsafendas denied ever knowing Russian, there is some evidence in the recently released archive records that suggests otherwise. Indeed, Tsafendas himself had admitted to a cleric that he had attended training school in Russia. Key also uncovered the testimony of individuals who were astonished by the precision of the stab wounds, which they argued could have been the work of a "trained assassin." Key's research raises some interesting questions about the changing views of "mental illness" in relation to political environments. The "conspiracy theory" that Key advocates not only raises the question as to whether Tsafendas was as "mentally insane" as many made him out to be, but also gives an interesting example of how a "crazed madman" can transform into an "unsung hero" over time. Interestingly, Tsafendas himself left a final request for a postmortem into whether his deed was a reasonable

political act or merely a "mindless killing"—his request was unfortunately not honoured. "Hell in a cell alongside the gallows," *Electronic Mail & Guardian* (4 November 1997), 2 [electronic journal], http://www.mg.co.za/mg/news/97nov1/4nov-assassin3.html (accessed 13 June 2000); and Own Correspondent and AFP, "Verwoerd's assassin dies," *ZA Now Daily Mail & Guardian* (10 October 1999), 7 [electronic journal], http://www.mg.co.za/mg/archive/99oct/10oct-news.html (accessed 13 June 2000).

19. SAPA, "Handful Attend Tsfandas Funeral" (9 October 1999) *Independent Online* http://www.iol.co.za/index.php?set_id=1&click_id=13&art_id=qw939462540347B232 (accessed 9 March 2009).

20. Mervyn Susser, a South African doctor and one of the early advocates of community psychiatry, argues that it originated in post-war America and Britain when declining levels of poverty and advances in curative medicine meant declining mortality rates and increased longevity. As a result, public health began to shift away from the earlier preoccupation with prevention of infectious disease and toward the problems of aging and degenerative conditions. Because of this change in approach towards medical care, Susser argues that society became more aware of mental illnesses that it previously had ignored. He bases his argument on the view that the United States and Europe's social medicine movement after World War II promoted the rise of community psychiatry and these trends in turn influenced South African practitioners. However, there is some difficulty in adopting Susser's view, especially when placed in light of recent discussions of social medicine in South Africa. For example, Shula Marks points out that South African doctors did not simply adopt their notions of social medicine from Europe or the United States, but after World War II South Africa was briefly at the forefront of the social medicine movement. The social medicine movement, much like community psychiatry, focused on a preventative and publicly funded national health system that moved away from the large hospital and promoted smaller community-based centres. Sidney and Emily Kark were at the forefront of this movement, establishing a community-oriented primary health care centre in Pholela that formed the foundation for their future initiatives in Israel and their later work with the World Health Organisation. It is therefore not correct to state that social medicine was simply imported from the United States and Europe.

    Nor is it correct to state that community psychiatry was simply an offshoot of the social medicine movement. Whereas Susser himself was directly involved with the social medicine movement and worked for a short span at Pholela, it is unlikely that many South African psychiatrists were influenced by social medicine, particularly as once those who promoted social medicine in South Africa left to work elsewhere, the medical profession as a whole rejected it. Moreover, as we have seen, psychiatry had always been administratively separate from the health system—the national government managed mental health services while provincial governments administered public hospitals. This meant that the majority of practitioners practiced outside of the general hospitals in separate mental hospitals.

    As Diana Ralph, who has studied community psychiatry in the United States and Europe, has pointed out, the emergence of community psychiatry was also due to changing economic and political conditions. She argues that community psychiatry developed as a means of social control in response to labour force alienation caused by increased economic competitiveness that began in the 1900s and had its peak in the 1940s and thereafter. She suggests that instead of focusing on the unemployable patients that had been housed in mental institutions, Western psychiatrists after 1945 began to address the needs of the employable, that is responsive and less-critical patients, through their adoption of community psychiatry. Ralph's argument is applicable to South Africa as well, for as we have seen, in the post-war years increased urbanisation in South Africa placed a large burden on an already overcrowded mental health structure and practitioners began focusing on the treatment of less acutely sick white men, while long-term and/or black patients were neglected. However, this view that community psychiatry was simply a form of labour control is too narrow, for it fails to recognize the element of human rights advocacy and criticism of custodial practices that were intrinsic to the movement, even if it has to be added that the main beneficiaries of these practices were whites. It also ignores the impact of innovations in psychopharmacological drugs, and the influence, albeit minimal, of the social medicine movement. Melvyn Susser, *Community Psychiatry: Epidemiologic and Social Themes* (New York: Random House, 1968), 3; Shula Marks, "Public Health Then and Now: South Africa's Early Experiment in Social Medicine: Its Pioneers and Politics," *American Journal of Public Health* 87, no. 3 (1997): 452. See also Alan Jeeves, "Health, Surveillance and Community: South Africa's Experiment with Medical Reform in the 1940s and 1950s," *South African Historical Journal* 44 (2001): 244–266; Sidney L. Kark and Guy Steuart, *A Practice of Social Medicine: A South African Team's Experiences in Different African Communities* (Edinburgh: E&S Livingstone, 1962); Sidney L. Kark, *The Practice of Community-Oriented Primary Health Care* (New York: Appleton-Century-Crofts, 1981); and Sidney and Emily Kark, *Promoting Community Health: From Pholela to Jerusalem* (Johannesburg, Witwatersrand University Press, 1999).

21. B. Crowhurst Archer, "Correspondence: Psychiatry and General Practice: Congress Symposium," *South African Medical Journal* 26, no. 44 (1952): 886.
22. A. McE Lamont, "The Place of the Mental Hospital in the Health of the Community," *South African Medical Journal* 28, no. 51 (1954): 1083.
23. Alice Cox, "Psychological Illness in South Africa: the Problems of Treatment and Care. The Psychiatrists Point of View," *South African Medical Journal* 27 no. 38 (1953): 814.
24. G.A. Elliott, "Psychiatry in a General Hospital," *South African Medical Journal* 28, no. 27 (1954): 561–567.
25. H. Moross, *Tara, The H. Moross Centre* (Johannesburg, Smith Mitchell Organisation, n.d.), 10.
26. H. Moross, "Thoughts on the Planning of Mental Health Services for South Africa," *South African Medical Journal* 34, no. 9 (1960): 173.
27. Martha Maria Le Roux, "Die Wordingsweg van Psigiatriese Maatskaplike Werk in Staatspsigiatriese Inrigtings in die Republiek van Suid-Afrika" (D. Soc. Sc. diss., Universiteit van die Oranje-Vrystaat, 1985), 277–283.
28. H. Moross, "The Development of Community Resources for Mental Health Care," *South African Medical Journal* 38 no. 20 (1964): 416–419.
29. Indeed, Alistair Lamont, the Commissioner of Mental Health, argued that mental illnesses simply "melted away" when patients were administered anti-psychotic drugs. Alistair McE. Lamont, "Man's Hidden Madness or Defence Against Insanity," *South African Medical Journal* 44 no. 24 (1970): 711.
30. Indian patients were mostly neglected and there were never any discussions for the creation of separate Indian-only institutions.
31. Don Foster and Sally Swartz, "Introduction: Policy Considerations," in *Mental Health Policy Issues*, 18.

32. Louis F. Freed, "Correspondence: Nativity and the Incidence of Mental Disorder in South Africa," *South African Medical Journal* 27, no. 16 (1953): 355–356.
33. R. W. S. Cheetham, "Society, the Legislator, Mental Health and Ourselves," *South African Medical Journal* 38, no. 31 (1964): 717.
34. Moross, "Thoughts on the Planning," 171.
35. Toker, 55–56.
36. Hansard, House of Assembly Debates (HAD), Vol. 98 (9 September 1958), col. 3257.
37. Parliamentary Correspondent, "The Treatment of Mentally Ill Patients," *South African Medical Journal* 35, no. 10 (1961): 216.
38. A. Kruger, *Mental Health Law in South Africa* (Durban: Butterworth, 1980), 24. Although in the 1970s and thereafter black patients seemed to have a higher discharge rate than white patients, this outcome was because the government began contracting out their care to Smith Mitchell & Co. For a more detailed discussion about Smith Mitchell institutions, see Chapter 6.
39. A. M. Lamont, "Report by an Inter-Departmental Study Group Regarding Accommodation Requirements at Mental Hospitals and Institutions for Mental Defectives in the Republic of South Africa" (Cape Town, 1969), 8.
40. Wilhelm Bodemer, interview by author, tape recording, Pretoria, Gauteng, 29 May 2002.
41. M. Minde, "The Mental Hospital and the Community," *South African Medical Journal* 32, no. 28 (1958), 710. It is unlikely that schizophrenia was in reality more prevalent in blacks than whites, but there are many reasons why it could have continued to be the main diagnosis. Blacks were less likely during apartheid to consult psychiatrists for minor symptoms, and services for black patients were so inadequate that only those that imposed a danger to society were institutionalized. The prevalence of schizophrenia as a diagnosis among blacks also stemmed, however, from the prejudiced views of some practitioners.
42. Wulf Sachs, *Black Hamlet* (Johannesburg: Witwatersrand University Press, 1996), 71.
43. B. J. F. Laubscher, *Sex, Custom and Psychopathology: A Study of South African Pagan Nations* (London: George Routledge & Sons Ltd., 1937), xi.
44. Laubscher, 220.
45. Jock McCulloch, "The Empire's New Clothes: Ethnopsychiatry in Colonial Africa," *History of the Human Sciences* 6, no. 2 (1993): 37–38.
46. G. G. Minaar, *The Influence of Westernization on the Personality of a Group of Zulu Men* (Pretoria: Human Sciences Research Council), 1976; R. W. S. Cheetham and J. A. Griffiths, "Sickness and Medicine—an African Paradigm," *South African Medical Journal* 62, no. 25 (1982): 954–956. Leslie Swartz, "Transcultural Psychiatry in South Africa: Part I," *Transcultural Psychiatric Research Review* 23, no. 4 (1986): 274–275.
47. W. David Hammond-Tooke, "African World-View and its Relevance for Psychiatry," *Psychologia Africana* 16 no. 1 (1975): 25–32 and 145; and W. David Hammond-Tooke, *Rituals and Medicines: Indigenous Healing in South Africa* (Johannesburg: Ad. Donker, 1989), 12–20.
48. Hammond Tooke, *Rituals and Medicines*, 8.
49. A. I. Berglund, *Zulu Thought-Patterns and Symbolism* (London: C. W. Hurst and Co., 1976).
50. Jean Comaroff, "Healing and Cultural Transformation: The Tswana of Southern Africa," *Social Science and Medicine—Part B, Medical Anthropology* 15, no. 3 (1981): 367–378; J. Mills, "The Posession State *Intwaso*: An Anthropological Re-Appraisal," *South African Journal of Sociology* 16,

no. 1 (1985): 9–13; Swartz, "Transcultural Psychiatry in South Africa: Part I," 279.

51. M. C. O'Connell, "The Aetiology of Thwasa," *Psychotherapeia* 6, no. 4 (1980): 18–23; M. C. O'Connell, "Spirit Possession and Role of Stress among the Xisibe of Eastern Transkei," *Ethnology* 21 (1982): 21–37.
52. A. G. Le Roux, "Psychological Factors in the Health of South African Blacks," *South African Medical Journal* 56, no. 13 (1979): 532–534; T. L. Holdstock, "Psychology in South Africa Belongs to the Colonial Era: Arrogance of Ignorance?" *South African Journal of Psychology* 11, no. 4 (1981): 123–129.
53. Leslie Swartz, "Transcultural Psychiatry in South Africa: Part I," *Transcultural Psychiatric Research Review* 23, no. 4 (1986): 274.
54. Her italics. M. Vera Bührmann, *Living in Two Worlds: Communication between a White Healer and her Black Counterparts* (Cape Town and Pretoria: Human & Rousseau, 1984), 13.
55. Bührmann, 15.
56. S. G. Lee, "Spirit Possession among the Zulu," in *Spirit Mediumship and Society in Africa*, eds. J. Beattie and A. G. Le Roux (London: Routledge and Kegan Paul, 1969).
57. Swartz, "Transcultural Psychiatry, Part I", 275, 277; N. C. Manganyi, *Being Black in the World* (Johannesburg: SPRO-CAS/Ravan, 1973).
58. Patrick J. Bracken, "Post-Empiricism and Psychiatry: Meaning and Methodology in Cross-Cultural Research," *Social Science and Medicine* 36, no. 3 (1993): 265–272.
59. C. W. Allwood, "Psychiatry in Primary Health Care in South Africa," (M. Med. diss., University of Witwatersrand, 1979); Jan H. Robbertze, "Mental Health Priorities in South Africa," in *Economics of Health in South Africa, Volume II: Hunger Work and Health*, eds. Francis Wilson and Gill Westcott (Johannesburg: Ravan Press, 1980), 312–328; Jan H. Robbertze, interview by author, tape recording, Stellenbosch, Cape, 14 May 2002.
60. Swartz, 289.
61. Dolly Nkosi, interview with Godfrey Dlulane, 6 July 2002, Katlehong, Gauteng, tape recording.
62. Editorial, "Herbalists, Diviners and even Witchdoctors," *South African Medical Journal* 50, no. 19 (1976): 721.
63. Leslie Swartz, "Transcultural Psychiatry in Context, Part II: Cross Cultural Issues in Mental Health Practice," *Transcultural Psychiatric Research Review* 24, no. 1 (1987): 27.
64. Republic of South Africa, *Report of the Commission of Inquiry into the Responsibility of Mentally Deranged Persons and Related Matters* (Pretoria: Government Printer, 1967), 66
65. Republic of South Africa, *Report of the Commission of Inquiry into the Responsibility of Mentally Deranged Persons*, 60–61.
66. Republic of South Africa, *Report of the Commission of Inquiry into the Responsibility of Mentally Deranged Persons*, 17.
67. Republic of South Africa, *Report of the Commission of Inquiry into the Responsibility of Mentally Deranged Persons*, 8.
68. Indeed, the difficulty of defining exactly what made an individual "criminally insane," or, as some psychiatrists called it, "psychopathic," had been a difficult issue for the South African government for many years. For example, the Class VI of the 1916 Mental Disorders Act had originally defined the "psychopathic" patient, or as it was termed, the "moral imbecile" as "a person who from early age displays some permanent mental defect coupled with strong vicious or criminal propensities on which punishment has had little or

no deterrent effect." In 1944, the government revised this section to delete the term "moral imbecile" and replace it with "socially defective person." Thereafter a "socially defective person" was defined as "a person who suffers from mental abnormality associated with anti-social conduct, and who by reason of such abnormality and conduct requires care, supervision and control for his own protection or in the public interest." The inclusion of Class VI in the Mental Disorders Act meant that "moral imbeciles" or "socially defective persons" could not be tried in criminal cases and had to be sent to institutions. However, in 1957, the government deleted Class VI and decided to insert nothing in its place. Many believed that "psychopaths" could understand the proceedings and were perfectly capable of defending themselves. Republic of South Africa, *Report of the Commission of Inquiry into the Mental Disorders Act* (Pretoria: The Government Printer, 1972), 38–39.

69. J. J. de Villiers, "Correspondence: Mental Disorder, Crime and Sin," *South African Medical Journal* 24, no. 23 (1950): 455.
70. "Dit is dus nie 'n ongewone verskynsel dat Blanke verhoorafwagtendes probeer om sielsiek verklaar te word nie. Dit verskaf gewoonlik nie moeite nie, want die pleidooi is: ‚dit het skielik swart geword en toe ek weer sien het dít of dát gebeur'. Die gedraf van die mense is verder as 'n reël heeltemal normaal. Die Bantoepasiënte, met wie ek in die Transvaal in aanraking gekom het, het geen nabootsingsprobleme opgelewer nie." P. H. Henning, "Die Nabootsing van Geesteskrankheid onder Bantoe Verhoorafwagtende Mans van af Durban Gevangenis (Natal)," *South African Medical Journal* 40, no. 38 (1966): 937.
71. Henning, "Die Nabootsing van Geesteskrankheid," 937–941.
72. Editorial, '"The Criminal's Responsibility," *South African Medical Journal* 25, no. 1 (1951): 6–7.
73. M. Ginsburg, "The Psychopath and the Mental Hospital," *South African Medical Journal* 32, no. 12 (1958): 318.
74. Ginsburg, "The Psychopath," 321.
75. The South African National Council for Mental Health changed its name to the National Council for Mental Health in 1986. Lage Vitus, "The Role of the National Council for Mental Health and Government Agencies in Developing Mental Health Policy" (M.A. diss., University of South Africa, 1987), 214.
76. Welfare Organizations Act No. 40 of 1947, W.O. 72; Vitus, 42.
77. Vitus, 43–44.
78. My emphasis. Jan H. Robbertze, interview by author, tape recording, Stellenbosch, Cape, 14 May 2002.
79. Hendrika Gesina Moutinho, "Planning and Policy Formulation in the Field of Mental Health" (M.A. diss., University of South Africa, 1988), 89–96.
80. In 1969, when the fears of drug abuse among whites were receiving much media attention, the Secretary of Health transferred the operations of these clinics to the Department of Health and ensured that nursing staff were resident at these clinics. Moutinho, 22.
81. Vitus, 85–86.
82. Republic of South Africa, *Report of the Commission of Inquiry into the Responsibility of Mentally Deranged Persons and Related Matters.*
83. Republic of South Africa, *Report of the Commission of Inquiry into the Responsibility of Mentally Deranged Persons*, 51.
84. Republic of South Africa, *Report of the Commission of Inquiry into the Responsibility of Mentally Deranged Persons*, 27.
85. Republic of South Africa, *Report of the Commission of Inquiry into the Responsibility of Mentally Deranged Persons*, 51.
86. Republic of South Africa, *Report of the Commission of Inquiry into the Responsibility of Mentally Deranged Persons, 51.*

87. Republic of South Africa, *Report of the Commission of Inquiry into the Responsibility of Mentally Deranged Persons*, 27.
88. Republic of South Africa, *Report of the Commission of Inquiry into the Responsibility of Mentally Deranged Persons*, 40–41.
89. Republic of South Africa, *Report of the Commission of Inquiry into the Responsibility of Mentally Deranged Persons*, 48–49.
90. Republic of South Africa, *Report of the Commission of Inquiry into the Responsibility of Mentally Deranged Persons*, 54.
91. Republic of South Africa, *Report of the Commission of Inquiry into the Responsibility of Mentally Deranged Persons*, 55.
92. Republic of South Africa, *Report of the Commission of Inquiry into the Responsibility of Mentally Deranged Persons*, 30.
93. Robert Ross, *A Concise History of South Africa* (Cambridge: Cambridge University Press), 135.
94. Deborah Posel, *The Making of Apartheid 1948–1961: Conflict and Compromise* (Oxford: Clarendon Press, 1991), 231.
95. Hermann Giliomee and Lawrence Schlemmer, *From Apartheid to Nation-Building* (Cape Town: Oxford University Press, 1989), 102.
96. Bantu Homelands Citizens Act of 1970.
97. Bantu Homelands Constitution Act (National States Constitutional Act) no. 21 of 1971; Kevin Solomons, "Chapter 11: The Development of Mental Health Facilities in South Africa, 1916–1976," in *Economics of Health in South Africa, Volume II: Hunger Work and Health*, eds. Francis Wilson and Gill Westcott (Johannesburg: Ravan Press, 1980), 306.
98. For the most part, however, those living in these areas consulted with healers with respect to their emotional distress.
99. "Psychiatry," 31.
100. Tom Sharpe's novel, *Riotous Assembly*, contains a comical parody of these "cultural therapy" practices in mental institutions during apartheid. The superintendent of Fort Rapier mental hospital (likely a pseudonym for Fort Napier), allows the re-enactment of the Battle of Blood River and Isandhlwana by the patients as a form of therapy. The novel highlights the white-male main concerns of practitioners. When one practitioner expresses unease with the organization of the re-enactment, another responds:

    'Our chief responsibility is to the whites . . . and it can only help them to see the great events of the past re-enacted here. I have every hope that by participating in them our patients will come to see that there is still a place for the mentally sick in modern South Africa. I like to think of this pageant as drama therapy on a vast scale.'

    To the music of *1812 Overture* and in costume, patients re-enacted the battles. However, the performance goes horribly awry and white and black patients actually end up massacring each other. Tom Sharpe, *Riotous Assembly* (London: Martin Secker and Warburg, 1971), 220 and 217–232.
101. "Psychiatry," 29.
102. Proclamation by the State President of the Republic of South Africa, Rehabilitation Institutions in the Bantu Homelands, No. R. 133, 1975, *Government Gazette* (6 June 1975), No. 4735.
103. H. C. J. Van Rensburg and A. Mans, *Profile of Disease and Health Care in South Africa* (Pretoria, Cape Town and Johannesburg: 1982), 271–293.
104. Solome Malebele, "Problems in Mental Health Care," in *Proceedings of Two Symposia: Mental Health Care for a New South Africa Held at the University of Witwatersrand, May 1990 and Rural Community Mental Health Care Held at Tintswalo Hospital, June 1990*, ed. Melvyn Freeman (Johannesburg: Centre for the Study of Health Policy, 1990), 62.

105. Malebele, 66.
106. Mamphele Rampele, "Health and Social Welfare in South Africa Today" (paper presented at the American Association for the Advancement of Science Annual Meeting, Philadelphia, 25–30 May 1986), 3.
107. Sean O'Donoghue, "Health and Politics: An Appraisal and Evaluation of the Provision of Health, and Mental Health Services for Blacks in South Africa" (M.A. diss., Rhodes University, 1989), 124.
108. Melvyn Freeman, "The Challenges Facing Mental Health Care in South Africa" in *Proceedings of Two Symposia*, 5.
109. Freeman, "The Challenges Facing Mental Health Care," 5.
110. Muriel Horrell, *A Survey of Race Relations in South Africa 1959–1960* (Johannesburg, South African Institute of Race Relations, 1961), 133.
111. Constitution of the Republic of South Africa Act no. 110 of 1983.
112. V. Sewpaul, "Fragmentation of Psychiatric Service Delivery in Natal consequent upon the Policy of Apartheid," *Social Work* 26, no. 2 (1990): 109–114.
113. Bantu Authorities Act, No. 68 of 1951.
114. Cliff Allwood, "Problems in Institutional and Hospital Care of Psychiatric Patients," in *Proceedings of Two Symposia*, 21; Cliff Allwood, interview with author, tape recording, Johannesburg, Gauteng, 25 July 2002.
115. Ashwin Valjee, interview with author, tape recording, Durban, Kwazulu-Natal, 11 June 2002.
116. George Hart, interview with author, tape recording, Randburg, Gauteng, 27 June 2002.
117. G. W. Gale, "The Durban Medical School: A Progress Report," *South African Medical Journal* 29, no. 19 (1955): 438.
118. Pam Christie and Colin Collins, "Bantu Education: Apartheid Ideology and Labour Reproduction," in *Apartheid and Education: The Education of Black South Africans*, ed. Peter Kallaway (Johannesburg: Ravan Press, 1991), 174.
119. Editorial, "Medical Journals and International Hate," *South African Medical Journal* 55, no.15 (1979): 572.

NOTES TO CHAPTER 5

1. Tom Sharpe, *Indecent Exposure* (London: Secker & Warburg, 1973), 78–120, 162.
2. Glen Elder, "Of Moffies, Kaffirs and Perverts: Male Homosexuality and the Discourse of Moral Order in the Apartheid State," in *Mapping Desire: Geographies of Sexualities*, eds. D. Bell and G. Valentine (London and New York, Routledge, 1995), 56.
3. Glen Elder, *Hostels, Sexuality, and the Apartheid Legacy: Malevolent Geographies* (Athens, Ohio: Ohio University Press, 2003).
4. Glen Retief, "Keeping Sodom Out of the Laager," in *Defiant Desire*, eds. Mark Gevisser and Edwin Cameron (Johannesburg: Ravan Press), 100.
5. There are many studies that in the last decade have argued that queer identity is an ever-changing and unstructured concept. It is not my intention to recreate these debates, which have been well documented. For further information regarding the changing nature of homosexual identity, see Kim Phillips and Barry Reay, eds., *Sexualities in History*; M. H. Kirsch, *Queer Theory and Social Change* (London and New York, Routledge, 2000); A. Jagose, *Queer Theory: An Introduction* (New York, New York University Press, 1998); and G. Isaacs and B. McKendrick, *Male Homosexuality in*

South Africa: Identity Formation, Culture, and Crisis (Cape Town, Oxford University Press, 1992).

6. Immorality Amendment Act, no. 23 of 1957.
7. See D. Joubert, ed., *Tot Dieselfde Geslag: Debat oor Homoseksualiteit in 1968* (Cape Town: Tafelberg, 1974), 34–72, for a collection of articles in *Die Burger.*
8. Kevin Botha and Edwin Cameron, "South Africa," in *Sociolegal Control of Homosexuality: A Multi-Nation Comparison,* eds. Donald J. West and Richard Green (New York and London, Plenum Press, 1997), 5–42.
9. For further description of laws regulating homosexual activities before 1966, see Botha and Cameron, "South Africa."
10. Richard Green, "The United States," and Rainer Hoffmann, Jörg Hutter, and Rüdiger Lautmann, "Germany," in *Sociolegal Control of Homosexuality*, 145 and 261. Not all states repealed their sodomy laws and it was only in November, 2003, that the American Supreme Court ruled that individuals in Texas could not be punished for partaking in homosexual activities. Thirteen U.S. states still have sodomy laws. According to a CNN report, four states, "Texas, Kansas, Oklahoma and Missouri prohibit oral and anal sex between same-sex couples. The other nine ban consensual sodomy for everyone: Alabama, Florida, Idaho, Louisiana, Mississippi, North Carolina, South Carolina, Utah and Virginia." "Supreme Court Strikes Down Texas Sodomy Law," 18 November 2003, http://www.cnn.com/2003/LAW/06/26/scotus.sodomy/, (accessed 19 July 2004).
11. "Submission from the South African Police," in Republic of South Africa (RSA), *Report of the Select Committee on the Immorality Amendment Bill: Original Evidence,* S.C. 7-'68 (Pretoria: Government Printer, 1968), 11–12.
12. Similarly, Sander Gilman has suggested that "individual perversion is seen as a proof of the potential perversion of the group." Indeed in South Africa, fears that seemingly "normal" heterosexual men and women could be "perverted" to becoming homosexuals were prevalent. Gilman, *Difference and Pathology,* 192.
13. RSA, S.C. 7-'68, 38.
14. RSA, S.C. 7-'68, 38.
15. Elder also notes that "the bulk of the discussion [during the select committee investigation] revolved around the control and regulation of white homosexuality exclusively." Elder, "Of Moffies," 58 and 60.
16. See T. Dunbar Moodie, "Mine Cultures and Miners' Identity on the South African Gold Mines," in *Town and Countryside in the Transvaal: Capitalist Penetration and Popular Response,* ed. Belinda Bozzoli (Johannesburg: Raven Press, 1983), 176–197; T. Dunbar Moodie with Vivienne Ndatshe and British Sibuyi, "Migrancy and Male Sexuality on the South African Gold Mines," *Journal of Southern African Studies* 14, no. 2 (1988): 228–256; T. Dunbar Moodie with Vivienne Ndatshe, *Going for Gold: Men, Mines and Migration* (Johannesburg: Witwatersrand University Press, 1994).
17. Meaghan E. Campbell, "Discourse Analysis of Rape in South African Townships (1948–1994): A Case for 'Policing the Penis'," (M.A. diss., Dalhousie University, 2000), 45 and 150–151.
18. RSA, S.C. 7-'68, 71.
19. See Carol E. Kaufman, "Reproductive Control in Apartheid South Africa," *Population Studies,* 54, no. 1 (2001): 105–114.
20. See, for example, Q. Rahman, "Fluctuating Asymmetry, Second to Fourth Finger Length Ratios and Human Sexual Orientation," *Psychoneuroendocrinology* 30, no. 4 (2005): 382–391; A. Camperio-Ciani, F. Corna, C. Capiluppi, "Evidence for Maternally Inherited Factors Favouring Male Homosexuality and Promoting Female Fecundity," *Proceedings of the Royal*

Society of London. Series B. Biological Sciences 271, no. 1554 (2004): 2217–2221; A. A. Howsepian, "Sexual Modification Therapies: Ethical Controversies, Philosophical Disputes, and Theological Reflections," *Christian Bioethics* 10, no. 2–3 (2004): 117–135; W. H. James, "The Cause(s) of the Fraternal Birth Order Effect in Male Homosexuality," *Journal of Biosocial Science* 36, no. 1 (2004): 51–59, 61–62.; D. F. Swaab, "Sexual Differentiation of the Human Brain: Relevance for Gender Identity, Transsexualism and Sexual Orientation," *Gynecological Endocrinology* 19, no. 6 (2004): 301–312; M. Yarhouse, "Homosexuality, Ethics and Identity Synthesis," *Christian Bioethics* 10, no. 2–3 (2004): 239–257; and V. L. Quinsey, "The Etiology of Anomalous Sexual Preferences in Men," *Annals of the New York Academy of Sciences* 989 (2003): 105–117, 144–153.

21. See, for example, A. M. Don, "Transvestism and Transsexualism: A Report of 4 Cases and Problems Associated with their Management," *South African Medical Journal* 37 (1963): 479–485.
22. Louis F. Freed, "Medico-Sociological Data in the Therapy of Homosexuality," *South African Medical Journal* 28, no. 48 (1954): 1022–1023.
23. Freed, "Medico-Sociological," 1023.
24. Louis F. Freed, "The Summarised Findings of Medico-Sociological Investigation into the Problem of Prostitution in Johannesburg," *South African Medical Journal* 22, no. 2 (1948): 52; K. Moodie, "Ducktails, Flick-Knives and Pugnacity," *Journal of Southern African Studies* 24, no. 4 (1998): 759.
25. Don, 483.
26. Gillis, RSA, S.C. 7-'68, 152.
27. Simonz, RSA, S.C. 7-'68, 95.
28. S. Dubow, "Afrikaner Nationalism, Apartheid and the Conceptualisation of Race," *Journal of African History,* 33 (1992): 209–237.
29. S. L. Gilman, *Freud, Race, and Gender* (Princeton, Princeton University Press, 1993), 135–136.
30. J. F. Ritchie, *The African As Suckling And As Adult: A Psychological Study* (Livingstone: Rhodes-Livingstone Institute, 1943), 42. See M. Epprecht, "'Bisexuality' and the Politics of Normal in African Ethnography," *Anthropologica* 48, no. 2 (2006): 187–201, for further discussion of Ritchie's arguments.
31. Don, 482.
32. Cilliers, RSA, S.C. 7-'68, 225. These views contradict those of many prominent African leaders, such as Robert Mugabe, who, like van Zyl, has suggested that homosexuality was an imported perversion from Europe. Indeed, as Marc Epprecht has shown, "[m]any black Zimbabweans believe that homosexuality was introduced to the country by white settlers and is now mainly propagated by 'the West'." M. Epprecht, "The 'Unsaying' of Indigenous Homosexualities in Zimbabwe: Mapping a Blindspot in an African Masculinity," *Journal of Southern African Studies* 24, no. 4 (1998): 631.
33. B. J. B. Laubscher, *Sex, Custom and Psychopathology; a Study of South African Pagan Natives* (London: Routledge, 1937), 271.
34. A. McE. Lamont, "Predictability of Behaviour Disturbance in Patients Presenting with Psychiatric Symptoms," *South African Medical Journal* 40, no. 5 (1966): 87–90.
35. M. Epprecht, "'Bisexuality' and the Politics of Normal."
36. Gay and Lesbian Archives (GALA), A. Levin to the Secretary of Parliament, 28 February 1968, Immorality Amendment Bill of 1968 (AM2656), B106.
37. Don, "Transvestism and Transsexualism."
38. Don.
39. Fourie, RSA, S.C. 7-'68, 294.

40. Psychoanalysis today has been rejected by many practitioners as a viable treatment option for homosexuality, yet many continue to use it to treat their patients. For a detailed assessment of the relationship between psychoanalysis and homosexuality, see T. Dean and C. Lane, eds. *Homosexuality and Psychoanalysis* (Chicago, University of Chicago Press, 2001).
41. Zabow suggests that the Society of Neurologists, Psychiatrists and Neurosurgeons became the SPSA in 1966. However, neurologists were still part of the organization in 1968. It is unclear as to exactly when neurologists left the group and the SPNSA was renamed as the SPSA. Department of Justice Archives (DJA), Pretoria, Truth and Reconciliation Commission Records (TRC), T. Zabow, "Submission to Health Sector of Truth and Reconciliation Committee by the Society of Psychiatrists of South Africa," 1.
42. Louis F. Freed, "Homosexuality and the Bill" *South African Medical Journal* 42, no. 22 (1968): 567.
43. GALA, Levin.
44. Zabow, RSA, S.C. 7-'68, 163.
45. Sakinofsky, RSA, S.C. 7-'68, 147.
46. GALA, Society of Psychiatrists and Neurologists of South Africa, "Memorandum to the Select Parliamentary Committee Enquiring into the Immorality Amendment Bill," 28 March 1968, AM2656, B180.
47. B. Tholfsen, "Cross Gendered Longings and the Demand for Categorization: Enacting Gender Within the Transference-Countertransference Relationship," *Journal of Gay and Lesbian Psychotherapy* 4, no. 2 (2000): 27–46.
48. As Glen Retief points out, there has been limited investigation into the effects of the amendments to the Immorality Act, although there are indications that the police raided parties and clubs in the 1970s. Immorality Amendment Bill of 1969; and G. Retief, "Keeping Sodom Out of the Laager", in *Defiant Desire*, eds. Mark Gevisser and Edwin Cameron (Johannesburg: Ravan Press, 1994), 103.
49. Retief, 102.
50. Stanley E. Harris, "Military Policies Regarding Homosexual Behavior: An International Survey," *Journal of Homosexuality* 21, no. 4 (1991): 67–74.
51. Policy Directive No HSAW/1/13/82. Translated and quoted in Mikki Van Zyl et al., "The Aversion Project: Human Rights Abuses of Gays and Lesbians in the SADF by Health Workers during the Apartheid Era," (Cape Town: Simply Said and Done, 1999), 46.
52. Van Zyl et al.
53. Van Zyl et al.
54. Robert M. Kaplan, 45–92.
55. Truth and Reconciliation Commission of South Africa (TRC), *Truth and Reconciliation Commission of South Africa Report* (Basingstoke and Oxford, Macmillan Reference Limited, 1998), vol. 4; G. Kraak, dir. and J. Kruger, prod., *Property of the State: Gay Men in the Apartheid Military,* 52 min. (Cape Town, Stargate Distribution, 2002), videocassette; and R. M. Kaplan, "Treatment of Homosexuality During Apartheid," *British Medical Journal,* 329, no. 7480 (2004): 1415–1416.
56. Van Zyl et al., 46.
57. Allison D. Newton, "The Application of Brief Psychotherapy in Military Psychiatry" MA thesis, (Pretoria: University of Pretoria, 1981), 3.
58. Curriculum Vitae of Prof. Aubrey Levin, MD, GALA Archives.
59. Letter from Dr. Aubrey Levin to The Secretary of Parliament, 28 February 1968, AM2656 B106 GALA Archives.
60. Van Zyl et al., 64.
61. Resister No. 47: 15, quoted in Van Zyl et al., 73.

62. "Calgary Psychiatrist Faces 21 Sex Assault Charges Involving Patients" *The Globe and Mail* (Friday, 30 July 2010) http://www.theglobeandmail.com/news/national/prairies/calgary-psychiatrist-faces-21-sex-assault-charges-involving-patients/article1657274/ (accessed 12 August 2010).
63. Staff at AFP, "Apartheid Army did Sex Changes on Gays: News Report," 31 July 2000, http://www.gfn.com/tools/printstory.phtml?sid=6921, (accessed 29 June 2004).
64. Interview IV1:2, quoted in Van Zyl et al., 76.
65. Van Zyl et al., 77.
66. Interview IV5 and 5B, quoted and translated in Van Zyl et al., 78–79.
67. Rebecca Sinclair, "The Official Treatment of White, South Africa, Homosexual Men and the Consequent Reaction of Gay Liberation from the 1990s to 2000" (Ph.D. diss., University of Johnnesburg, 2007), 162.
68. Van Zyl et al., 59.
69. Barry Fowler, "1 Mil" Sentinel Projects http://sadf.sentinelprojects.com/1mil/introtoc.html (accessed 29 May 2009).
70. Van Zyl et al., 79–85.
71. Barry Fowler, "1 Mil—Chapter One, The Psychologists" Sentinel Projects, http://sadf.sentinelprojects.com/1mil/introtoc.html (accessed 28 May 2009).
72. Transcript of Interview 8. Interview with Grobler for "The Aversion Project." In Newton, 152.
73. Sinclair, 133.
74. Personal email from Barry Fowler to Tiffany Jones, 12 Aug 2010.
75. Barry Fowler, "1 Mil—Chapter One, The Psychologists" Sentinel Projects, http://sadf.sentinelprojects.com/1mil/introtoc.html (accessed 28 May 2009).
76. Newton, 28–29.
77. *Aanhangsel A by Beleidsdirektief HSAW/1/13/82* quoted in Sentinel Projects, Fowler, "1-Mil" http://sadf.sentinelprojects.com/1mil/introtoc.html (accessed 28 May 2009).
78. Clive Wells, "Doctor: 1 Mil Psychiatry & Border" Sentinel Projects, http://sadf.sentinelprojects.com/propat/5cw.html (accessed 28 May 2009).
79. "Psychologist at 5SAI (1988)" http://sadf.sentinelprojects.com/bg1/5saibf.html (accessed 28 May 2009).
80. Personal email from Barry Fowler to Tiffany Jones, 12 Aug 2010.

NOTES TO CHAPTER 6

1. Memo from David Tabatznik, "Lifecare History," Lifecare Archives (LCA), c1996, 5, Annexure B.
2. Discussions about the relationship between private commercial interests and the colonial state in African countries have become increasingly popular since the 1970s. South African studies on the role of business during apartheid focus on the collusion between companies and the apartheid state. They also, however, highlight the effect of forces such as labour resistance or the economic profligacy of apartheid policies on company practices. Therefore, they show the somewhat paradoxical position that companies held within apartheid—at times supporting the apartheid government, at other times directly opposing it, and sometimes doing both. See, for example, Andrew Torchia, "The Business of Business: An Analysis of the Political Behaviour of the South African Manufacturing Sector under the Nationalists," *Journal of Southern African Studies* 14, no. 3 (April 1988): 421–455; Jock McCulloch, *Asbestos Blues: Labour Capital, Physicians & the State in South Africa* (Oxford: James Currey, 2002). For a discussion on studies of the role of both local and multinational

companies in Africa since the end of colonisation, see A. G. Hopkins, "Big Business in African Studies," *Journal of African History* 21, no. 1 (1987): 129–130.

3. In the late 1940s, when TB had become endemic in the country, Smith Mitchell obtained a contract with the Johannesburg municipality to provide care for the large number of white TB patients crowding Rietfontein hospital, the one central government hospital in Johannesburg that accepted TB patients. Smith Mitchell opened a few TB hospitals that catered to white patients. By 1954, however, doctors were also looking for beds for black TB patients. Smith Mitchell, under the precincts of the apartheid government, utilized abandoned mining compounds in rural areas for black TB hospitals. The company continued to expand so that by 1963, Smith Mitchell was providing 3,342 TB beds for different municipalities. As tuberculosis drugs improved and TB became less endemic, many of these TB hospitals closed or were converted into mental sanatoria. However, with many individuals with Acquired Immune Deficiency Syndrome (AIDS) today contracting tuberculosis, TB beds are once again required. Smith Mitchell, now known as Lifecare Inc., still provides TB beds for various provincial governments and in 1994 opened a new TB hospital known as Lifemed that has 175 beds for TB patients. Memo from David Tabatznik.
4. This number of mental sanatoria includes Randwest, Randmore, Millsite, Randaf, Randfontein, and Homelake, each part of the larger Randfontein Complex. This number excludes all Smith Mitchell TB sanatoria and elderly care facilities. Memo from David Tabatznik, 5, Annexure B.
5. Memo from David Tabatznik, 5.
6. Departmental responsibility for contracted institutions was not always clear. In 1977 Lage Vitus, Deputy Director of the South African National Council for Mental Health and Chairman of the Society of Social Workers, complained that "the Council had been running into a brick wall for years trying to get some action [for black mentally disabled individuals], but there were at least three Departments involved: Department of Bantu Administration, of Health and Social Welfare, and the buck is passed to and fro." "AG Africa," Citizens Commission of Human Rights Archives (CCHRA), Johannesburg, 1977.
7. All amounts are in US dollars and are based on the nominal annual exchange rates for the stated year (R0.68 to US$1). Records of daily rates per patient prior to 1973 no longer exist. Hansard, Debates of the House of Assembly (HAD), Vol. 56 (2 May 1975), col. 860.
8. If patients had to be transferred to public hospitals for general medical care, they were officially discharged and their file sent to the provincial general hospital. This arrangement was necessary to enable the national government to pay the medical costs to the provincial hospital. Once treatment in the provincial hospital was complete, patients were then returned to Smith Mitchell institutions as new admissions. In this way, the government only paid for the days that a patient stayed in a Smith Mitchell facility. However, the continuous discharge and readmission of patients together with the sheer numbers involved meant that keeping track of patients was difficult. Cases where patients became lost were common. One such case was of a woman who went to visit her brother in the state-run Sterkfontein hospital in Pretoria in 1974. Upon her arrival, she was told that her brother had been transferred to Randwest Sanatorium. At Randwest, however, she was told that her brother had died in a fire. However, the body shown to her was not that of her brother. She never found her brother. Staff Reporter, "'Hospitals lost my son,' court told," *Rand Daily Mail* (Johannesburg), 25 March 1977.

Transvaal Archives Depot (TAD), Pretoria, Registrar of the Supreme Court of South Africa Records, Witwatersrand Local Division (WLD) Illiquid case 10948/1976.

Platman also reports of "a mother who was looking for her child, who had apparently been transferred to Kirkwood . . . when 54 patients from the children's unit had been sent. They had apparently sent children who had addresses in the Cape. This child had apparently been sent inspite [*sic*] of the mother visiting on a two weekly basis." Parents were rarely informed of their children's transferral and doctors regularly reported that families lost track of their relatives. Stanley Platman, "Randfontein," LCA, 1984, 5 and 11.

9. P. H. Henning, Letter to The South African Institute of Race Relations, Department of Mental Health Archives (DMHA) A12/2/1 vol. 7 (17 July 1976).
10. In 1977, Mulder was implicated in a financial scandal that entailed the irregular use of secret state funds through the Department of Information. He was alleged to have issued funds in order to control the opposition English-language press and establish *The Citizen* daily newspaper on behalf of the National Party. Although the investigation, headed up by Judge R. P. B. Erasmus, initially cleared the State President, J. P. Vorster, of any wrongdoing, the scandal ultimately ended up causing Vorster to resign after Mulder argued in the *Rapport* newspaper that Vorster had indeed known about the use of funds. Rodney Davenport and Christopher Saunders, *South Africa: A Modern History,* 5th ed. (London; New York: MacMillan Press and St. Martin's Press, 2000), 454–458.
11. Sean O'Donoghue, "Health and Politics: An Appraisal and Evaluation of the Provision of Health, and Mental Health Services for Blacks in South Africa" (M.A. diss., Rhodes University, 1989), 23–24.
12. Lin Menge, Mike Engelbrecht, and Mervyn Rees, "The men in the business . . . ," *Rand Daily Mail,* 27 May 1975.
13. Jan H. Robbertze, interview by author, tape recording, Stellenbosch, Cape, 14 May 2002.
14. Alistair McE. Lamont, "Report by an Inter-departmental Study Group Regarding Accommodation Requirements at Mental Hospitals and Institutions for Mental Defectives in the Republic of South Africa" (Cape Town, 1969), 5.
15. Lin Menge, Mike Engelbrecht, and Mervyn Rees, "Life at the End of the Road: Inside SA's Mental Hospitals," *Rand Daily Mail,* 27 May 1975.
16. Francis Wilson, *Migrant Labour* (Johannesburg: The South African Council of Churches and SPRO-CAS, 1972), 10. For further descriptions about the living conditions in mining compounds, see Patrick Harries, *Work, Culture and Identity: Migrant Labourers in Mozambique and South Africa c1960–1910* (Portsmouth: Heinemann, 1994); Elaine Katz, *White Death: Silicosis on the Witwatersrand Gold Mines, 1886–1910* (Johannesburg, Witwatersrand University Press, 1994); and Dunbar Moodie, *Going for Gold: Men, Mines and Migration* (Johannesburg: Witwatersrand University Press, 1994).
17. Lin Menge, Mike Engelbrecht, and Mervyn Rees, "Life at the End of the Road: Inside SA's Mental Hospitals," *Rand Daily Mail,* 27 May 1975.
18. Stanley Platman, "Ekuhlengeni," LCA, 1984, 3; Stanley Platman, "Waverley," LCA, 1984, 21.
19. Charles Pinderhughes, Jeanne Spurlock, Jack Weinberg, Alan Stone, "Report of the Committee to Visit South Africa," American Psychiatric Association, 1978, 16.
20. Randfontein issued shoes to all of their patients. This meant that the predominance of athlete's foot and warts that existed in those institutions that did

not have shoes for all their patients was not found at Randfontein. "Minutes of a Meeting of Divisional Superintendents Held at Waverley Sanatorium on 11 August 1982 at 09h00," LCA, 7; and Stanley Platman, "Randfontein," LCA, 1982, 3.

21. Stanley Platman, "Poloko," LCA, 1982, 7; "Memo. Poloko Sanatorium," LCA, 1982.
22. Stanley Platman, "Randwest," LCA, 1982, 5; Stanley Platman, "Millsite Complex," LCA, 1984, 26.
23. Jan H. Robbertze, interview by author, tape recording, Stellenbosch, Cape, 14 May 2002.
24. Stanley Platman, "East Rand," LCA, 1982, 4; Platman, "Randfontein," 1984, 19.
25. Platman, "Randfontein," 1982, 6; 1984, 10.
26. Platman, "Millsite," 1984, 26.
27. Pinderhughes et al., 15; Platman, "Poloko," 1982, 7; and Stanley Platman, "Poloko," LCA, 1984, 3–4.
28. Stanley Platman, "Ekuhlengeni," LCA, 1982, 3; Platman, "Poloko," 1982, 3.
29. The shoe shop at Millsite later closed down due to the poor quality of shoes that the patients produced. Platman, "Millsite," 1984, 17.
30. Platman, "East Rand," 1982, 4; Platman, "Randfontein," 1982, 2; Platman, "Poloko," 1984, 12; Platman, "Waverley," 1984, 22; Platman, "Millsite," 1984, 17.
31. Platman, "Randfontein," 1984, 10; Platman, "Millsite," 1984, 7; Andre Cronje, "Comments by Mr. Cronje on Dr. Platman's Report on Randwest Sanatorium" LCA, (1982), 1.
32. See, for example, at Waverley in 1984 where 277 adult patients worked out of a total of 553. Platman, "Waverley," 1984, 12. At Randwest in 1975 over 400 patients worked in the hospital and in the industrial areas. By 1984, this number had increased to 877, so that over thirty percent of all patients were working. Menge et al., "Life at the End of the Road." In 1984 at Ekuhlengeni, over forty-three percent of all patients worked within the institution itself. The Allanridge superintendent estimated in 1984 that the company saved R19,176 ($16,395.04) a year by having patients work in the institution. As Allanridge was one of the smaller institutions with only 350 patients, larger institutions that had a larger patient base from which to draw its labour, saved considerably more. Stanley Platman, "Allanridge," LCA, 1984, 13.
33. Poloko began paying patients who worked around the hospital R2 a month. As patients worked five and a half hours a day, six days a week, this meant that patients were paid approximately 1.5 cents an hour. Platman, Poloko, 1984, 6 and 12. Patients who worked in industrial therapy at Waverley in 1984 could earn anywhere from as little as 50 cents to R5 a month, depending on productivity. Therefore, on average, patients at Waverley earned R2.16 a month. Platman, Waverley, 1984, 12 and 23. At Millsite, average patient wages were R1 a month, ranging from 50 cents to R8 a month in 1984. Platman, Millsite, 1984, 3–4. This meant that patients were earning four cents a day on average. In 1984, patients at Randfontein who made dresses for other facilities were paid between R1 and R6 a month. As it was estimated that fifteen patients could make thirty dresses a day, and the institution charged about 85 cents per dress, if the institutions paid patients the maximum amount of R6 a month, it made a minimum profit of approximately R675 a month. Platman, Randfontein, 1984, 17; Andre Cronje, "Randfontein Sanatorium: Comments on Dr. S. Platman's report," LCA, 1984, 3; and "Page 17,

Paragraph 5." Unpublished note, Stanley Platman Personal Archives (SPPA), 1984.

34. Platman, "Waverley," 1984, 30; Stanley Platman, "Witpoort," LCA, 1984, 2.
35. See, for example, Platman, "Ekuhlengeni," LCA 1984, 4; Platman, "Poloko," 1984, 2–4.
36. One case of a staff member sexually assaulting a patient was at Allanridge in 1982 when a male assistant sexually assaulted two female patients. After the general practitioner conducted examinations of the women and found evidence of sexual assault, the company called the police. While it is not known whether criminal charges were placed, the staff member was fired. Superintendents at other institutions also complained about of sexual activities in the institutions and while some may have been consensual, power relations between staff and patient made consensual sex highly problematic. Platman, "Allanridge," 1984, 12.
37. Platman, "Poloko," 1982, 2.
38. "Minutes of a Meeting of Divisional Superintendents Held at Waverley Sanatorium on 11 August 1982 at 09h00," LCA, 2; Platman, "Randwest," 1982, 3.
39. Platman, "Poloko," 1982, 3.
40. Platman, "Randwest," 1982, 3.
41. Death rates were higher in winter and for black patients. Randwest reported a death rate as high as 7.2 percent. Mentally challenged children also had a high death rate at 7.8 percent at Randwest and 6.5 percent at Ekuhlengeni. The high death rate among children was most likely due to the terrible conditions in which they lived and their more vulnerable immune systems. For psycho-geriatric institutions, these statistics were obviously higher at 15.3 percent, but as the APA Committee put it, "many of these deaths cannot be attributed simply to old age or to allowing old patients to die comfortably . . . we saw charts of black patients in their forties and fifties who were apparently allowed to die. . . ." Pinderhughes et al., 11–12. The general practitioner at Poloko admitted that many deaths had "no apparent reason." Platman, Poloko, 1984, 23. At Allanridge, Platman examined five charts of some of the younger individuals who had died in 1983, and was confused as to how determinations of deaths were established. He stated: "I believe all these deaths are strange and that the death certificates at best were guess work. It must concern us when young patients die and they either have no prior history of a physical problem or the prior illness is at best difficult to understand." Platman, "Allanridge," 1984, 6. Death rates in Smith Mitchell institutions were probably higher than those stated as many of the more serious cases were transferred to local hospitals where surgery was performed.
42. Pinderhughes et al., 11.
43. Platman, "Waverley," 1984, 27.
44. Platman, "Randfontein," 1982, 14.
45. Andre Cronje, "Comments by Mr. Cronje on Dr Platman's Report on Randfontein Sanatorium (Female)," LCA, 1982, 3.
46. Platman, "Ekuhlengeni," 1984, 28.
47. Smith Mitchell, "Meeting of Representatives of the Department of Health and Messrs Smith, Mitchell and Company Held at 9 a.m." DMHA, A12/2/1 vol. 1, 10 December 1974.
48. Letter from J. Gilliand, Secretary of Health to The Secretary S. A. Association of Private Hospitals (19 July 1976) DMHA, A12/2/1 vol. 6; and Andre Cronje, "Comments by Mr. Cronje on Dr. Platman's Report on Waverley Sanatorium," LCA, 1982.

49. Platman, "Poloko," 1984, 12.
50. Platman, "Randfontein," 1984, 13.
51. Interestingly, these categories were designed by Dr. H. Moross, formerly the South African psychiatrist who headed up Tara. In his retirement, he became advisor to Smith Mitchell. "Guide for the Management of Long-Term Psychiatric and Psychogeriatric Patients in the Smith Mitchell Group of Hospitals: (A Manual on Grading and Grouping)" (1978), DMHA, A12/2/1 Vol 9.
52. The CCHR claimed that there were many political dissidents housed in Smith Mitchell facilities. While a few patients were burdensome prisoners and some were perhaps political agitators, numerous investigations by international bodies found no evidence of dissidents in Smith Mitchell institutions and the housing of political dissidents in South Africa's mental hospitals was the exception to the rule.
53. Platman, "Poloko," 1982, 1; Platman, "Ekuhlengeni," 1982, 1; Platman, "East Rand," 1984, 6; Platman, "Poloko," 1984, 6; Platman, "Witpoort," 1984, 2; Platman, "Randfontein," 1984, 21.
54. Stanley Platman, "Kirkwood," LCA, 1984, 4; Platman, "East Rand," 1984, 6.
55. The MASA subgroup, the South African Society of Psychiatrists (SASOP) was only established in 1990.
56. Truth and Reconciliation Commission, Health Sector Hearings, Cape Town, 18 June 1997, <http://www.truth.org.za/HRVtrans/health/health02.htm> (22 February 2000), 78.
57. Republic of South Africa, Truth and Reconciliation Commission of South Africa, *Truth and Reconciliation Commission of South Africa Report,* Vol. 4 (1998), 146.
58. See, for example, Dr. Brett's comments in Platman, "Waverley," 1984, 3.
59. Smith Mitchell, "Responsibilities of Part-Time Medical Practitioners Employed in Private Psychiatric Hospitals and Sanatoria Conducted by Messrs Smith, Mitchell and Co," DMHA, A12/2/1 vol. 2 (1975).
60. Platman, Waverley, 1984, 28.
61. Black men also worked within Smith Mitchell institutions as nurses, but were a minority. Smith Mitchell argued that male nurses were essential within these chronic care facilities as they were able to control patients and perform some of the heavy labour that came with care of mentally "disabled" patients. The shortage of black male nurses in South Africa, however, did not enable the company to hire the numbers of male nurses it would have liked. Thus, the majority of nurses caring for patients were female, although many male domestics assisted them with patient care.
62. Shula Marks, *Divided Sisterhood: Race, Class and Gender in the South African Nursing Profession* (New York: St Martin's Press, 1994), 10.
63. Marks, 166.
64. Platman, "Allanridge," 1984, 3.
65. Stanley Platman, "Preliminary General Recommendations," LCA and SPPA, 1982.
66. *Source*: Compiled from LCA, "Management Structure," 1 August 1982.
67. Koena Botsane, a psychiatric nurse, points out that "working as a psychiatric nurse in a psychiatric hospital shares a number of similarities with being a psychiatric patient." She points out four areas where they share similar circumstances: "1. Monotonous and inferior meals. 2. Cold Conditions. Most institutions do not have adequate heating. Thus when it is cold for the patients it is also cold for the nurses. 3. Financial exploitation. Patients doing industrial therapy receive as little as R2.00 per month. Nurses increments are unstable and irregular. 4. The patients in institutions are at the mercy of the

health workers. Nurses too have little autonomy as the 'merit system' is used to promote conformity, fear and disunity amongst the nurses." Koena Botsane, "The Crisis for Psychiatric Nurses" in *Proceedings of Two Symposia: Mental Health Care for a New South Africa Held at the University of Witwatersrand, May 1990 and Rural Community Mental Health Care Held at Tintswalo Hospital, June 1990,* ed. Melvyn Freeman (Johannesburg: Centre for the Study of Health Policy, 1990), 38.

68. Fleur de Villiers, "Millions out of Madness," *Sunday Times,* 27 April 1975.
69. De Villiers.
70. Lin Menge, Mike Engelbrecht, and Mervyn Rees, *Rand Daily Mail,* 24–28 May 1975.
71. Hansard, HAD, Vol. 60 (18 February 1976), col. 1520.
72. "A New Kind of Concentration Camp Inside South Africa," *New York Voice,* 21 May 1976, 6; Peter Deeley, "Scandal of the Money-Making Mental Homes," *The Observer* (London) 3 June 1979; and Per Wästberg, "De Mentalsjuka privat guldgruva," "Det är polisen som förser lägren med ny arbetskraft" and "Mentalsjukhus I Sydafrika privat guldgruva," *Das Nyheter* (Sweden) 18 February 1976; and O'Donoghue, 23–24.
73. See *Peace and Freedom,* vol. 3, suppl., January, 1976.
74. Mental Health Amendment Act, 1976, Act No. 48, 1976, *Government Gazette* (7 April 1976), No. 5074; Prisons Act No. 8 of 1959.
75. One needs only to look at newspaper articles in the 1990s for the degree of staff discontent that actually existed. When many staff members no longer felt the threat of the act, they began expressing their discontent to both local and international reporters. Some nurses even wrote letters to the DOH, voicing their opinions about the substandard conditions in which they and patients work and lived. See Ciska Matthes, Linda Rulahe, and Gavin Evans "Behind the Asylum Walls," *Weekly Mail* 7, no. 22, 7 June to 13 June 1991; Corlia Erwee, "'n Kykie Na Sanatoriums vir Swartmense," *Beeld* (Johannesburg) 13 June 1991; and unpublished article by Ciska Matthes for the *Weekly Mail,* "Homosexual Rape is Allegedly a Daily Occurrence in the Sick Bay of Millsite," 1991.
76. Shortly after the publication of the *Observer* articles, the government denied entry visas to all *Observer* journalists and the South African embassy in London reportedly tried to pressure the newspaper to withdraw its allegations. "PR's TA Time Track," CCHRA, 13 May 1977; O'Donoghue, 23–24.
77. Politieke Beriggewer, "Rooi Kruis kom in SA kyk," *Die Transvaler* (Johannesburg) 22 October 1976; Korrespondent, "Minister Reageer: Sielsikes Kry Goie Sorg," *Die Burger* (Cape) 20 April 1976.
78. International Committee of the Red Cross, "Annual Report 1976" (Geneva, 1977), 18; and "Annual Report 1977" (Geneva, 1978), 17.
79. United Nations Centre Against Apartheid, "Report by WHO," Geneva, 22 March 1977 in *Notes and Documents* 11/77 (April, 1977), 25.
80. Our Correspondent, "Multi-Million Project Includes One Near City: Five Black Mental Hospitals to be Built," *Pretoria News,* 24 June 1977; "Adams Welcomes State Decision," *Cape Times,* 29 June 1977.
81. Pinderhughes et al., 5–6.
82. Pinderhughes et al., 5–6
83. O'Donoghue, iii.
84. Platman describes his recruitment as being somewhat curious as he was approached by Bernard Tabatznik at a party after hearing that he had lived briefly in South Africa in the 1960s and was married to a South African. At first he thought it was a joke, but then realizing that it was serious, he

accepted under the condition that he was given full access and his expenses were paid. Over the years, Platman's mandate grew to conduct evaluations of all the Smith Mitchell facilities, give some training to staff on areas of concern, build relationships with medical staff and universities, and attempt to create a "nucleus of a community program that would assist in the discharge of patients and the prevention of hospitalization when possible." He was also asked to consult on various administrative activities, such as the creation of a form for new admissions and the implementation of computer programmes at some institutions. When I asked Platman why Tabatznik would continue to enlist his services over the years despite his criticisms, he stated that he believed that Tabatznik genuinely wanted to upgrade the facilities. Stanley Platman, interview by author, tape recording, Baltimore, MD, 29 March 2003; "Letter from Stanley Platman to A.S. Cronje," SPPA, 4 December 1983.

85. Platman writes: "Mr Tabatznik . . . committed himself to do all that was economically possible to improve the facilities and public mental health . . . Much to my surprise my report was received with a positive concern and I was provided detailed reports on how they were reacting to each finding and recommendation." "A Follow-up on the 'Report of the Committee to Visit South Africa'" SPPA, c1986, 2–4. See also Platman "Preliminary General Recommendations," c1982, 2.
86. "Letter to Vera Thomas from Rian Venter," SPPA, 12 November 1982.
87. "Letter to Vera Thomas from Rian Venter."
88. Stanley Platman, "Thabamoopo," LCA, 1985, 11.
89. Platman, "East Rand," 1982, 4 and 17; Stanley Platman, "Thabamoopo," LCA, 1982, 11.
90. Platman, "Poloko," 1982, 2; "Allanridge," 1984, 18.
91. Sidney Bloch, "Report on Visit to Smith Mitchell Hospital," November 1978, LCA, 1.
92. Platman, "Randfontein," 1984, 7; and Platman, "Allanridge," 1984, 2.
93. Platman, "Poloko," 1982, 2.
94. "Meeting of Representatives of the Department of Health and Messrs Smith, Mitchell and Company Held at 9 a.m.," DMHA, A12/2/1, vol. 1, 10 December 1974, 3; and Platman, "Poloko," 1982, 2.
95. Platman, "Poloko," 1984; Platman, "Randfontein," 1984, 19; and Platman, "Waverley," 1984, 17.
96. "Minutes of a Meeting of Divisional Superintendents Held at Waverley Sanatorium at 09h00," LCA, 11 August 1982; and Platman, "Poloko," 1984, 34.
97. Platman, "Waverley," 1984, 20.
98. Platman, "Thabamoopo," 1985, 1.
99. "Letter to Mr. Richard Lurie, Smith Mitchell Institutions from Helen Suzman," SPPA, 30 June 1987.
100. "Letter to Mr D Tabatznik from Marius Barnard MD," SPPA, 13 July 1987.
101. "Letter to Dick Walt, American Medical News from Ralph Crawshaw," SPPA, 19 June 1987.
102. Kimberley A. Porteus et al., Centre for Health Policy, *Cost and Quality of Care: A Comparative Study of Public and Privately Contracted Chronic Psychiatric Hospitals* (Johannesburg: Centre for Health Policy, Department of Community Health, University of Witwatersrand, August 1998), 211 and 219.
103. Porteus et al., 218.

104. Platman, "Poloko," 1982, 4.
105. Platman, "Kirkwood," 1984, 3.
106. Platman, "Poloko," 1982, 3.
107. Platman, "Randwest," 1982, 5.

NOTES TO CHAPTER 7

1. Dr. P. J. Van B. Viljoen in Hansard, House of Assembly Debates (HAD), (1 June 1977), col. 8887.
2. Citizens Commission on Human Rights, *Betraying Society: Psychiatry Cases of Fraud* (Los Angeles: CCHR, 1999), 48.
3. Bryan R. Wilson, *The Social Dimensions of Sectarianism. Sects and New Religious Movements in Contemporary Society* (Oxford: Clarendon Press, 1990), 288
4. This builds on the arguments of Stephen Kent, who has clearly articulated why Scientology should be discussed as "a multi-faceted transnational corporation that has religion as only one of its many components." He argues that those that promote Scientology as a religious organization fail to recognize the historical data that suggests that its founder, Ron L. Hubbard, only claimed Scientology to be a religion for marketing and tax reasons. He also argues that Scientology has objectives other than religion such as "political aspirations, business operations, cultural productions, pseudo-medical practice, pseudo-psychiatric practice, social services (some of which are of dubious quality), and alternative family structures." Stephen A. Kent, "Scientology—Is This a Religion?" *Marburg Journal of Religion* 4, no. 1 (1999): 1 and 3.
5. The Church of Scientology claims that their first office opened in Johannesburg in 1957, but the South African Commission of Enquiry into Scientology states that they opened in 1959. Republic of South Africa, *Commission of Enquiry into Scientology for 1972*, (Pretoria, Government Printer, 1972); Ron L. Hubbard, "HCO Policy Letter—Religion", 29 October 1962, Hubbard Communications Office, East Grinstead, Sussex, England.
6. Republic of South Africa, Commission of Enquiry, 17.
7. "Memorandum: Hubbard Association of Scientologists International (H.A.S.I.)," MPO 30 MP 7/1
8. Quoted in Letter to the Minister of Justice from the Commissioner of Police" 29, 3, 1966 MPO 30 M.P. 7/1
9. Stephen A. Kent, "Scientology—Is This a Religion?," 3
10. Republic of South Africa, Commission of Enquiry, 32.
11. Republic of South Africa, Commission on Enquiry, 16.
12. "Letter to the Hon. B. J. Vorster from P. Dallas," 16 June 1966, MPO 30 M.P. 7/1 .
13. Letter from Joy Ollemans to P. C. Pelser, 4 October 1967, MPO 30 M.P. 7/1.
14. Letter to the Hon. S. L. Muller, Minister of the Interior, from Jan Lacey, Public Relations Chief for Africa," 4 November 1968, MPO 30 M.P 7/1 Polisie-Scientology.
15. Ron L. Hubbard, *Dianetics: The Modern Science of Mental Health* (Los Angeles: Bridge Publications, 1992), 174.
16. Ron L. Hubbard, Professional Auditor's Bulletin No. 119, 1 September 1957, quoted in Chris Owen, "Scientology's Fight *For* Apartheid," 1997, http://www.solitarytrees.net/cowen/misc/aparth.htm (accessed 29 May 2009).
17. See Chris Owen, "Miscellaneous Writings on Scientology" http://www.solitarytrees.net/cowen/misc/index.htm (accessed 29 May 2009); Ted Mayette

and Keshet, eds. "L. Ron Hubbard: Scientology, Dianetics and Racism" http://www.solitarytrees.net/racism/ (accessed 19 Aug 2008) and Andreas Heldal-Lund, "Operation Clambake: Undressing the Church of Scientology Since 1996" http://www.xenu.net/ (accessed 19 Aug 2008); and Lilly von Marcab "Scientology Cult: Hubbard's Extreme Racism OK With Us" *International* (29 Jun 2008) (accessed 19 Aug 2008).

18. Ron L. Hubbard, *Scientology: The Fundamentals of Thought* (Los Angeles: Bridge Publications, 2007), 30.
19. *Total Freedom Scientology: International Edition*, No. 1. (1969), 7.
20. Memorandum: Lafayette Ronald Hubbard (Scientology) (1966), MPO 30 MP7/1.
21. Ron L. Hubbard, "Confidential Report to the Prime Minister from L Ron Hubbard" (1966), MPO 30 MP 7/1.
22. Charles Stickley, *Brain-Washing: A Synthesis of the Russian Textbook on Psychopolitics* (Sussex: Hubbard College of Scientology, c1955), 6.
23. Ron Hubbard, "South African Broadsheet" Issue No. 1 (1968) WLO O 5310/1968.
24. Ron Hubbard, "South African Broadsheet" Issue No. 1 (1968) WLO O 5310/1968.
25. "Submission B" MPO 30 MP 7/1 (c1967).
26. Ron L. Hubbard, "HCO Information Letter of 4 April 1969" MPO 30 MP7/1.
27. *Total Freedom Scientology: International Edition*, No. 1. (1969), 1.
28. *Total Freedom* (1969), 1.
29. *Total Freedom* (1969), 1.
30. "Letter from Sachs, Berman & Schneider" to the Hon. St. L. Muller," 9 September 1969 and "Letter from Hubbard Scientology Organisation in South Africa to Dr. E. L. Fisher," 8 September 1969, MPO 30 M.P. 7/1 Polisie-Scientology
31. Executive Council for Africa Church of Scientology, "Telegram to the Hon SL Muller Minister of Police," 15 April 1969, MPO30 MP7/1.
32. "Court Told of Inquiry by Scientology," *Cape Argus* 1969; Republic of South Africa, *Commission of Enquiry*, Addendum 1.
33. "Action by Scientology Adjourned," *Cape Argus*, February 1969.
34. Poster, MPO 30 M.P 7/1 Polisie-Scientology.
35. "Letter to hon. D. de Wet, Minister of Health from O. W. K. Jackson," 12 December 1968. MGE 114 G16/3.
36. Welfare Organizations Act No. 40 of 1947, W. O. 72; Lage Vitus, "The Role of the National Council for Health and Government Agencies in Developing Mental Health Policy," M. A. diss., University of South Africa, 1987, 42.
37. Vitus, 85–86.
38. Republic of South Africa, *Commission of Enquiry*, 232.
39. *HAD*, (19 February 1976), col. 1576.
40. *HAD*, (9 May 1975), cols. 5738–5739.
41. *HAD*, (2 March 1976), col. 2312.
42. *HAD*, (19 February 1976), col. 1595.
43. Robert Ross, *A Concise History of South Africa* (New York: Cambridge University Press, 1999), 134.
44. Kent has assessed the way in which Scientology attempts to achieve "international dominance" and exert "global influence if not control over resources and opponents" (147). He shows how Scientology launches pre-emptive attacks and sometimes overtakes its so-called enemies in order to facilitate its growth. Kent argues that the game plan of Scientology and its subsidiaries, such as the Citizens Commission of Human Rights, is to eliminate their

enemies, in this case, psychiatrists. Kent has looked at the international efforts of CCHR against its opponents. In its anti-psychiatric campaign, Scientology has had some success in at least highlighting the questionable tactics of psychiatry worldwide, from Canada, where in 1981, they exposed the detention of a psychiatric patient, Henry Kowalski, who "was confined with the criminally insane while receiving heavy drug treatments and electroshocks" (150). They also publicized the use of sleep/sedation therapy in Australia in the 1990s. They also have a campaign against the abuse of prescriptions in pharmaceutical drugs, such as its Ritalin (150–151). Because they are scrutinizing the psychiatric and pharmaceutical industry, they are usually the first to begin asking questions about practices. Indeed, they are initiating some much needed discussion of these issues. Although its more prominent followers such as John Travolta and Tom Cruise, among other American actors, who promote Scientology, are making Scientology a much more well-known entity, especially with incidents such as Cruise's recent criticism of Brooke Shields of her taking anti-depressants for her post-partum depression, Scientology has been active in the political sphere worldwide since the 1950s. Stephen A. Kent, "The Globalization of Scientology: Influence, Control and Opposition in Transnational Markets," *Religion* 29 (1999): 147–169.

45. Dr. G. De V. Morrison in HAD, (19 February 1976), col. 1593.
46. Quoted in HAD, (18 February 1976), col. 1522.
47. Own Correspondent, "Congress Row over Black Mental Patients," *Rand Daily Mail*, 16 Jan 1979.
48. Ian Morgan, "Big Three in Drug Tender 'Collusion'," *Sunday Times: Business Times*, 25 March 1977.
49. Republic of South Africa, WJF Steenkamp, "Report of the Commission of Inquiry into the Pharmaceutical Industry" (Pretoria: Government Printer, 1978).
50. *Financial Mail* (6 April 1984), 24–26.
51. "Minister Puts Down Bribery Allegations" *Rand Daily Mail*, 24 February 1983; Mervyn Rees, "The New Drug Pushers: What a Commission of Inquiry said Five Years Ago about Gifts to Doctors," *Sunday Express*, 27 February 1983; Arlene Getz, Martin Welz, and Wilmar Utting, "Professors Named on Kaye Gift List," *Sunday Express*, 27 February 1983; A Doctor, "Chandeliers are Chickenfeed!", *Sunday Express*, 27 February 1983.
52. See "Minister Puts Down Bribery Allegations," *Rand Daily Mail*, 24 February 1983; "Professors Named on Kaye Gift List," *Sunday Express* (Johannesburg), 27 February 1983; A doctor, "Chandeliers are Chickenfeed!", *Sunday Express*, 27 February 1983; Mervyn Rees, "The New Drug Pushers: What a Commission of Inquiry Said Five Years ago About Gifts to Doctors," *Sunday Express*, 27 February 1983; Wilmar Utting and Arlen Getz, "Kaye Backed Nat Losers," *Sunday Express*, 13 March 1983; and Geoffrey Allen, "Bitter-Sweet Pills 'Vir Volk and Vaderland,'" *Rand Daily Mail*, 14 June 1983.
53. "Drug firm Admits Funding 6-week Trip," *Sunday Express*, 27 February 1983.
54. Philip McIntosh, "Cost or Safety: the Drug Dilemma" and "The South African Connection in the Supply of Generic Drugs," *The Age* (Australia), 3 June 1987; Letter to Mr. Philip McIntosh from David Tabatznik, 11 June 1987; and "Salesmen Sent to Hospitals to Seek out the Deadly Medicine," *Sunday Express*, 20 February 1983.
55. Citizens Commission on Human Rights, "Psychiatric Human Rights Abuses in South Africa: Links to Australian Drug Industry" (1987), 14.

56. Stanley Platman, interview by author, tape recording, Baltimore, MD, March 2003. Citizens Commission on Human Rights, "Psychiatric Human Rights Abuses in South Africa: Links;" Deborah Smith, "South African Denies Drug Company Holding," *Times on Sunday*, 15 February 1987.
57. David Carte, "Tabatznik—Aussie TV's Smear Victim," *Sunday Times, Business Times*, 24 May 1987.
58. Today, Smith Mitchell is known as Lifecare Inc. and is owned and operated by Afrox Healthcare. It has approximately 10,000 beds for chronically ill, elderly, and mental patients all contracted by the South African government. Afrox Healthcare website <http://www.afroxhealthcare.co.za/index.html> (29 December 2002).
59. "Dit werk fantasties en daarmee is die sielkundiges die eens. Op alle vlakke van ons samelewing het ons vandag hierdie probleem van verslaafdes en die gepaardgaande verlies aan mannekrag hetsy vakkundig of geskool op 'n laer peil. Narconon help hulle almal en bring hulle terug op 'n vlak waar hulle weer gelukkig en gesond is. Wat meer is, dit is permanent en geen opvolg behandeling is nodig nie." "Letter to the hon. S. L. Muller", 19 Feb 1973. MPO 30 M.P 71 Polisie-Scientology.
60. See Narconon International Website: http://www.narconon.org/narconon_centers/narconon_africa (accessed 8 April 2009).
61. HAD, (1 June 1977), cols. 8948–8949 and "Apartheid and Mental-Health Care," *The Lancet*, II: 8036 (1977), p. 491.
62. "Letter to Dr. John Dommissee from Dr. Alan A Stone," 3 December 1982, Stanley Platman Archives.
63. Rachel Jewkes, "The Case for South Africa's Expulsion From International Psychiatry," United Centre Against Apartheid, 1984.
64. American Psychiatric Association, Position Statement, Resolution Against Apartheid, 1985.
65. "South Africa Dropped as WMA Meeting Site," *Psychiatric News*, (17 May 1985).
66. Lyford Cay Nassau, "The Commonwealth Accord on Southern Africa (The 'Nassau Accord')" in *Mission to South Africa—the Commonwealth Report*, The Commonwealth Group of Eminent Persons, Penguin Books, 1986.
67. S. P. Sashidharan, "Correspondence: South African Psychiatry," *Bulletin of the Royal College of Psychiatrists*, 9 (1985), 202; and "Apartheid and Psychiatry," *Lancet* (29 December 1984).
68. Editorial, "Medical Journals and International Hate," *South African Medical Journal* 55, no.15 (1979): 572.
69. L. A. Hurst, "Correspondence: Advances in Contemporary Psychiatry," *South African Medical Journal* 50, no. 27 (1976): 1036.
70. L. S. Gillis, "Letters to the Editor: Mental-Health Care in South Africa," *The Lancet* II, no. 8044 (1977): 920.
71. Gillis, 920.
72. Cliff Allwood, interview with author, tape recording, Johannesburg, Gauteng, 25 July 2002.
73. George Hart, interview with author, tape recording, Johannesburg, Gauteng, 27 June 2002.
74. SPSA Declaration, 31 Jan 1985.
75. Society of Psychiatrists of South Africa (MASA), "Position Statement," Department of Justice Archives (DJA) Truth and Reconciliation Commission (TRC) Submission, 31 January 1985.
76. Lage Vitus, "The Role of the National Council for Mental Health and Government Agencies in Developing Mental Health Policy" (M.A. diss., University of South Africa, 1987), 87 and 182.

77. CCHR, "Report on Meeting with L. Vitus," 14 April 1977, CCHR Archives, Gauteng, South Africa.
78. Metín Başoğlu, *Torture and its Consequences* (Cambridge and New York: Cambridge University Press, 1992), 465.
79. Hart.
80. Cliff Allwood, interview with author, tape recording, Johannesburg, Gauteng, 25 July 2002.
81. Ashwin Valjee, interview with author, tape recording, Durban, KwaZulu-Natal, 11 June 2002.
82. Simpson, "Executive Summary," 2.
83. Valjee.
84. Michael Simpson, interview with author, Pretoria, Gauteng, 23 April 2002; and Michael Simpson, "Executive Summary of the Evidence to be Given by Professor Michael A. Simpson to the Truth & Reconciliation Commision's Health Sector Hearings, Cape Town, June 1997," Department of Justice Archives.
85. Allwood and Hart.
86. Jan H. Robbertze, interview by author, tape recording, Stellenbosch, Cape, 14 May 2002.
87. D. Gilbert, "Psychiatrists Resign Top Jobs Over Apartheid," *Sunday Tribune*, 3 February 1985.
88. Allwood.
89. Chris Owen, "Scientology's Fight for Apartheid: The Secret History of Racism in Scientology," "Africa, Clear Continent," *Solitary Trees* http://www.solitarytrees.net/cowen/misc/index.htm (accessed 12 June 2006).
90. See, for example, Ted Mayette and Keshet, eds. "L. Ron Hubbard: Scientology, Dianetics and Racism" http://www.solitarytrees.net/racism/ (accessed 19 Aug 2008) and Andreas Heldal-Lund, "Operation Clambake: Undressing the Church of Scientology Since 1996" http://www.xenu.net/ (accessed 19 Aug 2008); and Lilly von Marcab "Scientology Cult: Hubbard's Extreme Racism OK With Us" *International* (29 Jun 2008) (accessed 19 Aug 2008).
91. Mayette and Keshet, http://www.solitarytrees.net/racism/legacy.htm (accessed 19 Aug 2008).
92. Chris Owen, "Africa, Clear Continent: How the Church of Scientology has tried to 'win' South Africa" (c1997) http://www.solitarytrees.net/cowen/essays/southafrica.html (accessed 21 April 2006).
93. Stefaans Brummer, "Scientology's IFP Links," *Daily Mail & Guardian* (28 Feb 1997): http://www.mg.co.za/articledirect.aspx?articleid=207551&area=%2farchives__print_edition%2f (accessed 21 April 2006).
94. "News in Brief," *Daily Mail & Guardian (07 Mar 1997)*, (accessed 21 April 2006): http://www.mg.co.za/articledirect.aspx?articleid=179779&area=%2farchives__print_edition%2f.
95. "March 28—Expansion for Scientology in South Africa, " http://www.scientology.org.za/articles/803261435582.vm (accessed 14 June 2008).
96. "January 25—Scientology Volunteer Ministers Leave Behind a Legacy of Help" http://www.scientology.org.za/articles/701251313121.vm (accessed 14 June 2008).
97. Ben Ngubane, "Keynote Address at the Grand Opening of the Church of Scientology Johannesburg" (2003) http://www.scientology.org.za/community/opening/page06.html (accessed June 4, 2008).
98. David Miscavige, "Keynote Address at the Grand Opening of the Church of Scientology Johannesburg" (2003) http://www.scientology.org.za/community/opening/index2.html (accessed June 14, 2008).

NOTES TO THE CONCLUSION

1. Kim M. Phillips and Barry Reay, "Introduction" in *Sexualities in History: A Reader* (London and New York: Routledge, 2002), 15.
2. Deborah Posel, "Whiteness and Power in the South African Civil Service: Paradoxes of the Apartheid State," *Journal of Southern African Studies* 25, no. 1 (1999): 99.
3. Shula Marks, *Divided Sisterhood: Race, Class, and Gender in the South African Nursing Profession* (New York: St. Martin's Press, 1994).
4. On 30 August 2004, the government presented its Traditional Health Practitioner's Bill, that will gradually enable South Africa's estimated 200,000 healers to be integrated into the health care system through registration. This bill, however, has taken some time to implement. See "Law Catches up with Traditional Medicine," *Daily Mail & Guardian*, 30 August 2004, <http://www.mg.co.za/> (30 August 2004).
5. See Karen Flint, *Healing Traditions: African Medicine, Cultural Exchange, and Competition in South Africa, 1820–1948* (Athens: Ohio University Press, 2008), for a discussion of traditional healers in the KwaZulu-Natal area before apartheid.
6. Constitution of the Republic of South Africa, 1996.
7. Mental Health Care Bill, 2001.
8. Kimberley A. Porteaus, et. al., *Cost and Quality of Care: A Comparative Study of Public and Privately Contracted Chronic Psychiatric Hospitals* (Johannesburg: Centre for Health Policy, Department of Community Health, University of Witwatersrand, 1998), 188.
9. Robert Kohn et al., "Race and Psychiatric Services in Post-Apartheid South Africa: A Preliminary Study of Psychiatrists' Perceptions," *International Journal of Social Psychiatry* 50, no. 1 (2004): 18–24.
10. Karyn Maughan, "Crippling Backlogs in Psychiatric Testing of Rape, Murder Suspects," *The Star* (4 July 2006), 6.
11. Maughan, 6.
12. See, for example, *Saturday Star,* 18 Dec 1998; *Daily News,* 22 July 1999; *Sunday Times*, 4 Feb 2001; *Pretoria News,* 10 Mar 2005; and *Pretoria News,* 1 Feb 2005.
13. See Ethics Institute of South Africa, http://www.ethicsa.org.za/index.php?page=who_are_we (accessed 26 May 2009).
14. Quoted in "The Sun-City Hypothesis—An Alternative Hypothesis to Mental Illness," *Mindfreedom*. 1 August 2007, http://www.mindfreedom.org/as/act/inter/mfsouthafrica/sun-city-hypothesis (accessed 26 May 2009).

Bibliography

ARCHIVES

1/TSO	Tsolo Magistrate Records
A272	Public Servants' Association Collection
AM2656	Immorality Amendment Bill of 1968
CAD	Central Archives Depot, Pretoria
CCHRA	Citizens Commission on Human Rights Archives, Johannesburg
DJA	Department of Justice Archives, Pretoria
DMHA	Department of Mental Health Archives, Pretoria
GALA	Gay and Lesbian Archives of South Africa, University of Witwatersrand, Johannesburg
KAB	Cape Town Archives Repository, Cape Town
LCA	Lifecare Archives, Ferndale, Gauteng
MPO	Private Secretary of the Minister of Police Records
NAD	Natal Archives Depot, Pietermaritzburg
NTS	Secretary of Native Affairs Records
GG	Governor General's Records
PM	Prime Minister Records
RSC	Supreme Court Registrar Records
SPPA	Stanley Platman's Personal Archives, Baltimore, Maryland
TAD	Transvaal Archives Depot, Pretoria
TRC	Truth and Reconciliation Commission Records
WLD	Registrar of the Supreme Court of South Africa, Witwatersrand Local Division

GOVERNMENT LEGISLATION

Bantu Authorities Act No. 68 of 1951

Bantu Homelands Citizens Act of 1970

Bantu Homelands Constitution Act (National States Constitutional Act) No. 21 of 1971

Constitution of the Republic of South Africa Act No. 110 of 1983

Immorality Amendment Act No. 23 of 1957

Immorality Amendment Bill of 1968

Mental Disorders Act No. 38 of 1916

Mental Health Act No. 18 of 1973

Mental Health Care Bill of 2001

Prisons Act No. 8 of 1959

Welfare Organizations Act No. 40 of 1947

SOUTH AFRICAN GOVERNMENT REPORTS

Annual Reports for the Commissioner for Mental Hygiene/Health, 1939–1970
Department of Health and Welfare, Codified Instructions: Mental Health Act, 1973
Commission of Enquiry into Scientology RP 55/1973
Commission of Inquiry to inquire into the Responsibility of Mentally Deranged Persons and Related Matters (Rumpff Commission) RP 69/1967
Commission of Inquiry into the Mental Disorders Act, 1916 (Act No. 38 of 1916, as amended) and Related Matters (Van Wyk Commission) RP 80/1972
Committee of Inquiry into the Care of Mentally Deficient Persons, 1967
House of Assembly Debates, 1939–1979
Lamont, A. M. Report by an Inter-Departmental Study Group Regarding Accommodation Requirements at Mental Hospitals and Institutions for Mental Defectives in the Republic of South Africa, 1969
Report of the Select Committee on the Immorality Amendment Bill: Original Evidence, S.C. 7-'68 (Pretoria: Government Printer, 1968)
Statistics South Africa, "The People of South Africa Population Census, 1996" http://www.statssa.gov.za/census01/Census96/HTML/default.htm
Truth and Reconciliation Commission of South Africa. *Truth and Reconciliation Commission of South Africa Report*, Vol. 4. Basingstoke and Oxford: Macmillan Reference Limited, 1998

NEWSPAPERS

The Age (Australia)
Daily Mail and Guardian (South Africa)
The Globe and Mail (Canada)
Independent Online
New York Voice
The Observer (London)
Peace and Freedom
Rand Daily Mail (Johannesburg)
The Star (Johannesburg)
Sunday Express (Johannesburg)
Sunday Times (South Africa)

BOOKS, ARTICLES, AND OTHER REPORTS AND PAPERS

"Die Hantering Van Persone Met Psigopatiese Neigings." *South African Medical Journal* 40, no. 45 (1966): 1079.
"First National Congress of Psychiatry: Abstracts of Papers." *South African Medical Journal* 49, no. 24 (1975): 920–986.
"The Mental Disorders Amendment Act 1957." *South African Medical Journal* 31, no. 31 (1957): 785–786.
"Mental Hospital Services in the Union: An Interview With the Minister of Health." *South African Medical Journal* 20, no. 13 (1946): 390–391.
"Poisoning by Arsenic in South Africa." *South African Medical Journal* 14, no. 18 (1940): 383–384.
"Psychiatry." *Bantu* 21, no. 7 (1974): 7.
"Psychiatry and South Africa." In *Creating Racism: Psychiatry's Betrayal: In the Guise of Help*. Los Angeles: Citizens Commission on Human Rights, 1995, 6–19.

Ackerknecht, Erwin Heinz. *A Short History of Psychiatry.* 2nd revised ed. New York: Hafner, 1968.

Adhikari, M., M. Mackenjee, R. Green-Thompson, W. Loening, A. Moosa, Y. K. Seedat, and J. W. Downing. "Correspondence: Medical Journals and International Hate." *South African Medical Journal* 56, no. 1 (1979): 6.

Adler, Patricia A., and Peter Adler. "General Introduction." In *Constructions of Deviance: Social Power, Context, and Interaction,* eds. Patricia A. Adler and Peter Adler. Belmont, California: Wadsworth Publishing Company, 1993, 1–5.

Alexander, Franz, and Sheldon T. Selesnick. *The History of Psychiatry: An Evaluation of Psychiatric Thought and Practice From Prehistoric Times to the Present.* New York: Harper & Row, 1966.

Allwood, Cliff W. "Problems in Institutional and Hospital Care of Psychiatric Patients." In *Proceedings of Two Symposia: Mental Health Care for a New South Africa Held at the University of Witwatersrand, May 1990 and Rural Community Mental Health Care Held at Tintswalo Hospital, June 1990,* ed. Melvyn Freeman. Johannesburg: Centre for the Study of Health Policy, 1990, 12–25.

———. "Psychiatry in Primary Health Care in South Africa." M. Med. diss., University of Witwatersrand, 1979.

American Association for the Advancement of Science and Physicians for Human Rights in conjunction with the American Nurses Association and the Committee for Health in Southern Africa. *Human Rights and Health: The Legacy of Apartheid.* Washington: American Association for the Advancement of Science, 1998.

Andersson, Neil, and Shula Marks. "Apartheid and Health in the 1980s." *Social Science & Medicine* 27, no. 7 (1988): 667–681.

Archer, B. Crowhurst. "Correspondence: Psychiatry and General Practice: Congress Symposium." *South African Medical Journal* 26, no. 44 (1952): 886–887.

———. "Mental Health and Public Health." *South African Medical Journal* 32, no. 41 (1958): 1004–1007.

———. "A Mental Health Service for South Africa." *South African Medical Journal* 39, no. 43 (1965): 1095–1098.

———. "Psychiatry in South Africa: A Short History and Review." *South African Medical Journal* 37, no. 17 (1963): 467–468.

Asuni, Tolani, Friderun Schoenberg, and Charles R Swift. *Mental Health and Disease in Africa.* Ibadan: Spectrum Books, 1994.

Barrett, Robert J. "Clinical Writing and the Documentary Construction of Schizophrenia." *Culture, Medicine and Psychiatry* 12 (1988): 265–299.

Baruch, Geoff, and Andrew Treacher. *Psychiatry Observed.* London, Boston: Routledge & K. Paul, 1978.

Başoğlu, Metín. *Torture and its Consequences.* Cambridge and New York: Cambridge University Press, 1992.

Bayer, Ronald. *Homosexuality and American Psychiatry: The Politics of Diagnosis.* New York: Basic Books, 1981.

Berglund, A. I. *Zulu Thought-Patterns and Symbolism.* London: C. W. Hurst and Co., 1976.

Berrios, German, and Roy Porter. *A History of Clinical Psychiatry: The Origin and History of Psychiatric Disorders.* London: Athlone, 1995.

Beuschel, Gail C. "Shutting Africans Away: Lunacy, Race and Social Order in Colonial Kenya, 1910–1964." Ph.D. diss., School of Oriental and African Studies, 2001.

Bloch, Sidney, and Peter Reddaway. *Russia's Political Hospitals: the Abuse of Psychiatry in the Soviet Union.* London: Gollancz, 1977.

Bolland, O. Nigel. "Mannoni and Fanon: The Psychology of Colonization and the Decolonization of the Personality." *New Scholar* 4, no. 1 (1973): 29–47.

Bonner, Phillip, Peter Delius, and Deborah Posel. "The Shaping of Apartheid: Contradiction, Continuity and Popular Struggle." In *Apartheid's Genesis: 1935–1962*. Johannesburg: Wits University Press, 1993, 1–41.

Botha, Kevan, and Edwin Cameron. "South Africa." In *Sociolegal Control of Homosexuality: A Multi-Nation Comparison*, eds. Donald J. West and Richard Green. New York and London: Plenum Press, 1997, 5–42.

Botsane, Koena. "The Crisis for Psychiatric Nurses." In *Proceedings of Two Symposia: Mental Health Care for a New South Africa Held at the University of Witwatersrand, May 1990 and Rural Community Mental Health Care Held at Tintswalo Hospital, June 1990*, ed. Melvyn Freeman. Johannesburg: Centre for the Study of Health Policy, 1990, 37–43.

Bracken, Patrick J. "Post-Empiricism and Psychiatry: Meaning and Methodology in Cross-Cultural Research." *Social Science and Medicine* 36, no. 3 (1993): 265–272.

Bradford, Helen. *A Taste of Freedom: The ICU in Rural South Africa, 1924–1930*. New Haven and London: Yale University Press, 1987.

Breggin, Peter R. *Toxic Psychiatry: Psychiatry's Assault on the Brain With Drugs, Electroshock, Biochemical Diagnoses, and Genetic Theories*. New York: St. Martin's Press, 1991.

Brink, C. D. "Psychosomatic Disorders." *South African Medical Journal* 19, no. 1 (1945): 11–14.

Buchan, T. "Some Problems in the Hospital Management of Criminal Mental Patients." *South African Medical Journal* 50, no. 32 (1976): 1252–1256.

———. "The Treatment of Depression in African Patients." *South African Medical Journal* 45, no. 36 (1971): 1001–1004.

Bührmann, M. Vera. *Living in Two Worlds: Communication Between a White Healer and Her Black Counterparts*. Cape Town: Human & Rousseau, 1984.

———. "Western Psychiatry and the Xhosa Patient." *South African Medical Journal* 51, no. 14 (1977): 464–466.

Bulhan, Hussein Abdilahi. *Frantz Fanon and the Psychology of Oppression*. New York: Plenum, 1985.

Burman, Sandra, and Margaret Naude. "Bearing a Bastard: The Social Consequences of Illegitimacy in Cape Town, 1896–1939." *Journal of Southern African Studies* 17, no. 3 (1991): 373–413.

Burrows, Edmund H. *A History of South Africa Up to the End of the Nineteenth Century*. Cape Town : A. A. Balkema, 1958.

Busfield, Joan. *Managing Madness: Changing Ideas and Practice*. London; Dover, N.H.: Hutchinson, 1996.

———. *Men, Women and Madness: Understanding Gender and Mental Disorder*. London: Macmillan, 1996.

Butchart, Alex, Brandon Hamber, Martin Terre Blanche, and Mohammed Seedat. "Violence, Power and Mental Health Policy in Twentieth Century South Africa." In *Mental Health Policy Issues for South Africa*. Edited by Don Foster, Melvyn Freeman, and Yogan Pillay. Pinelands: Medical Association of South Africa, 1997.

Butchart, Alexander. *The Anatomy of Power: European Constructions of the African Body*. London; New York: Zed Books, 1998.

———. "The 'Bantu Clinic': A Genealogy of the African Patient As Object and Effect of South African Clinical Medicine, 1930–1990." *Culture, Medicine and Psychiatry* 21 (1997): 405–441.

Caldwell, Bill S. "The Impact of French Colonialism on the Colonized: Three Experiences." *Indiana Social Studies Quarterly* 30, no. 1 (1977): 84–93.

Calloway, Paul. *Russian/Soviet and Western Psychiatry: A Contemporary Comparative Study*. New York: Wiley, 1993.

Campbell, Chloë. "Eugenics, Race and Empire: The Kenya Casebook." Ph.D. diss., School of Oriental and African Studies, University of London, 2000.

Campbell, Meaghan E. "Discourse Analysis of Rape in South African Townships (1948–1994): A Case for 'Policing the Penis'." M.A. thesis, Dalhousie University, 2000.

Camperio-Ciani, A., F. Corna, and C. Capiluppi. "Evidence for Maternally Inherited Factors Favouring Male Homosexuality and Promoting Female Fecundity." *Proceedings of the Royal Society of London. Series B. Biological Sciences* 271, no. 1554 (2004): 2217–2221.

Carothers, John Colin. *The African Mind in Health and Disease: A Study in Ethnopsychiatry*. Geneva: World Health Organization, 1953.

Caunce, Stephen. *Oral History and the Local Historian*. London: Longman, 1994.

Chapman, Audrey R., and Leonard Rubenstein. *Human Rights and Health: The Legacy of Apartheid*. Washington, DC: American Association for the Advancement of Science, 1998.

Cheetham, R. W. S. "Commission of Inquiry into the Mental Disorders Act in Relation to the Problems of Today." *South African Medical Journal* 44, no. 48 (1970): 1371–1372.

———. "Society, the Legislator, Mental Health and Ourselves." *South African Medical Journal* 38, no. 31 (1964): 716–720.

Cheetham, R. W. S., and J. A. Griffiths. "Sickness and Medicine: An African Paradigm." *South African Medical Journal* 62, no. 25 (1982): 954–956.

Chesler, Phyllis. *Women and Madness*. New York: Avon, 1983.

Christie, Pam, and Colin Collins. "Bantu Education: Apartheid Ideology and Labour Reproduction." In *Apartheid and Education: The Education of Black South Africans*, ed. Peter Kallaway. Johannesburg: Ravan Press, 1991, 160–183.

Citizens Commission on Human Rights. "Psychiatric Human Rights Abuses in South Africa: Links to Australian Drug Industry." 1987.

———. *Betraying Society: Psychiatry Cases of Fraud*. Los Angeles: CCHR, 1999.

Citizens Commission on Human Rights (South Africa & International). "Submission to the South African Truth & Reconciliation Commission: 'The Tragedy of Psychiatry Creating Apartheid'." 1997.

Cluver, E. H. *Social Medicine*. South Africa: Central News Agency, 1951.

Cluver, P. F. "Some Technical Problems in Electro-Convulsive Therapy." *South African Medical Journal* 16, no. 19 (1942): 350.

Cohen, Morris J. "The New Hope in Mental Disorders." *South African Medical Journal* 14, no. 21 (1941): 434.

Comaroff, Jean. "Healing and Cultural Transformation: The Tswana of Southern Africa." *Social Science and Medicine—Part B, Medical Anthropology* 15, no. 3 (1981): 367–378.

Comaroff, John, and Jean Comaroff. "The Madman and the Migrant." In *Ethnography and the Historical Imagination*, eds. John Comaroff and Jean Comaroff. Boulder: Westview Press, 1992, 155–180.

Comaroff, John L. "Reflections on the Colonial State in South Africa and Elsewhere: Factions, Fragments, Facts and Fictions." *Social Identities* 4, no. 3 (1998): 321–361.

Cooper, Frederick, and Ann L. Stoler. "Introduction: Tensions of Empire: Colonial Control and Visions of Rule." *American Ethnologist* 16, no. 4 (1989): 609–621.

Cornwell, Gareth. "George Webb Hardy's *The Black Peril* and the Social Meaning of 'Black Peril' in Early Twentieth Century South Africa." *Journal of Southern African Studies* 22, no. 3 (1996): 441–454.

Corrigan, Phillip, and Derek Sayer. *The Great Arch: English State Formation As Cultural Revolution.* Oxford; New York: Blackwell, 1985.

Cox, Alice. "Psychological Illness in South Africa: The Problems of Treatment and Care. The Psychiatrist's Point of View." *South African Medical Journal* 27, no. 38 (1953): 813–814.

Dain, Norman. "Anti-psychiatry." In *American Psychiatry After World War II (1944–1994)*, eds. Roy W. Menninger and John C. Nemiah, 277–298. Washington: American Psychiatric Press, 2000.

Daneel, M. H., E. Du Pisani, B. T. Jackson, A. Levin, S. J. Olivier, L. Strydom, and L. R. Uys. "Some Perceptions of Disease Among the Urban Blacks of Mangaung, Bloemfontein, South Africa: A Preliminary Report." Paper presented at the Conference on African Healing Strategies, Florida, 9 March 1984.

Davenport, Rodney, and Christopher Saunders. *South Africa: A Modern History.* Fifth ed. New York: St. Martin's Press, 2000.

Davies, Kerry. "'Silent and Censured Travellers'? : Patients' Narratives and Patients' Voices : Perspectives on the History of Mental Illness Since 1948." *Social History of Medicine* 14, no. 2 (2001): 267–292.

Daynes, G., and N. P. Msengi. "'Why Am I Ill? Who Made Me Ill?': The Relevance of Western Psychiatry in Transkei." *South African Medical Journal* 56, no. 8 (1979): 307–308.

De Beer, Cedric. *The South African Disease: Apartheid, Health and Health Services.* Trenton, NJ: Africa World Press, 1986.

de la Rey, Cheryl. "On Political Activism and Discourse Analysis in South Africa." In *Culture, Power and Difference: Discourse Analysis in South Africa*, eds. Ann Levett, Amanda Kottler, Erica Burman, and Ian Parker. Cape Town: University of Cape Town Press, 1997, 189–197.

De Luca, V., H. Wang, A. Squassina, G. W. Wong, J. Yeomans, and J. L. Kennedy. "Linkage of M5 Muscarinic and Alpha7-Nicotinic Receptor Genes on 15q13 to Schizophrenia." *Neuropsychobiology* 50, no. 2 (2004): 124–127.

de Villiers, J. J. "The Aetiology of Mental Illness." *Edinburgh Medical Journal* 57 (1950): 276.

———. "Correspondence: Mental Disorder, Crime and Sin." *South African Medical Journal* 24, no. 23 (1950): 455–456.

———. "Letter to the Editor: Psycho-Analysis." *South African Medical Journal* 25, no. 36 (1951): 36.

de Vos, P. J. G. "Some Aspects Concerning Research in Psychiatry." *South African Medical Journal* 19, no. 10 (1945).

de Wet, J. S. du T. "Convulsive Therapy and Analytical Psycho-Therapy in a Case of Psychoneurosis." *South African Medical Journal* 18, no. 18 (1944): 317.

Deacon, Harriet. "Racial Categories and Psychiatry in Africa: The Asylum on Robben Island in the Nineteenth Century." In *Race, Science and Medicine, 1700–1960*, eds. Waltraud Ernst and Bernard Harris. London; New York: Routledge, 1999, 101–122.

Dean, T., and Lane, C., eds. *Homosexuality and Psychoanalysis.* Chicago, University of Chicago Press, 2001.

Dommisse, John. "Apartheid As a Public Mental Health Issue." *International Journal of Health Services* 15, no. 3 (1985): 501–510.

———. "Health and Health Care in Post-Apartheid South Africa: A Future Vision." *Journal of the National Medical Association* 80, no. 3 (1988): 325–333.

———. "The Psychiatry and the Psychosocial Pathology of Apartheid, 1948–1982." *United Nations Centre Against Apartheid Notes and Docs*, 3/83 (1983).

Don, A. M. "Transvestism and Transsexualism: A Report of 4 Cases and Problems Associated with the Management." *South African Medical Journal* 37 (1963): 479–485.

Dreyfus, Hubert, and Paul Rabinow. *Michel Foucault: Beyond Structuralism and Hermeneutics*. Chicago: University of Chicago Press, 1983.

Dubow, Saul. "Afrikaner Nationalism, Apartheid and the Conceptualisation of Race." *Journal of African History*, 33 (1992): 209–237.

———. "Ethnic Euphemisms and Racial Echoes." *Journal of Southern African Studies* 20, no. 4: 355–370.

———. *Scientific Racism in South Africa*. Cambridge: University of Cambridge Press, 1995.

Duffin, Jacalyn. *History of Medicine: A Scandalously Short Introduction*. Toronto: University of Toronto Press, 2000.

Edelstein, Ilana, Vaughan Weber, and Yogan Pillay. "The Role of the Private Sector." In *Mental Health Policy Issues for South Africa*, eds. Don Foster, Melvyn Freeman, and Yogan Pillay. Pinelands: Medical Association of South Africa, Multimedia Publications, 1997, 132–142.

Edgar, Robert R., and Hilary Sapire. *African Apocalypse: The Story of Nontetha Nkwenkwe, a Twentieth-Century South African Prophet*. Johannesburg: Witwatersrand University Press, 1999.

Editorial. "Medical Journals and International Hate." *South African Medical Journal* 55, no. 15 (1979): 572–573.

———. "Mental Health." *South African Medical Journal* 44, no. 27 (1970): 774.

———. "Mental Health Services." *South African Medical Journal* 35, no. 21 (1961): 423–424.

———. "The Non-European Medical School." *South African Medical Journal* 25, no. 27 (1951): 469–470.

———. "Psychiatric Services in South Africa." *South African Medical Journal* 32, no. 41 (1958): 996–997.

———. "Why South Africa Is Short of Psychiatrists." *South African Medical Journal* 35, no. 8 (1961): 147–148.

Edwards, Graham A., and Bruce Flaherty. "Electro-Convulsive Therapy: A New Era of Controversy." *Australian & New Zealand Journal of Psychiatry* 12, no. 3 (1978): 161–164.

Edwards, S. D., P. W. Grobbellaar, N. V. Makunga , P. T. Sibaya, L. Nene, S. T. Kunene, and A. S. Magwaza. "Traditional Zulu Theories of Illness in Psychiatric Patients." *Journal of Social Psychology* 121, no. 2 (1983): 213–221.

Elder, Glen S. *Hostels, Sexuality, and the Apartheid Legacy: Malevolent Geographies*. Athens, Ohio: Ohio University Press, 2003.

———. "Of Moffies, Kaffirs and Perverts: Male Homosexuality and the Discourse of Moral Order in the Apartheid State." In *Mapping Desire: Geographies of Sexualitie*, eds. David Bell and Gill Valentine. London and New York: Routledge, 1995, 56–65.

Elliott, G. A. "The Integration of Medicine With Mental Health Activities." *South African Medical Journal* 38, no. 8 (1964): 148–151.

———. "The Mind-Body Relationship." *South African Medical Journal* 27, no. 38 (1953): 817–818.

———. "Psychiatry in a General Hospital." *South African Medical Journal* 28, no. 27 (1954): 561–567.

Epprecht, Marc. "'Bisexuality' and the Politics of Normal in African Ethnography." *Anthropologica* 48, 2 (2006): 187–201.

———. "The 'Unsaying' of Indigenous Homosexualities in Zimbabwe: Mapping a Blindspot in an African Masculinity." *Journal of Southern African Studies* 24, no. 4 (1998): 631–651.

Fancher, R. E. "Freud's Attitudes Towards Women: A Survey of His Writings." *Queen's Quarterly* 82, no. 3 (1975): 368–393.

Fanon, Frantz. *Black Skin, White Masks.* Translated by Charles Lam Markmann. New York: Grove Press, 1952, 1967.

———. *The Wretched of the Earth.* Translated by Constance Farrington. New York: Grove Press, 1963.

Farrand, D. "Is a Combined Western and Traditional Health Service for Black Patients Desirable?" *South African Medical Journal* 66, no. 20 (1984): 779–780.

Felman, Shoshana. "Women and Madness: The Critical Phallacy." *Diacritics* (1975): 2–10.

Fernando, Suman. *Mental Health, Race, and Culture.* New York: St. Martin's Press, 1991.

Fink, Max. *Electroshock: Healing Mental Illness.* New York: Oxford University Press, 1999.

Finnane, Mark. "The Ruly and the Unruly: Isolation and Inclusion in the Management of the Insane." In *Isolation: Places and Practices of Exclusion,* eds. Carolyn Strange and Alison Bashford. London and New York: Routledge, 2003, 90–103.

Fireside, Harvey. *Soviet Psychoprisons.* New York: Norton, 1979.

Fischer, P. J. "Cultural Aspects of Bantu Psychiatry." *South African Medical Journal* 36, no. 8 (1962): 133–138.

Fleisch, Brahm David. "Social Scientists As Policy Makers: E. G. Malherbe and the National Bureau for Educational and Social Research, 1929–1943." *Journal of Southern African Studies* 21, no. 3 (1995): 349–372.

Flint, Karen. *Healing Traditions: African Medicine, Cultural Exchange, and Competition in South Africa, 1820–1948.* Athens: Ohio University Press, 2008.

Fontenot, Deborah B. "A Vision of Anarchy: Correlate Structures of Exile and Madness in Selected Works of Doris Lessing and Her South African Contemporaries." Ph.D. diss., University of Illinois, 1988.

Foster, Don, Melvyn Freeman, and Yogan Pillay, eds. *Mental Health Policy Issues for South Africa.* Pinelands: Medical Association of South Africa, 1997.

Foucault, Michel. *The Birth of the Clinic: An Archaeology of Medical Perception.* New York: Pantheon Books, 1973.

———. *Discipline & Punish: The Birth of the Prison.* New York: Pantheon Books, 1977.

———. "Govermentality." In *The Foucault Effect: Studies in Governmentality, With Two Lectures by and an Interview With Michael Foucault,* eds. Graham Burchell, Colin Gordon, and Pete Miller. London: Harvester Wheatsheaf Press, 1991.

———. *Madness and Civilization: a History of Insanity in the Age of Reason.* New York: Pantheon Books, 1965.

Freed, Louis F. "Correspondence: Nativity and the Incidence of Mental Disorder in South Africa." *South African Medical Journal* 27, no. 16 (1953): 355–356.

———. "Homosexuality and the Bill." *South African Medical Journal* 42, 22, (1968): 567.

———. "Medico-Sociological Data in the Therapy of Homosexuality." *South African Medical Journal* 28, 48 (1954): 1022–1023.

———. "The Summarised Findings of Medico-Sociological Investigation into the Problem of Prostitution in Johannesburg." *South African Medical Journal* 22, no. 2 (1948): 52–56.

Freeman, Hugh L. *A Century of Psychiatry.* London: Mosby, 1999.

Freeman, Melvyn. "The Challenges Facing Mental Health Care in South Africa." *Proceedings of Two Symposia: Mental Health Care for a New South Africa*

Held at the University of Witwatersrand, May 1990 and Rural Community Mental Health Care Held at Tintswalo Hospital, June 1990. Johannesburg: Centre for the Study of Health Policy, 1990, 3–11.

Freud, Sigmund. "Obsessive Acts and Religious Practices." In *The Collected Papers*. Vol. 2. London: Hogarth Press, 1924.

———. *Totem and Taboo: Resemblances Between the Psychic Lives of Savages and Neurotics*. Translated by A. A. Brill. New York: 1946.

Gale, G. W. "The Durban Medical School: A Progress Report." *South African Medical Journal* 29, no. 19 (1955): 436–440.

Gelfand, Michael. *The Sick African: A Clinical Study*. Third ed. Cape Town: Juta, 1957.

Geller, Jeffrey L., and Maxine Harris. *Women of the Asylum: Voices From Behind the Walls, 1840–1945*. New York: Anchor Books, 1994.

Gendzier, Irene L. "Psychology and Colonialism: Some Observations." *Middle East Journal* 30, no. 4 (1976): 501–515.

Geuter, Ulfried. *The Professionalization of Psychology in Nazi Germany*. New York: Cambridge University Press, 1992.

Geyer, Felix, ed. *Alienation, Ethnicity, and Postmodernism*. Westport: Greenwood Press, 1996.

Gibson, Nigel C. *Fanon: The Postcolonial Imagination*. Oxford: Polity, 2003.

Giliomee, Hermann, and Lawrence Schlemmer, *From Apartheid to Nation-Building*. Cape Town: Oxford University Press, 1989.

Gillis, L. S. "Education for Appropriate Psychiatry." *South African Medical Journal* 49, no. 4 (1975): 112–116.

———. *Guidelines in Psychiatry*. Cape Town: D. Philip, 1977.

———. "Letters to the Editor: Mental-Health Care in South Africa." *The Lancet* 310, no. 8044 (1977): 920–921.

———. "The Prevention of Mental Illness-Myth or Mandatory." *South African Medical Journal* 40, no. 38 (1966): 923–930.

———. "The Psychiatric Day Hospital: An Evaluation of 4 Years' Experience." *South African Medical Journal* 32, no. 36 (1958): 881–884.

———. "Social and Community Psychiatry in South Africa." *South African Medical Journal* 36, no. 8 (1962): 141–148.

Gillis, L. S., R. Elk, O. Ben-Arie, and A. Teggin. "The Present State Examination: Experiences With Xhosa-Speaking Psychiatric Patients." *British Journal of Psychiatry* 141 (1982): 143–147.

Gillis, Lynn, and Stella Egert. *The Psychiatric Outpatient: Clinical and Organizational Aspects*. London: Faber, 1973.

Gilman, Sander L. *Difference and Pathology: Stereotypes of Sexuality, Race, and Madness*. Ithaca: Cornell University Press, 1985.

———. *Disease and Representation: Images of Illness From Madness to AIDS*. Ithaca: Cornell University Press, 1988.

———. *Freud, Race, and Gender*. Translated by A. A. Brill. Princeton, NJ: Princeton University Press, 1993.

Gittins, Diana. *Madness in Its Place: Narratives of Severalls Hospital, 1913–1997*. London; New York: Routledge, 1998.

Gochman P. A., D. Greenstein, A. Sporn, N. Gogtay, R. Nicolson, A. Keller, M. Lenane, F. Brookner , and J. L. Rapoport. "Childhood Onset Schizophrenia: Familial Neurocognitive Measures." *Schizophrenia Research* 71, no. 1 (2004): 43–47.

Goffman, Erving. *Asylums: Essays on the Social Situation of Mental Patients and Other Inmates*. Chicago: Aldine Publishing Company, 1962.

Green, Richard. "The United States." In *Sociolegal Control of Homosexuality: a Multi-Nation Comparison*, eds. Donald J. West and Richard Green. New York and London: Plenum Press, 1997, 145–167.

Greenstein, Ran. "The Study of South African Society: Towards a New Agenda For Comparative Historical Inquiry." *Journal of Southern African Studies* 20, no. 4 (1994): 641–661.

Grob, Gerald N. *The Mad Among Us: A History of the Care of America's Mentally Ill.* New York, Toronto: Free Press. Maxwell Macmillan Canada. Maxwell Macmillan International, 1994.

———. "World War II and American Psychiatry." *Psychohistory Review* 19, no. 1 (1990): 41–69.

Gronfein, William. "Psychotropic Drugs and the Origins of Deinstitutionalization." *Social Problems* 32, no. 5 (1985): 437–454.

Gross, Herbert S., Myrna R. Herbert, Genell L. Knatterrund, and Lawrence Donner. "The Effect of Race and Sex on the Variation of Diagnosis and Disposition in a Psychiatric Emergency Room." *Journal of Nervous and Mental Disease* 148, no. 6 (1969): 638–642.

Hall, J. K. *One Hundred Years of American Psychiatry.* New York: Published for the American Psychiatric Association by the Columbia University Press, 1944.

Hamber, Brandon, and Brian Rock. "Mental Health and Human Rights: In Search of Context, Consequence and Effective Care." *Rethinking Rights* 1 (1993): 73–91.

Hammond-Tooke, W. David. "African World-View and Its Relevance for Psychiatry." *Psychologia Africana* 16, no. 1 (1975): 25–32.

———. *Rituals and Medicines: Indigenous Healing in South Africa.* Johannesburg: Ad. Donker, 1989.

Harries, Patrick. *Work, Culture and Identity: Migrant Labourers in Mozambique and South Africa, c1860–1910.* Johannesburg: Witwatersrand University Press, 1994.

Harris, Stanley E. "Military Policies Regarding Homosexual Behavior: An International Survey" *Journal of Homosexuality* 21, no. 4 (1991): 67–74.

Hayes, Grahame. "The Struggle for Mental Health in South Africa: Psychologists, Apartheid and the Story of Durban OASSSA." *Journal of Community & Applied Social Psychology* 10, no. 4 (2000): 327–341.

Health and Human Rights Project. "Professional Accountability in South Africa." 1997.

Heldal-Lund, Andreas. "Operation Clambake: Undressing the Church of Scientology Since 1996" http://www.xenu.net/. Accessed 19 August 2008.

Hemphill, R. E. "The Council of the College and Sanctions Against South Africa." *Bulletin of the Royal College of Psychiatrists* 12 (1988): 142–143.

Henderson, Sir David, and Ivor R. C. Batchelor. *Henderson and Gillespie's Textbook of Psychiatry for Students and Practitioners.* 9th ed. London: Oxford University Press , 1962.

Henige, David. *Oral Historiography.* London: Longman, 1982.

Henning, P. H. "Die Nabootsing Van Geesteskrankheid Onder Bantoe Verhoorafwagtende Mans Vanaf Durban Gevangenis (Natal)." *South African Medical Journal* 40, no. 38 (1966): 937–944.

Higgs, J. A. "Insulin Therapy." *South African Medical Journal* 12, no. 16 (1938): 590–593.

Hocoy, Dan. "Apartheid, Racism, and Black Mental Health in South Africa, and the Role of Racial Identity." Ph.D. diss., Queen's University, 1997.

Hoffmann, Rainer, Jörg Hutter, and Rüdiger Lautmann. "Germany." In *Sociolegal Control of Homosexuality: A Multi-Nation Comparison,* eds. Donald J. West and Richard Green. New York and London: Plenum Press, 1997, 255–268.

Holdstock, T. L. "Psychology in South Africa Belongs to the Colonial Era: Arrogance of Ignorance?" *South African Journal of Psychology* 11, no. 4 (1981): 123–129.

Hopkins, A. G. "Big Business in African Studies." *Journal of African History* 21, no. 1 (1987): 119–140.

Horrell, Muriel. *A Survey of Race Relations in South Africa 1950–1960*. Johannesburg: South African Institute of Race Relations, 1961.

Howells, John G., ed. *World History of Psychiatry*. New York: Brunner/Mazel, 1975.

Howsepian, A. A. "Sexual Modification Therapies: Ethical Controversies, Philosophical Disputes, and Theological Reflections," *Christian Bioethics* 10, no. 2–3 (2004): 117–135.

Hubbard, Ron L. *Dianetics: The Modern Science of Mental Health*. Los Angeles: Bridge Publications, 1992.

———. *Scientology: The Fundamentals of Thought*. Los Angeles: Bridge Publications, 2007.

Hubert, Susan J. *Questions of Power: The Politics of Women's Madness Narratives*. Newark, NJ; London: University of Delaware Press: Associated University Press, 2002.

Hughes, John S. *The Letters of a Victorian Madwoman*. Columbia: University of South Carolina Press, 1993.

Hull, John M. "Religion, Education and Madness: A Modern Trinity." *Educational Review* 43, no. 3 (1991): 347–362.

Hurst, Lewis A. "Electroencephalography in Mental Hospital Practice." *South African Medical Journal* 20, no. 3 (1946): 54–55.

———. "Electroencephalography in Mental Hospital Practice." *South African Medical Journal* 20, no. 4 (1946): 87–89

———. "Hereditary Factors in Mental Disorder and Mental Defect." *South African Medical Journal* 18, no. 23 (1944): 397–401.

———. "Heredito-Constitutional Research in Psychiatry." *South African Medical Journal* 14, no. 18 (1940).

Hurst, Lewis A., and Mary B. Lucas. "South Africa." In *World History of Psychiatry*, ed. John G. Howells. New York: Brunner/Mazel, 1975

Illich, Ivan. *Disabling Professions*. London: Marion Boyers Publishers, 1977.

Isaacs, Gordon, and Brian McKendrick. *Male Homosexuality in South Africa: Identity Formation, Culture, and Crisis*. Cape Town: Oxford University Press, 1992.

Jackson, Lynette Aria. "Narratives of 'Madness' and Power: A History of Ingutsheni Mental Hospital and Social Order in Colonial Zimbabwe, 1908–1959." Ph.D. diss., Columbia University, 1977.

———. *Surfacing Up: Psychiatry and Social Order in Colonial Zimbabwe*. History of Psychiatry Series. New York: Cornell University Press, 2005.

Jagose, A. *Queer Theory: An Introduction*. New York: New York University Press, 1998.

James, Theodore. "The First Fifty: A Review of the South African Medical Congress." *South African Medical Journal* 49, no. 32 (1975): 1313–1316.

James, W. H. "The Cause(s) of the Fraternal Birth Order Effect in Male Homosexuality." *Journal of Biosocial Science* 36, no. 1 (2004): 51–59, 61–62.

Jansen, F. E. "The Medical System As an Aspect of Culture and Some Acculturative Effects of Western Cross-Cultural Medical Services." *South African Journal of Ethnology* 6 (1983): 11–17.

Jeeves, Alan. "Health, Surveillance and Community: South Africa's Experiment With Medical Reform in the 1940s and 1950s." *South African Historical Journal* 43 (2000): 244–266.

Jones, Tiffany F. "Contradictions and Constructions: Psychiatric Perceptions in Apartheid South Africa, 1948–1979." M.A. diss., Dalhousie University, 2000.

Joubert, D., ed. *Tot Dieselfde Geslag: Debat oor Homoseksualiteit in 1968*. Cape Town: Tafelberg, 1974.

Kaplan, Bert. *The Inner World of Mental Illness. A Series of First Person Accounts of What It Was Like*. New York: Harper and Row, 1964.

Kaplan, Robert M. "Treatment of Homosexuality During Apartheid." *British Medical Journal*, 329, no. 7480 (2004): 1415–1416.

Kark, Sidney L. *The Practice of Community-Oriented Primary Health Care*. New York: Appleton-Century-Crofts, 1981.

Kark, Sidney L., and Emily Kark. *Promoting Community Health: From Pholela to Jerusalem*. Johannesburg: Witwatersrand University Press, 1999.

Kark, Sidney L., and Guy W. Steuart. *A Practice of Social Medicine: A South African Team's Experiences in Different African Communities*. Edinburgh: E. & S. Livingstone, 1962.

Katz, Elaine. *White Death: Silicosis on the Witwatersrand Gold Mines, 1886–1910*. Johannesburg: Witwatersrand University Press.

Kaufman, Carol E. "Reproductive Control in Apartheid South Africa." *Population Studies*, 54, no. 1 (2001): 105–114.

Keegan, Timothy. "Gender, Degeneration and Sexual Danger: Imagining Race and Class in South Africa ca.1912." *Journal of Southern African Studies* 27, no. 3 (2001): 459–477.

Kellett, Peter. "Attempted Suicide in Durban: A General Hospital Study." *South African Medical Journal* 40, no. 5 (1966): 90–95.

Kent, Stephen A. "The Globalization of Scientology: Influence, Control and Opposition in Transnational Markets." *Religion* 29 (1999): 147–169.

———. "Scientology—Is This a Religion?" *Marburg Journal of Religion* 4, no. 1 (1999): 1–23.

Khanna, Ranjana. *Dark Continents: Psychoanalysis and Colonialism*. Durham and London: Duke University Press, 2003.

Kirsch, M. H. *Queer Theory and Social Change*. London and New York: Routledge, 2000.

Klausen, Susanne. "'For the Sake of Race': Eugenic Discourses in the South African Medical Record, 1903–1926." *Journal of Southern African Studies* 23, no. 1 (1997): 27–50.

Kneeland, Timothy W., and Carol A. B. Warren. *Pushbutton Psychiatry: A History of Electroshock in America*. Westport, CT: Praeger Publishers, 2002.

Kohn, Robert et al. "Race and Psychiatric Services in Post-Apartheid South Africa: A Preliminary Study of Psychiatrists' Perceptions." *International Journal of Social Psychiatry*, 50, no. 1 (2004): 18–24.

Koty, John. *Die Behandelung Der Alten Und Kraken Bei Dun Naturvölken*. Stuttgart: C. L. Hirschfeld, 1934.

Kruger, Albert. *Mental Health Law in South Africa*. Durban: Butterworth, 1980.

Laidler, Percy Ward. *South Africa: Its Medical History 1652–1898: A Medical and Social Study*. Cape Town: C. Struik, 1971.

Laing, R. D. *The Divided Self: An Existential Study of Sanity and Madness*. Hammondsworth: Penguin, 1965.

———. *Mad to Be Normal: Conversations with R. D. Laing*, ed. Bob Mullan. London: Free Association Books, 1995.

Lamont, Alistair McE. "Affective Types of Psychotic Reaction in Cape Coloured Persons." *South African Medical Journal* 25, no. 3 (1951): 40–42.

———. "Man's Hidden Madness or Defence Against Insanity." *South African Medical Journal* 44, no. 24 (1970): 708–712.

———. "The Place of the Mental Hospital in the Health of the Community." *South African Medical Journal* 28, no. 51 (1954): 1082–1085.

Lamont, Alistair McE, and Willem J. Blignault. "A Study of Male Bantu Admissions at Weskoppies During 1952." *South African Medical Journal* 27, no. 31 (1953): 637–639.

Langschmidt, G. F. "Mental Health." *South African Medical Journal* 15, no. 18 (1941): 360–361.

Laubscher, B. J. F. *Sex, Custom and Psychopathology: a Study of South African Pagan Natives*. London: G. Routledge & Sons, 1937.

Le Roux, A. G. "Psychological Factors in the Health of South African Blacks." *South African Medical Journal* 56, no. 13 (1979): 532–534.

Le Roux, Martha Maria. " Die Wordingsweg Van Psigiatriese Maatskaplike Werk in Staatspsigiatriese Inrigtings in Die Republiek Van Suid-Afrika." D. Soc. Sc. diss., Universiteit van die Oranje-Vrystaat, 1985.

Lee, S. G. "Spirit Possession Among the Zulu." In *Spirit Mediumship and Society in Africa*. eds. J. Beattie and A. G. Le Roux. London: Routledge and Kegan Paul, 1969.

Lewis, Mindy. *Life Inside: A Memoir*. New York: Atra Books, 2002.

Livni, S. "Reflections on the Psychosomatic Approach in General Practice." *South African Medical Journal* 21, no. 22 (1947): 857–863.

Lloyd, Genevieve. *The Man of Reason: "Male" and "Female" in Western Philosophy*. Minneapolis: University of Minnesota Press, 1984.

Louw, Johann, and Sally Swartz. "An English Asylum in Africa: Space and Order in Valkenberg Asylum." *History of Psychology* 4, no. 1 (2001): 3–23.

Lund, Crick et al. "Mental Health Policy Development and Implementation in South Africa: A Situation Analysis" (Mental Health and Poverty Project, 31 January 2008) http://workhorse.pry.uct.ac.za:8080/MHAPP (accessed 5 June 2009).

Malebele, Solome. "Problems in Rural Mental Health Care." In *Proceedings of Two Symposia: Mental Health Care for a New South Africa Held at the University of Witwatersrand, May 1990 and Rural Community Mental Health Care Held at Tintswalo Hospital, June 1990*, ed. Melvyn Freeman. Vol. 61–67. Johannesburg: Centre for the Study of Health Policy, 1990.

Malzberg, B. *The Mental Health of the Negro*. New York: Research Foundation for Mental Hygiene, 1963.

Mamdani, Mahmood. *Citizen and Subject: Contemporary Africa and the Legacy of Late Colonialism*. Princeton, NJ: Princeton University Press, 1996.

Manganyi, N. C. *Being Black in the World*. Johannesburg: SPRO-CAS/Ravan, 1974.

Manicom, Linzi. "Ruling Relations: Rethinking State and Gender in South African History." *Journal of African History* 33 (1992): 441–465.

Mannoni, O. *Prospero and Caliban: The Psychology of Colonization*. Translated by Pamela Powesland. New York, Frederick A. Praeger, 1964.

Marks, Shula. *Divided Sisterhood: Race, Class, and Gender in the South African Nursing Profession*. New York: St. Martin's Press, 1994.

———, ed. *Not Either an Experimental Doll: The Separate Worlds of Three South African Women*. London: The Women's Press, 1987.

———. "Public Health Then and Now: South Africa's Early Experiment in Social Medicine: Its Pioneers and Politics." *American Journal of Public Health* 87, no. 3 (1997): 452–560.

Mayette, Ted and Keshet, eds. "L. Ron Hubbard: Scientology, Dianetics and Racism" http://www.solitarytrees.net/racism/. Accessed 19 August 2008.

Mazzoni, Christina. *Saint Hysteria: Neurosis, Mysticism, and Gender in European Culture*. Ithaca, NY: Cornell University Press, 1996.

McClintock, Anne. *Double Crossings: Madness, Sexuality and Imperialism: The 2000 Garnett Sedgewick Memorial Lecture*. Vancouver: Ronsdale Press, 2001.

McCulloch, Jock. *Asbestos Blues: Labour Capital, Physicians & the State in South Africa*. Oxford: James Currey, 2002.

———. *Black and White Artifact: Fanon's Clinical Psychology and Social Theory.* New York: Cambridge University Press, 1983.

———. *Colonial Psychiatry and 'the African Mind'.* Cambridge, New York: Cambridge University Press, 1995.

———. "The Empire's New Clothes: Ethnopsychiatry in Colonial Africa." *History of the Human Sciences* 6, no. 2 (1993): 35–52.

Memmi, Albert. *The Colonizer and the Colonized.* Translated by Howard Greenfeld. Boston: Beacon Press, 1965.

Menninger, Roy W., and John C. Nemiah. *American Psychiatry After World War II (1944–1994).* Washington, DC: American Psychiatric Press, 2000.

Menzies, Robert. "Historical Profiles of Criminal Insanity." *International Journal of Law and Psychiatry* 25 (2002): 379–404.

Micale, Mark, and Paul Lerner. *Traumatic Pasts: Histories, Psychiatry and Trauma in the Modern Age 1870–1930.* Cambridge: Cambridge University Press, 2001.

Micale, Mark S. "Hysteria and Its Historiography: The Future Perspective." *History of Psychiatry* 1, no. 1 (1990): 33–124.

Millett, Kate. *Sexual Politics.* New York: Avon, 1971.

Mills, J. "The Possession State *Intwaso*: An Anthropological Re-Appraisal." *South African Journal of Sociology* 16, no. 1 (1985): 9–13.

Minaar, G. G. *The Influence of Westernization on the Personality of a Group of Zulu Men.* Human Sciences Research Council, Pretoria, 1976.

Minde, M. "Correspondence: Psychiatric Education." *South African Medical Journal* 51, no. 19 (1977): 652.

———. "The History of Mental Health Services in South Africa: Part I. In the Days of the Dutch East India Company." *South Africa Medical Journal* 48, no. 29 (1974): 1270–1272.

———. "History of Mental Health Services in South Africa: Part II. During the British Occupation." *South African Medical Journal* 48, no. 38 (1974): 1629–1632.

———. "History of Mental Health Services in South Africa: Part III. The Cape Province." *South African Medical Journal* 48, no. 53 (1974): 2230–2234.

———. "History of Mental Health Services in South Africa: Part IV. The Orange Free State." *South African Medical Journal* 48, no. 38 (1974): 2327–2330.

———. "History of Mental Health Services in South Africa: Part IX. The Protection and Care of the Feebleminded." *South African Medical Journal* 49, no. 41: 1716–1720.

———. "History of Mental Health Services in South Africa: Part VI. The Transvaal." *South African Medical Journal* 49, no. 10 (1975): 367–374.

———. "History of Mental Health Services in South Africa: Part VII. Services Since Union." *South African Medical Journal* 49, no. 11 (1975): 405–409.

———. "History of Mental Health Services in South Africa: Part XIII. The National Council for Mental Health." *South African Medical Journal* 50, no. 37 (1976): 1452–1456.

———. "History of Mental Health Services in South Africa: Part XIV. Psychiatric Education." *South African Medical Journal* 51, no. 7 (1977): 210–214.

———. "History of the Mental Health Services in South Africa: Part V. Natal." *South African Medical Journal* 49, no. 9 (1975): 322–326.

———. "Intestinal Parasites in Bantu Mental Patients." *South African Medical Journal* 36, no. 28: 559–562.

———. "Mental Health—Past, Present and Future." *South African Medical Journal* 29, no. 47 (1955): 1124–1127.

———. "The Mental Hospital and the Community." *South African Medical Journal* 32, no. 28 (1958): 709–712.

Mitchell, Juliet. *Psychoanalysis and Feminism*. London: Allen Lane, 1974.
Mitchell, Timothy. "The Limits of the State: Beyond Statist Approaches and the Critics." *The American Political Science Review* 85, no. 1 (1991): 77–96.
Moffson, A. "Schizophrenia in Male Bantu Admissions to Weskoppies Hospital." *South African Medical Journal* 28, no. 32 (1954): 662–666.
———. "A Study of 400 Consecutive Male Bantu Admissions to Weskoppies Mental Hospital." *South African Medical Journal* 29, no. 29 (1955): 689–692.
Moodie, Katie. "Ducktails, Flick-Knives and Pugnacity." *Journal of Southern African Studies* 24, no. 4 (1998): 753–774.
Moodie, T. Dunbar. "Mine Cultures and Miners' Identity on the South African Gold Mines." In *Town and Countryside in the Transvaal: Capitalist Penetration and Popular Response,* ed. Belinda Bozzoli. Johannesburg: Ravan Press, 1983, 176–197.
Moodie, T. Dunbar, with Vivienne Ndatshe. *Going for Gold: Men, Mines and Migration*. Johannesburg: Witwatersrand University Press, 1994.
Moodie, T. Dunbar, with Vivienne Ndatshe and British Sibuyi. "Migrancy and Male Sexuality on the South African Gold Mines." *Journal of Southern African Studies* 14, no. 2 (1988): 228–256.
Moross, H. "The Development of Community Resources for Mental Health Care." *South African Medical Journal* 38, no. 20 (1964): 415–419.
———. *Tara: The H. Moross Centre*. Johannesburg: Smith Mitchell Organisation, n.d.
———. "A Therapeutic Community in the Setting of a Psychiatric Teaching Hospital. I. Diagnostic and Treatment Resources and Modus Operandi." *South African Medical Journal* 41, no. 14 (1967): 351–355.
———. "A Therapeutic Community in the Setting of a Psychiatric Teaching Hospital. II. Psychiatric Occupational Therapy." *South African Medical Journal* 41, no. 15 (1967): 375–380.
———. "Thoughts on the Planning of Mental Health Services for South Africa." *South African Medical Journal* 34, no. 9 (1960): 171–174.
Moutinho, Hendrika Gesina. "Planning and Policy Formulation in the Field of Mental Health." M.A. diss., University of South Africa, 1988.
Naidoo, B. T. "A History of the Durban Medical School." *South African Medical Journal* 50, no. 41 (1976): 1625–1628.
Nassau, Lyford Cay. "The Commonwealth Accord on Southern Africa (The 'Nassau Accord')." In *Mission to South Africa—The Commonwealth Report*. The Commonwealth Group of Eminent Persons, Penguin Books, 1986.
Newton, Allison D. "The Application of Brief Psychotherapy in Military Psychiatry." MA thesis. Pretoria: University of Pretoria, 1981.
Ngubane, Harriet. "Aspects of Clinical Practice and Traditional Organization of Indigenous Healers in South Africa." *Social Science & Medicine* 15 (1981): 361–365.
———. *Body and Mind in Zulu Medicine: An Ethnography of Health and Disease in Nyuswa-Zulu Thought and Practice*. London; New York: Academic Press, 1977.
Nunes, Julia, and Scott Simmie. *Beyond Crazy: Journey Through Mental Illness*. Toronto: McClelland & Stewart, 2002.
O'Connell, M. C. "The Aetiology of Thwasa." *Psychotherapeia* 6, no. 4 (1980): 18–23.
———. "Spirit Possession and Role of Stress Among the Xisibe of Eastern Transkei." *Ethnography* 21 (1982): 21–37.
O'Donoghue, Sean B. "Health and Politics: An Appraisal and Evaluation of the Provision of Health, and Mental Health Services for Blacks in South Africa." M.A. diss., Rhodes University, 1989.

Owen, Chris. "Miscellaneous Writings on Scientology" http://www.solitarytrees.net/cowen/misc/index.htm. Accessed 29 May 2009.

———. "Scientology's Fight For Apartheid" 1997, http://www.solitarytrees.net/cowen/misc/aparth.htm. Accessed 29 May 2009.

Palomo, T., T. Archer, R. M. Kostrzewa, and R. J. Beninger. "Gene-Environment Interplay in Schizopsychotic Disorders." *Neurotoxicology Research* 6, no. 1 (2004): 1–9.

Parle, Julie. *States of Mind: Searching for Mental Health in Natal and Zululand, 1868–1918*. Scottsville: University of Kwa-Zulu Natal Press, 2007.

———. "Witchcraft or Madness? The Amandiki of Zululand, 1894–1914." *Journal of Southern African Studies* 29, no. 1 (2003): 105–132.

Parliamentary Correspondent. "Mental Illness in the Union: Debate in Parliament." *South African Medical Journal* 32, no. 38 (1958): 946–947.

———. "The Treatment of Mentally Ill Patients." *South African Medical Journal* 35, no. 10 (1961): 216–217.

Pearlman, T. "The Management of White Certified Schizophrenic Patients in the Community of the Witwatersrand." *South African Medical Journal* 44, no. 41 (1970): 1181–1182.

Peires, J. B. *The Dead will Arise: Nongqawuse and the Great Xhosa Cattle-Killing Movement of 1856–1857*. Johannesburg: Ravan Press, 1989.

Penfold, Susan P., and Gillian A. Walker. *Women and the Psychiatric Paradox*. Montreal: Eden Press, 1983.

Perk, David. "A Psychiatrists' Experience in the 2nd World War." *South African Medical Journal* 21, no. 23 (1947).

———. "Psychoneurosis in the Soldier: Its Psychopathology and Aetiology." *South African Medical Journal* 22, no. 16 (1948): 511.

Peterson, Dale. *A Mad People's History of Madness*. Pittsburgh: University of Pittsburgh Press, 1981.

Petronis, A. "The Origin of Schizophrenia: Genetic Thesis, Epigenetic Antithesis, and Resolving Synthesis." *Biological Psychiatry* 15, no. 55 (2004): 965–970.

Phillips, Kim M., and Barry Reay, eds. *Sexualities in History: A Reader*. London and New York: Routledge, 2002.

Pinderhughes, Charles, Jeanne Spurlock, Jack Weinberg, and Alan Stone. "Report of the Committee to Visit South Africa." American Psychiatric Association, 1978.

Pinderhughes, Charles A. "Letters to the Editor: Dr. Pinderhughes Replies for the Committee to Visit South Africa." *American Journal of Psychiatry* 137, no. 7 (1980): 867.

Porter, Roy. *Madness: A Brief History*. New York: Oxford University Press, 2002.

———. *A Social History of Madness: Stories of the Insane*. London: Weidenfeld and Nicolson, 1987.

Porteus, Kimberley A., Makhosazana Sibeko, Tennyson Lee, Neil Soderlund, Lucy Gilson, and Enoch Peprah. *Cost and Quality of Care: A Comparative Study of Public and Privately Contracted Chronic Psychiatric Hospitals*. Johannesburg: Centre for Health Polity, Department of Community Health, University of Witwatersrand, 1998.

Posel, Deborah. "The Assassination of Hendrik Verwoerd: The Spectre of Apartheid's Corpse." *African Studies* 68, no. 3 (2009): 331–350.

———. *The Making of Apartheid 1948–1961: Conflict and Compromise*. Oxford: Clarendon Press, 1991.

———. "Whiteness and Power in the South African Civil Service: Paradoxes of the Apartheid State." *Journal of Southern African Studies* 25, no. 1 (1999): 99–119.

Potts, Maggie, and Rebecca Fido. *"A Fit Person to Be Removed:" Personal Accounts of Life in a Mental Deficiency Institution.* Plymouth: Northcote House Publishers, 1991.

Quinsey, V. L. "The Etiology of Anomalous Sexual Preferences in Men." *Annals of the New York Academy of Sciences* 989 (2003): 105–117, 144–153.

Rahman, Q. "Fluctuating Asymmetry, Second to Fourth Finger Length Ratios and Human Sexual Orientation." *Psychoneuroendocrinology* 30, no. 4 (2005): 382–391.

Ralph, Diana S. *Work and Madness: The Rise of Community Psychiatry.* Montréal: Black Rose Books, 1983.

Rampele, Mamphele. "Health and Social Welfare in South Africa Today." Paper presented at the American Association for the Advancement of Science Annual Meeting, Philadelphia, 25–30 May 1986.

Razanajao, Cl., J. Postel, and D. F. Allen. "The Life and Psychiatric Work of Frantz Fanon." *History of Psychiatry* 7, no. 4 (1996): 499–524.

Reaume, Geoffrey. *Remembrance of Patients Past: Patient Life at the Toronto Hospital for the Insane, 1870–1940.* Don Mills, Ontario: Oxford University Press, 2000.

Reid, Graeme, Simon Lewin, Shiela Lapinsky, Jeanelle de Gruchy, and Mikki van Zyl. "The Aversion Project: Human Rights Abuses of Gays and Lesbians in the SADF by Health Workers During the Apartheid Era." 1999.

Retief, Glen. "Keeping Sodom Out of the Laager." In *Defiant Desire,* eds. Mark Gevisser and Edwin Cameron. Johannesburg: Ravan Press, 1994, 99–111.

Riley, B. "Linkage Studies of Schizophrenia." *Neurotoxicology Research* 6, no. 1 (2004): 17–34.

Ripa, Yannick. *Women and Madness: The Incarceration of Women in Nineteenth Century France.* Translated by Catherine du Peloux Menagé. Cambridge: Polity Press, 1990.

Ritchie, J. F. *The African As Suckling And As Adult: A Psychological Study.* Livingstone: Rhodes-Livingstone Institute, 1943.

Robbertze, Jan H. "Mental Health Priorities in South Africa." In *Economics of Health in South Africa, Volume II: Hunger Work and Health,* eds. Francis and Westcott Gill Wilson. Johannesburg: Ravan Press, 1980, 312–328.

Roberts, H. *The Patient Patients.* London: Pandora, 1985.

Rollin, Henry R. "Psychiatry at 2000: A Bird's-Eye View." *Psychiatric Bulletin* 24 (2000): 11–15.

Roos, Neil. "Homes Fit for (White) Heroes: Servicemen, Social Justice and the Making of Apartheid, 1939–1948." *Journal of the Georgia Association of Historians* 20 (1999): 25–52.

Rosenberg, Charles E. "Disease in History: Frames and Framers." *The Milbank Quarterly* 67, no. 1 (1989): 1–15.

———. "Framing Disease: Studies in Cultural History. Introduction. Framing Disease: Illness, Society, and History." *Hospital Practice* 27, no. 7 (1992): 179–182, 185–186, 191–192.

———. "Introduction: Framing Disease: Illness, Society and History." *Hospital Practice* 27, no. 7 (1992): 305–318.

Ross, Robert. *A Concise History of South Africa.* New York: Cambridge University Press, 1999.

Russell, Denise. *Women, Madness & Medicine.* Cambridge: Polity Press, 1995.

Sachs, Wulf. *Black Hamlet.* With a new introduction by Saul Dubow and Jacqueline Rose. Johannesburg: Witwatersrand University Press, 1996.

Sadowsky, Jonathan. "The Confinement of Isaac O.: A Case of 'Acute Mania' in Colonial Nigeria." *History of Psychiatry* 7, no. 1 (1995): 91–112.

———. *Imperial Bedlam: Institutions of Madness in Colonial Southwest Nigeria.* Berkeley: University of California Press, 1999.

———. "Psychiatry and Colonial Ideology in Nigeria." *Bulletin of the History of Medicine* 71, no. 1 (1997): 94–111.

Sagner, Andreas. "Ageing and Social Policy in South Africa: Historical Perspectives With Particular Reference to the Eastern Cape." *Journal of Southern African Studies* 26, no. 3 (2000).

Sapinsley, Barbara. *The Private War of Mrs. Packard.* New York: Paragon House, 1991.

Sashidharan, S. P. "Apartheid and Psychiatry." *Lancet* (29 December 1984).

———. "Correspondence: Psychiatrists and Detainees in South Africa." *The Lancet* 321, no. 8316 (1983): 128.

———. "Correspondence: South African Psychiatry." *Bulletin of the Royal College of Psychiatrists,* 9 (1985), 202.

Schaffer, R. "Psychosomatic Medicine." *South African Medical Journal* 22, no. 5 (1948): 167–169.

Schmitt, Richard. "Introduction: Why Is the Concept of Alienation Important?" In *Alienation and Social Criticisms: Key Concepts in Critical Theory,* eds. Richard Schmitt and Thomas E. Moody. New Jersey: Humanities Press, 1994, 1–20.

Schneck, Jerome Mortimer. *A History of Psychiatry.* Springfield, IL: Thomas, 1960.

Scull, Andrew T. *Madhouses, Mad-Doctors, and Madmen the Social History of Psychiatry in the Victorian Era.* Philadelphia: University of Pennsylvania Press, 1981.

———. *The Most Solitary of Afflictions: Madness and Society in Britain, 1700–1900.* New Haven; London: Yale University Press, 1993.

———. "Psychiatry and Its Historians." *History of Psychiatry* 2, no. 3 (1991): 239–250.

———. "Psychiatry and Social Control in the Nineteenth and Twentieth Centuries." *History of Psychiatry* 2, no. 2 (1991): 149–169.

———. "Somatic Treatments and the Historiography of Psychiatry." *History of Psychiatry* 5, no. 1 (1994): 1–12.

———. Charlotte MacKenzie, and Nicholas Hervey. *Masters of Bedlam the Transformation of the Mad-Doctoring Trade.* Princeton, NJ: Princeton University Press, 1996.

Searle, Charlotte. *The History of the Development of Nursing in South Africa, 1652–1960: A Socio-Historical Survey.* Cape Town: Struik, 1965.

Sewpaul, V. "Fragmentation of Psychiatric Service Delivery in Natal Consequent Upon the Policy of Apartheid." *Social Work* 26, no. 2 (1990): 109–114.

Sharpe, Tom. *Indecent Exposure.* London: Secker & Warburg, 1973.

———. *Riotous Assembly.* London: Martin Secker and Warburg, 1971.

Shepard, M. "From Social Medicine to Social Psychiatry: The Achievement of Sir Aubrey Lewis." *Psychological Medicine* 10, no. 2 (1980): 211–218.

Shorter, Edward. *A History of Psychiatry From the Era of the Asylum to the Age of Prozac.* New York: John Wiley & Sons, 1997.

———. "Mania, Hysteria and Gender in Lower Austria, 1891–1905." *History of Psychiatry* 1, no. 1 (1990): 3–31.

Showalter, Elaine. *The Female Malady Women, Madness, and English Culture, 1830–1980.* New York: Pantheon Books, 1985.

———. "Victorian Women and Insanity." In *Madhouses, Mad-Doctors and Madmen: The Social History of Psychiatry in the Victorian Era,* ed. Andrew Scull. Philadelphia, University of Pennsylvania Press, 1981, 313–336.

Sigerist, Henry. *A History of Medicine.* 2 vols. New York: Oxford University Press, 1951 and 1961.

Simpson Wells, A. "Notes on the Training of South African Doctors." *South African Medical Journal* 26, no. 4 (1952): 61–64.

Sinclair, Rebecca. "The Official Treatment of White South African, Homosexual Men and the Consequent Reaction of Gay Liberation from the 1960s to 2000." Ph.D. diss., Johannesburg: University of Johannesburg, 2005.

Smith, H. W. "Decline in the Requests for the Admission of High Grade Mental Defectives to the Alexandra Institution." *South African Medical Journal* 29, no. 38 (1955): 891–894.

———. "Valkenberg-Hospitaal: I. Beknopte Historiese Agtergrond." *South African Medical Journal* 31, no. 12 (1957): 272–277.

———. "Valkenberg-Hospitaal: II. Die Tydperk 1889–1890." *South African Medical Journal* 31, no. 13 (1957): 299–304.

Smith, Theresa C., and Thomas A Oleszczuk. *No Asylum: State Psychiatric Repression in the Former USSR*. New York: New York University Press, 1996.

Solomons, Kevin. "Chapter 11: The Development of Mental Health Facilities in South Africa, 1916–1976." In *Economics of Health in South Africa, Volume II: Hunger Work and Health,* eds. Francis Wilson and Gill Westcott. Johannesburg: Ravan Press, 1980, 265–311.

Spurlock, Jeanne, Charles Pinderhughes, Jack Weinberg, and Alan A. Stone. "Letters to the Editor: Dr Spurlock and Associates Reply for the Committee to Visit South Africa." *American Journal of Psychiatry* 137, no. 7 (1980): 865–866.

Stickley, Charles. *Brain-Washing: A Synthesis of the Russian Textbook on Psychopolitics*. Sussex: Hubbard College of Scientology, c1955.

Stone, Alan A. "Letters to the Editor: Dr. Stone Replies for the Committee to Visit South Africa." *American Journal of Psychiatry* 137, no. 7 (1980): 866.

Stoppard, Janet M, and Linda M. McMullen. *Situating Sadness: Women and Depression in Social Context.* New York: New York University Press, 2003.

Susser, Melvyn. "Apartheid and the Causes of Death: Disentangling Ideology and Laws From Class and Race." *American Journal of Public Health* 73, no. 5 (1983): 581–584.

———. *Community Psychiatry: Epidemiologic and Social Themes.* New York: Random House, 1968.

———. "Disease in South Africa." *Lancet* 325, no. 8423 (1985): 283.

Susser, Merlyn, and Violet Padayachi Cherry. "Health and Health Care Under Apartheid." *Journal of Public Health Policy* 3, no. 4 (1982): 455–475.

Swaab, D. F. "Sexual Differentiation of the Human Brain: Relevance for Gender Identity, Transsexualism and Sexual Orientation." *Gynecological Endocrinology* 19, no. 6 (2004): 301–312.

Swartz, Leslie. *Culture and Mental Health: A Southern African View.* Cape Town: Oxford University Press, 1998.

———. "Culture and Mental Health in the Rainbow Nation: Transcultural Psychiatry in a Changing South Africa." *Transcultural Psychiatric Research Review* 33 (1996): 119–136.

———. "On the Edge: Ward-Rounds in a South African Psychiatric Emergency Department." *Social Science & Medicine* 35, no. 9 (1992): 1115–1122.

———. "The Politics of Black Patients' Identity: Ward-Rounds on the 'Black Side' of a South African Psychiatric Hospital." *Culture, Medicine and Psychiatry* 15 (1991): 217–244.

———. "The Reproduction of Racism in South African Mental Health Care." *South African Journal of Psychology* 21, no. 4 (1991): 240–246.

———. "Transcultural Psychiatry in Context, Part II: Cross Cultural Issues in Mental Health Practice." *Transcultural Psychiatric Research Review* 24, no. 1 (1987): 5–30.

———. "Transcultural Psychiatry in South Africa: Part I." *Transcultural Psychiatric Research Review* 23, no. 4 (1986): 273–304.

Swartz, Sally. "The Black Insane in the Cape, 1891–1920." *Journal of Southern African Studies* 21, no. 3 (1995): 399–415.

———. "Changing Diagnoses in Valkenberg Asylum, Cape Colony, 1891–1920: A Longitudinal View." *History of Psychiatry* 6, no. 24, Pt 4 (1995): 431–451.

———. "Colonizing the Insane: Causes of Insanity in the Cape, 1891–1920." *History of the Human Sciences* 8, no. 4 (1995): 39–57.

———. "Lost Lives: Gender, History and Mental Illness in the Cape, 1891–1910." *Feminism & Psychology* 9, no. 2 (1999): 152–158.

———. "Shrinking: A Postmodern Perspective on Psychiatric Case Histories." *South African Journal of Psychology* 26, no. 3 (1996): 150–156.

Szasz, Thomas Stephen. *A Lexicon of Lunacy: Metaphoric Malady, Moral Responsibility, and Psychiatry*. New Brunswick, USA: Transaction Publishers, 1933.

———. *The Manufacture of Madness: A Comparative Study of the Inquisition and the Mental Health Movement*. New York: Harper & Row, 1970.

———. *The Myth of Mental Illness: Foundations of a Theory of Personal Conduct*. New York: Hoeber-Harper, 1961.

Tholfsen, B. "Cross Gendered Longings and the Demand for Categorization: Enacting Gender Within the Transference-Countertransference Relationship." *Journal of Gay and Lesbian Psychotherapy* 4, no. 2 (2000): 27–46.

Thom, Rita. *Mental Health Services: A Review of Southern African Literature, 1967–1999*, Centre for Health Policy, University of the Witwatersrand, Johannesburg, 2000.

Toker, Eugene. "Mental Illness in the White and Bantu Populations of the Republic of South Africa." *American Journal of Psychiatry* 123, no. 1 (1966): 55–65.

Torchia, Andrew. "The Business of Business: An Analysis of the Political Behaviour of the South African Manufacturing Sector Under the Nationalists." *Journal of Southern African Studies* 14, no. 3 (1988): 421–455.

United Nations Centre Against Apartheid. "Report by WHO." Geneva: 1977.

Ussher, Jane M. *Women's Madness: Misogyny or Mental Illness?* New York: Harvester Wheatsheaf, 1991.

Vail, David J. *Dehumanization and the Institutional Career*. Springfield, Illinois: Charles C. Thomas, 1966.

Vail, Leroy, and Landeg White. "Forms of Resistance: Songs and Perceptions of Power in Colonial Mozambique." In *Banditry, Rebellion and Social Protest in Africa*, ed. Donald Crummey. London: J. Currey, 1986, 193–227.

Van der Burgh, C. *Estimates of the Incidence of Physical and Mental Defects Among Indian South Africans, 1977*. Pretoria: South African Human Sciences Research Council, Institute for Sociological, Demographic and Criminological Research, 1978.

———. *Views of White, Coloured, and Indian South Africans on Mental Illness and the Mentally Ill* . Pretoria: Human Sciences Research Council, 1983.

van Rensburg, H. C. J., and A. Mans. *Profile of Disease and Health Care in South Africa*. Pretoria, Cape Town, Johannesburg: Academica, 1982.

Van Zyl, Mikki et al., "The Aversion Project: Human Rights Abuses of Gays and Lesbians in the SADF by Health Workers during the Apartheid Era." Cape Town: Simply Said and Done, 1999.

Vaughan, Megan. *Curing Their Ills: Colonial Power and African Illness*. Cambridge: Stanford University Press, 1991.

———. "Madness and Colonialism, Colonialism as Madness: Re-Reading Fanon. Colonial Discourse and the Psychotherapy of Colonialism." *Paideuma* 39 (1993): 45–55.

Vermooten, Ian R. "Facilities Available for Treatment in Mental Hospitals: With Brief Reference to Extra-Mural Work Done by Government Psychiatrists." *South African Medical Journal* 27, no. 38 (1953): 815–817.

Vitus, Lage. "Mental Health Facilities: Much Needs to Be Done." *Race Relations News* 38, no. 5 (1976): 1–3.

———. "The Role of the National Council for Mental Health and Government Agencies in Developing Mental Health Policy." M.A. diss., University of South Africa, 1987.

von Marcab, Lilly. "Scientology Cult: Hubbard's Extreme Racism OK With Us." *International* June 29, 2008.

Waddell, W. "Psychosomatic Aspects of Obstetrics and Gynaecology." *South African Medical Journal* 22, no. 2 (1948): 63–67.

Wallace, H. L. "Correspondence: Phasing Out of Admissions of Non-White Students to University of Natal Medical School." *South African Medical Journal* 50, no. 8 (1976): 235.

Walton, H. "Attempted Suicide in Cape Town." *South African Medical Journal* 24, no. 45 (1950): 933–935.

———. "Correspondence: Psychiatric Services in South Africa." *South African Medical Journal* 32, no. 29 (1958): 744.

Warheit, G. J., C. E. Holzer, and S. A. Arey. "Race and Mental Illness: an Epidemiological Update." *Journal of Health and Social Behavior* 16 (1975): 243–256.

Wells, A. Simpson. "Notes on the Training of South African Doctors." *South African Medical Journal* 26, no. 4 (1952): 61.

West, Donald J., and Andrea Wöelke. "England." In *Sociolegal Control of Homosexuality: a Multi-Nation Comparison*, eds. Donald J. West and Richard Green. New York and London: Plenum Press, 1997, 197–220.

Westcott, Gill, and Francis Wilson. *Economics of Health in South Africa*, Vol. 1. Johannesburg: Ravan Press, 1979.

White, Luise. "The Traffic in Heads: Bodies, Borders and the Articulation of Regional Histories." *Journal of Southern African Studies* 23, no. 2 (1997): 325–338.

Wilmsen, Edwin N., Saul Dubow, and John Sharp. "Introduction: Ethnicity, Identity and Nationalism in Southern Africa." *Journal of Southern African Studies* 20, no. 3 (1994): 347–353.

Wilson, Bryan R. *The Social Dimensions of Sectarianism. Sects and New Religious Movements in Contemporary Society.* Oxford: Clarendon Press, 1990.

Wilson, Francis. *Migrant Labour.* Johannesburg: The South African Council of Churches and SPRO-CAS, 1972.

Wong, A. H., J. Trakalo, O. Likhodi, M. Yusuf, A. Macedo, M. H. Azevedo, T. Klempan, M. T. Pato, W. G. Honer, C. N. Pato, H. H. Van Tol, and J. L. Kennedy. "Association Between Schizophrenia and the Syntaxin 1A Gene." *Biological Psychiatry* 56, no. 1 (2004): 24–29.

Wood, Mary Elene. *The Writing on the Wall: Women's Autobiography and the Asylum.* Urbana: University of Illinois Press, 1994.

Wylie, Diana. *Starving on a Full Stomach: Hunger and the Triumph of Cultural Racism in Modern South Africa.* Charlottesville and London: University Press of Virginia, 2001.

Yardley, Lucy, ed. *Material Discourses of Health and Illness.* London and New York: Routledge, 1997.

Yarhouse, M. "Homosexuality, Ethics and Identity Synthesis." *Christian Bioethics* 10, no. 2–3 (2004): 239–257.

Yolken, R. "Viruses and Schizophrenia: a Focus on Herpes Simplex Virus." *Herpes* 11, suppl. 2 (2004): 2004.

Youssef, Hanafy A. and Salah A. Fadl; Alan Beveridge, ed. "Frantz Fanon and Political Psychiatry." *History of Psychiatry* 7, no. 4 (1996): 525–532.

Zabow, A. A. "Correspondence: Certification of Mentally Disordered Patients." *South African Medical Journal* 44, no. 32 (1970): 936.

WEBSITES AND FILMS

"Afrox Healthcare Website." Web page [accessed 29 December 2002]. Available at http://www.afroxhealthcare.co.za/index.html.

Key, Liza. Director. *A Question of Madness: The Furiousus*. 52 min. Produced by Key Films. New York: Filmmakers Library, 1999. Videocassette.

Kraak, Gerald. Director. *Property of the State: Gay Men in the Apartheid Military*. Produced by Jill Kruger. 52 min. Cape Town: Stargate Distribution, 2002. Videocassette.

Schenk, A. "Tara, The H. Moross Centre." Web page [accessed 20 July 2003]. Available at http://www.health.wits.ac.za/psychiatry/tara.htm.

"Sentinel Projects Website." Web page [accessed 29 May 2009]. Available at http://www.geocities.com/sadfbook/gays.htm.

Truth and Reconciliation Commission of South Africa. "Human Rights Violations, Health Sector Hearings." 17 June 1997 and 18 June 1997. Cape Town. Web page [accessed 22 February 2000]. Available at http://www.truth.org.za/HRVtrans/health/.

INTERVIEWS

Allwood, Cliff W. Interview by author, 25 July 2002. Johannesburg, Gauteng, tape recording.

Bodemer, Wilhelm. Interview by author, 29 May 2002. Pretoria, Gauteng, tape recording.

Dlamini, Nomsa, Martha Mongoya, and Sipho Mndaweni. Interview by author, 27 June 2002. Johannesburg, Gauteng, tape recording.

Gqomfa, Joseph Nqaba. Interview by author, 22 June 2006. Fort Beaufort, Eastern Cape, tape recording.

Hart, George. Interview by author, 27 June 2002. Johannesburg, Gauteng, tape recording.

Makubela, Tolo. Interview by Godfrey Dlulane, 6 July 2002. Katlehong, Gauteng, tape recording.

Nkosi, Dolly. Interview by Godfrey Dlulane, 6 July 2002. Katlehong, Gauteng, tape recording.

Platman, Stanley. Interview by author, 29 March 2003. Baltimore, Maryland, M.D., tape recording.

Robbertze, Jan H. Interview by author, 14 May 2002. Stellenbosch, Cape, tape recording.

Sable, Dan (name has been changed). Interview by author, 31 March 2002. Springs, Gauteng, tape recording.

Simpson, Michael. Interview by author, 23 April, 2002. Pretoria, Gauteng.

Valjee, Ashwin. Interview by author, 11 June 2002. Durban, Kwazulu-Natal, tape recording.

Index

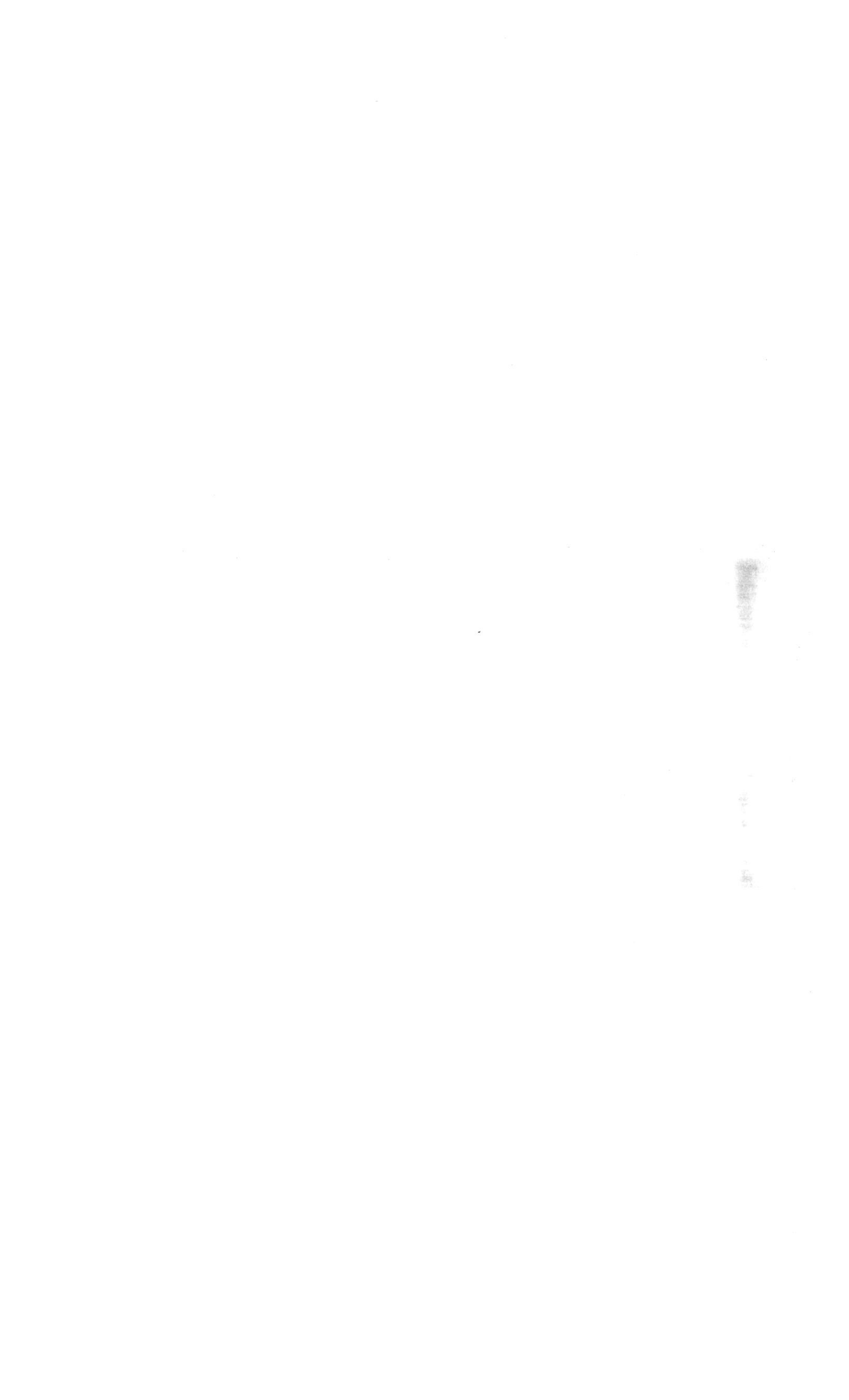